Thrombocytopenia

BASIC AND CLINICAL ONCOLOGY

Series Editor

Bruce D. Cheson
Professor of Medicine and Oncology
Head of Hematology
Georgetown University
Lombardi Comprehensive Cancer Center
Washington, D.C.

1. Chronic Lymphocytic Leukemia: Scientific Advances and Clinical Developments, *edited by Bruce D. Cheson*
2. Therapeutic Applications of Interleukin-2, *edited by Michael B. Atkins and James W. Mier*
3. Cancer of the Prostate, *edited by Sakti Das and E. David Crawford*
4. Retinoids in Oncology, *edited by Waun Ki Hong and Reuben Lotan*
5. Filgrastim (r-metHuG-CSF) in Clinical Practice, *edited by George Morstyn and T. Michael Dexter*
6. Cancer Prevention and Control, *edited by Peter Greenwald, Barnett S. Kramer, and Douglas L. Weed*
7. Handbook of Supportive Care in Cancer, *edited by Jean Klastersky, Stephen C. Schimpff, and Hans-Jörg Senn*
8. Paclitaxel in Cancer Treatment, *edited by William P. McGuire and Eric K. Rowinsky*
9. Principles of Antineoplastic Drug Development and Pharmacology, *edited by Richard L. Schilsky, Gérard A. Milano, and Mark J. Ratain*
10. Gene Therapy in Cancer, *edited by Malcolm K. Brenner and Robert C. Moen*
11. Expert Consultations in Gynecological Cancers, *edited by Maurie Markman and Jerome L. Belinson*
12. Nucleoside Analogs in Cancer Therapy, *edited by Bruce D. Cheson, Michael J. Keating, and William Plunkett*
13. Drug Resistance in Oncology, *edited by Samuel D. Bernal*
14. Medical Management of Hematological Malignant Diseases, *edited by Emil J Freireich and Hagop M. Kantarjian*
15. Monoclonal Antibody-Based Therapy of Cancer, *edited by Michael L. Grossbard*
16. Medical Management of Chronic Myelogenous Leukemia, *edited by Moshe Talpaz and Hagop M. Kantarjian*

17. Expert Consultations in Breast Cancer: Critical Pathways and Clinical Decision Making, *edited by William N. Hait, David A. August, and Bruce G. Haffty*
18. Cancer Screening: Theory and Practice, *edited by Barnett S. Kramer, John K. Gohagan, and Philip C. Prorok*
19. Supportive Care in Cancer: A Handbook for Oncologists: Second Edition, Revised and Expanded, *edited by Jean Klastersky, Stephen C. Schimpff, and Hans-Jörg Senn*
20. Integrated Cancer Management: Surgery, Medical Oncology, and Radiation Oncology, *edited by Michael H. Torosian*
21. AIDS-Related Cancers and Their Treatment, *edited by Ellen G. Feigal, Alexandra M. Levine, and Robert J. Biggar*
22. Allogeneic Immunotherapy for Malignant Diseases, *edited by John Barrett and Yin-Zheng Jiang*
23. Cancer in the Elderly, *edited by Carrie P. Hunter, Karen A. Johnson, and Hyman B. Muss*
24. Tumor Angiogenesis and Microcirculation, *edited by Emile E. Voest and Patricia A. D'Amore*
25. Controversies in Lung Cancer: A Multidisciplinary Approach, *edited by Benjamin Movsas, Corey J. Langer, and Melvyn Goldberg*
26. Chronic Lymphoid Leukemias: Second Edition, Revised and Expanded, *edited by Bruce D. Cheson*
27. The Myelodysplastic Syndromes: Pathology and Clinical Management, *edited by John M. Bennett*
28. Chemotherapy for Gynecological Neoplasms: Current Therapy and Novel Approaches, *edited by Roberto Angioli, Pierluigi Benedetti Panici, John J. Kavanagh, Sergio Pecorelli, and Manuel Penalver*
29. Infections in Cancer Patients, *edited by John N. Greene*
30. Endocrine Therapy for Breast Cancer, *edited by James N. Ingle and Mitchell Dowsett*
31. Anemia of Chronic Disease, *edited by Guenter Weiss, Victor R. Gordeuk, and Chaim Hershko*
32. Cancer Risk Assessment, *edited by Peter G. Shields*
33. Thrombocytopenia, *edited by Keith R. McCrae*

ADDITIONAL VOLUMES IN PREPARATION

Thrombocytopenia

Edited by

Keith R. McCrae

Case Western Reserve University

Cleveland, Ohio, U.S.A.

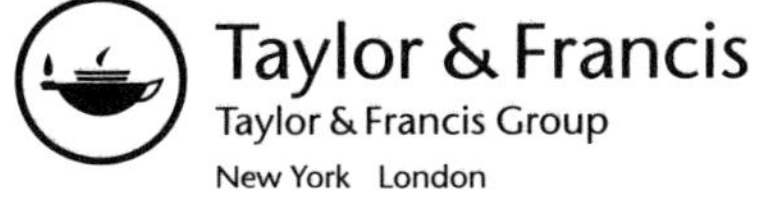

Published in 2006 by
Taylor & Francis Group
270 Madison Avenue
New York, NY 10016

Printed in the United States of America on acid-free paper
10 9 8 7 6 5 4 3 2 1

International Standard Book Number-10: 0-8247-2585-9 (Hardcover)
International Standard Book Number-13: 978-0-8247-2585-3 (Hardcover)
Library of Congress Card Number 2005046614

Library of Congress Cataloging-in-Publication Data

Thrombocytopenia / edited by Keith R. McCrae.
p. ; cm. -- (Basic and clinical oncology ; 33)
Includes bibliographical references and index.
ISBN-13: 978-0-8247-2585-3 (alk. paper)
ISBN-10: 0-8247-2585-9 (alk. paper)
1. Thrombocytopenia. I. McCrae, Keith R. II. Series.
[DNLM: 1. Thrombocytopenia. 2. Thrombocytopenia--etiology. WH 300 T5307 2006]

RC647.B5T47 2006
616.1'35--dc22 2005046614

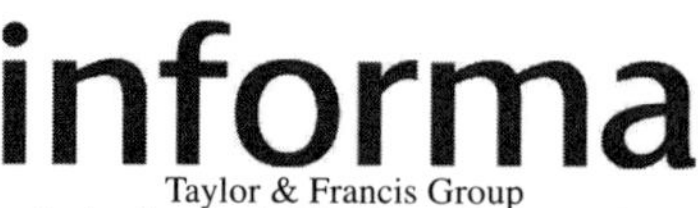

Taylor & Francis Group
is the Academic Division of Informa plc.

Visit the Taylor & Francis Web site at
http://www.taylorandfrancis.com

I would like to dedicate this book to the memory of my wife,
Jo Ann McCrae (1956–2002), whose unwavering
support throughout my career made this effort possible.

Preface

Thrombocytopenia is one of the most common hematologic problems encountered by physicians in any specialty. From the asymptomatic outpatient with mild thrombocytopenia to the bleeding, severely thrombocytopenic postoperative patient in the surgical intensive care unit (ICU), a myriad of disorders can cause a low platelet count. While many of these cause thrombocytopenia by accelerating the destruction or clearance of platelets in the peripheral blood, some are associated with decreased platelet production.

Thrombocytopenia attempts to provide a broad, but detailed overview of the syndromes associated with a low platelet count. Though most of the chapters are clinically focused, each also discusses relevant pathophysiology that enhances the reader's insight into current and emerging management strategies. Two chapters also provide an overview of the process of platelet production, with particular emphasis on the role of thrombopoietin and specific transcription factors required for normal megakaryocyte development. A timely discussion of emerging thrombopoietin analogs that will influence the management of thrombocytopenic states in years to come is also presented.

All contributors to this book are internationally recognized for their expertise in the diagnosis and management of platelet disorders.

For clarity, this book is divided into two major sections, the first of which reviews megakaryocyte biology and platelet production, as well as the congenital thrombocytopenias and miscellaneous thrombocytopenias resulting from marrow dysfunction and diminished platelet production. The second section reviews causes of thrombocytopenia resulting from enhanced peripheral platelet destruction, and reviews disorders such as immune thrombocytopenic purpura (ITP), thrombotic thrombocytopenic purpura (TTP) and the hemolytic uremic syndrome (HUS), heparin/induced thrombocytopenia (HIT), and pregnancy-associated thrombocytopenia. An important chapter on the appropriate use and potential complications of platelet transfusion is also included.

The breadth of this book should make it a useful reference for physicians from a variety of specialties, including adult and pediatric hematology-oncology, transfusion medicine, internal medicine and general pediatrics, and obstetrics. This book will also be of value to trainees in these areas, as well as medical students.

Keith R. McCrae

Contents

Contributors

Richard H. Aster Department of Medicine and Pathology, Medical College of Wisconsin, and Blood Research Institute, BloodCenter of Wisconsin, Milwaukee, Wisconsin, U.S.A.

Victor Blanchette Division of Haematology and Oncology, Department of Paediatrics, Hospital for Sick Children, Toronto, Ontario, Canada

James B. Bussel Platelet Disorders Center, Division of Pediatric Hematology-Oncology, Department of Pediatrics, Weill Medical College of Cornell University, New York, New York, U.S.A.

Douglas B. Cines Department of Pathology and Laboratory Medicine, University of Pennsylvania School of Medicine, Philadelphia, Pennsylvania, U.S.A.

James N. George Hematology-Oncology Section, Department of Medicine, College of Medicine, University of Oklahoma Health Sciences Center, Oklahoma City, Oklahoma, U.S.A.

Marc J. Kahn Section of Hematology/Medical Oncology, Department of Medicine, School of Medicine, Tulane University Health Sciences Center, New Orleans, Louisiana, U.S.A.

Cecile Kaplan Platelet Immunology Unit, Institut National de la Transfusion Sanguine, Paris, France

David J. Kuter MGH Cancer Center, Massachusetts General Hospital, Harvard Medical School, Boston, Massachusetts, U.S.A.

Cindy Leissinger Section of Hematology/Medical Oncology, Department of Medicine, School of Medicine, Louisiana Comprehensive Hemophilia Care Center, Tulane University Health Sciences Center, New Orleans, Louisiana, U.S.A.

Keith R. McCrae Division of Hematology-Oncology, Department of Medicine, Case Western Reserve University School of Medicine/University Hospitals of Cleveland, Cleveland, Ohio, U.S.A.

Janice McFarland Department of Pathology and Medicine, Medical College of Wisconsin, and BloodCenter of Wisconsin, Milwaukee, Wisconsin, U.S.A.

Steven E. McKenzie Cardeza Foundation for Hematologic Research, Thomas Jefferson University, Philadelphia, Pennsylvania, U.S.A.

Liyan Pang Department of Pediatrics, University of Pennsylvania School of Medicine, Children's Hospital of Philadelphia, Philadelphia, Pennsylvania, U.S.A.

Mortimer Poncz Department of Pediatrics, University of Pennsylvania School of Medicine, Children's Hospital of Philadelphia, Philadelphia, Pennsylvania, U.S.A.

Michael P. Reilly Cardeza Foundation for Hematologic Research, Thomas Jefferson University, Philadelphia, Pennsylvania, U.S.A.

J. Evan Sadler Department of Medicine and Department of Biochemistry and Molecular Biophysics, Washington University School of Medicine, and Howard Hughes Medical Institute, St. Louis, Missouri, U.S.A.

Theodore E. Warkentin Department of Pathology and Molecular Medicine and Department of Medicine, McMaster University, and Hamilton Regional Laboratory Medicine Program, Hamilton Health Sciences, General Site, Hamilton, Ontario, Canada

PART I: THROMBOCYTOPENIA DUE TO DISORDERED PLATELET PRODUCTION

1

Megakaryopoiesis and Platelet Formation

Liyan Pang and Mortimer Poncz

Department of Pediatrics, University of Pennsylvania School of Medicine, Children's Hospital of Philadelphia, Philadelphia, Pennsylvania, U.S.A.

INTRODUCTION

Megakaryocytes are hematopoietic precursors of platelets which in turn play an essential role in thrombosis and hemostasis (reviewed in Ref.1). Over the past 15 years, a great deal of new insight and information have been obtained concerning the various steps involved in the processes leading to a normal steady-state platelet level. The differentiation of hematopoietic stem cells to megakaryocytes will be presented below. The cytokines and receptors involved in this differentiation and the key hematopoietic transcription factors involved in the development of morphologically recognizable megakaryocytes are presented. Finally, the proteins and mechanisms involved in the formation of proplatelet processes and platelets will be presented. The growing insight into these processes has already led to understanding the molecular basis of a number of acquired and inherited hematologic disorders, and it is anticipated that further knowledge may lead to new insights into how to modulate both platelet numbers and thrombogenicity.

FORMATION OF MEGAKARYOCYTES FROM HEMATOPOIETIC STEM CELLS

Megakaryopoiesis is first noted in the yolk sac, so there appears to be an embryonic-fetal form of megakaryocyte formation that may or may not lead to distinct platelets from adult megakaryopoiesis (2). Megakaryocyte progenitors have been classified by the ability of the cells to give rise to mixed populations of cells containing morphologically recognizable megakaryocytes. Thus, individual cells that give rise to a mixture of granulocytes, erythrocytes, megakaryocytes, and macrophages have been termed CFU-GEMM; cells giving rise to erythrocytes and megakaryocytes have been termed CFU-EM; and cells giving rise to just megakaryocytes have been termed CFU-Meg (3). An attempt to understand the process of increased commitment from such colony studies has not been fruitful, but as seen below, it is likely that the 2N megakaryoblast arises (where 2N is the DNA content of a somatic cell) from a common erythroid-megakaryocytic progenitor, termed burst forming unit (BFU)-EM. Morphologically and immunologically recognizable megakaryocytes begin with the 2N megakaryoblasts, which in turn undergo endomitosis and cytoplasmic differentiation resulting in a pool of mature megakaryocytes. Typically in the normal human marrow, ~1:10,000 nucleated cells is a recognizable megakaryocyte, while in immune thrombocytopenia purpura (ITP), the number increases to ~1:1000 (4), similar to that seen normally in the murine marrow (5).

The hallmark of megakaryocyte development is the formation of a large cell of ~50–100 μM diameter containing a single, large, multi-lobulated, polyploid nucleus (6). Unlike other cells, megakaryocytes undergo an endomitotic cell cycle during which they replicate DNA but do not undergo cytokinesis and, as a result, acquire a DNA content of up to 128N (7). Cytoplasmic maturation occurs at the same time so that the cell accumulates surface markers such as the αIIb/β3 receptor (CD41), the cytoplasmic demarcation system, and the distinctive organelles and organelle granular proteins such as platelet factor 4 and Von Willebrand factor that are hallmarks of circulating platelets. All degrees of polyploidy are present in cells of each stage of cytoplasmic maturation, showing that a cell can mature cytoplasmically at any ploidy level, indicating that megakaryocyte proliferation and membrane demarcation and platelet formation are not strictly sequential events, so that it has been hard to decipher "early onset" megakaryocyte-specific genes from "late-onset" (8). Eventually, each megakaryocyte releases ~10^4 platelets (9).

General Cytokines

It had been clearly recognized for many years that there must be a mechanism that limits platelet count to an ~three-fold range ($150–450 \times 10^3/\mu^3$) and that results in increased platelet production in disorders such as ITP that are associated with increased peripheral destruction. A cytokine involved in this process was termed thrombopoietin (TPO) (10) as it was thought to be the equivalent of erythropoietin (EPO) which regulates red cell mass.

Historically, the study of megakaryocyte differentiation had been restricted by the rareness of these cells in the bone marrow, the difficulties associated with isolating and managing sufficient numbers of primary megakaryocytes, and the limited megakaryocytic potential of most established cell lines. Various growth factors regulate megakaryocyte differentiation on different levels (Fig. 1). Certain cytokines stimulate proliferation of megakaryocytic progenitors such as interlukin-3 (IL-3), IL-6, IL-11, IL-12, granulocyte-macrophage colony stimulating factor (GM-CSF), and EPO (11). Others have been reported to modulate megakaryocyte maturation and platelet development including IL-1α and leukemia inhibitory factor (LIF) (11,12). However, all of the above-mentioned growth factors and cytokines have very broad effects on all hematopoietic cell lines, although IL-11 (Neumega) is the only clinically approved cytokine for the treatment of thrombocytopenia at the moment (13). Below, we discuss the myeloproliferative (mpl) ligand that is also called TPO, as well as two chemokines, stromal-derived factor-1 (SDF-1; CXCL12) and platelet factor 4 (PF4; CXCL4).

Thrombopoietin (TPO)

The mpl oncogene was an orphan receptor that was homologically clearly similar to many GP130 cytokine receptors in structure, but had no known ligand and function until the use of antisense oligonucleotides showed that blocking the receptor led to a loss of megakaryocytes in marrow culture (14). This pivotal observation rapidly led to the cloning of its ligand TPO (15–17), which turned out to be highly related structurally to EPO in its N-terminal half. TPO was found to be a specific factor which controls megakaryocytic cell proliferation as well as maturation (5,18). Interestingly, abrogated expression of either the mpl receptor or TPO results in transgenic mice with approximately 85% fewer megakaryocytes in the bone marrow and circulating platelets, but not a complete absence (19,20). Furthermore, these studies also showed that the mpl:TPO axis was important for hematopoiesis in general, and that the mpl receptor is present on early hematopoietic cells (21,22). Thus, at the moment, the mpl:TPO axis appears to be important for hematopoiesis in general and megakaryopoiesis specifically (23).

How TPO normally regulates platelet counts is unclear. TPO is thought to be predominantly made in the liver (24). TPO then is absorbed by mpl on circulating platelets to negatively regulate the level of free TPO available to the marrow (25). In the marrow, TPO is also produced by stromal cells. The importance of circulating TPO versus local TPO production on platelet numbers is unclear. Do they satisfy separate hematopoietic pools as cells go through an orderly process of differentiation in the marrow? Clearly TPO regulation of thrombopoiesis is quite different from EPO regulation of erythropoiesis, where the kidneys are the sole source of EPO and there is no circulating sink regulating its level. Defects in mpl have been linked to the rare human disorder congenital amegakaryocytic thrombocytopenia (CAMT) (26,27). Whether these patients are at risk of developing more diffuse aplastic anemia is unclear at the moment (28). No disorder has yet to be linked to an absense of TPO, but patients with upregulating mutations in the TPO promoter have been described among the

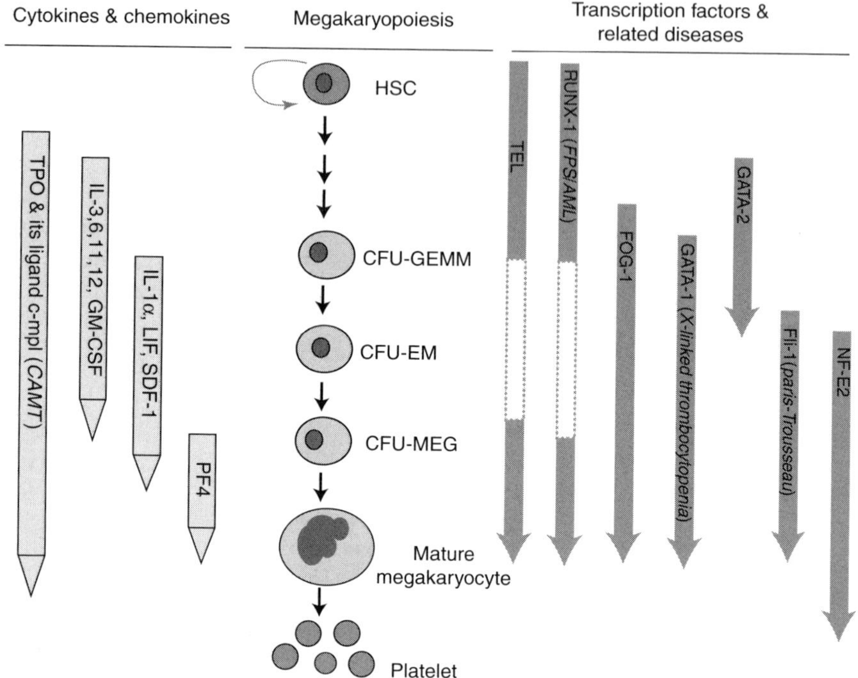

Figure 1 Regulation of the megakaryopoiesis by cytokines, chemokines, and transcription factors. Formation of megakaryocytes from the hematopoietic stem cells is a tightly regulated process in which both cytokines and chemokines (left side, light gray arrows), as well as transcription factors (right side, medium gray arrows) play important roles. Diseases in humans linked to the defects of those regulators are marked in italic characters.

familial forms of essential thrombocythemia. Finally, one of the great clinical hopes for TPO was its potential use for patient care. However, clinical trials did not show a significant decrease in the number of transfusions needed, but did suggest an increased risk of thrombosis (29), which may be due to TPO enhancing platelet reactivity directly by binding to the platelet mpl (30). Also, patients have developed antibodies to TPO.

Stromal-derived Factor-1 (SDF-1)

In addition to the role of the general cytokines and TPO in megakaryopoiesis, a great deal of attention has been paid to the biological effects of SDF-1 in this process. Initially it was thought that SDF-1 could enhance megakaryopoiesis (31). Further studies suggested that SDF-1 stimulates $CD34^+$ progenitor cells through its receptor CXCR4 by distinct pathways from TPO (32) and appears to enhance megakaryocyte precursor migration, which may be important in platelet formation in the appropriate hematopoietic niche (33–35). Utilization of the CXCR4 receptor on CD34+ progenitors may be one mechanism by which human immunodeficiency viruses lead to thrombocytopenia in affected patients (36).

PF4 and Other Chemokines

In the late 1980s, Platelet Factor 4 (PF4) was the first negative autocrine described in hematopoiesis (37). In vivo confirmation of this negative autocrine effect has recently been suggested in the initial analysis of platelet counts in the PF4 null mouse and a transgenic PF4 over expressing mouse (38). These studies with PF4 have since been extended to show that a number of additional CXC and CC subfamily chemokines can also negatively influence megakaryopoiesis (39). Subsequently, it has become clear that platelet α-granules contain not only large molar stores of the platelet-specific chemokines PF4 and the closely-related protein, platelet basic protein (PBP; CXCL7), but also RANTES (CCL5) and ENA-78 (CXCL5) (40–42). These chemokines are weak agonists of platelet activation through the presence of low levels of their receptors on the platelet surface, but may be important in linking thrombosis with the related process of inflammation.

TRANSCRIPTION FACTOR INVOLVED IN GENE REGULATION DURING MEGAKARYOPOIESIS

From the above discussion, it should be clear that the formation of megakaryocytes is the end result of multiple cytokines influencing a committed progenitor as it moves from one hematopoietic niche to another in an organized fashion (35). During this process, numerous tissue-specific genes are modified and spatially oriented in the nucleus to be primed for the eventual transcription of a series of megakaryocyte-specific genes (Fig. 1). Some of the events in the nucleus at the near-final stages of megakaryopoiesis are beginning to be understood with a focus on the hematopoietic-specific transcriptional factors involved. Below, the discussion is mostly focused on the GATA-1/FOG-1 complex as the best understood of such factors. Additionally, two Erythroblast transformation specific (Ets) family members, Fli-1, which clearly interacts with the GATA-1/FOG-1 complex and is specifically expressed during megakaryopoiesis, and Tel (Etv6), a related Ets family member that also affects megakaryopoiesis, will be discussed. In addition, nuclear factor-erythroid 2 (NF-E2 or p45) and the Runt domain transcription factor, RUNX-1 (AML1 or CBFA2), are two additional transcription factors with clear roles in megakaryopoiesis that will be discussed.

GATA-1/FOG-1

GATA-binding protein-1 (GATA-1) was first isolated as an erythroid-specific transcription factor with two zinc fingers that bind to a DNA sequence motif whose core is GATA (43). Subsequently, GATA-1 was shown to be expressed in megakaryocytes, mast cells, and eosinophils as well (44,45). Transient expression studies of a number of megakaryocyte-specific proximal promoters defined a number of functionally important GATA-binding sites (46–50). Furthermore, a point mutation in an in vitro functionally important GATA consensus binding site in the proximal promoter of the GPIbβ gene is the only described mutation in a megakaryocyte-specific promoter resulting in a clinically relevant defect, causing a Bernard-Soulier Syndrome phenotype in the affected patient (49).

While targeted disruption of the GATA-1 gene resulted in an embryonic lethal phenotype due to anemia (51), a tissue-specific knockdown of expression in a megakaryocyte-specific fashion had minimal anemia, but significant thrombocytopenia with increased numbers of immature and dysmorphic megakaryocytes in the marrow (52). GATA-2 is a related transcription factor to GATA-1 and is also hematopoietic-specific, but is expressed earlier on and also affects the aorta-gonad-mesonephros (AGM) differentiation into hematopoietic and vascular tissues (53). Continued GATA-2 expression during early megakaryopoiesis may explain the partial ability for platelet formation in the GATA-1 knockdown mouse (54).

FOG-1 (Friend of GATA-1) is a nine-zinc finger, hematopoietic-specific transcription factor isolated because of its ability to bind GATA-1 (55). Targeted disruption of the FOG-1 gene markedly prevented both erythroid and megakaryocytic development. Studies have shown that FOG-1 does not bind DNA directly, but binds only through GATA proteins. The only other hematopoietic lineages in which a member of the FOG family is expressed involve the lymphocytic lineages (56). Therefore, unlike with GATA-1 and GATA-2, there is not a partial FOG-1 rescue in the megakaryocyte/erythroid lineages when the FOG-1 gene is disrupted. The severity of the megakaryocyte defect in the FOG-1 gene targeted disruption mouse suggests that critical GATA-1-related activity requires its interactions with FOG-1. Recently, it had been shown that GATA-1 and FOG-1 synergistically enhance the expression of the megakaryocyte-specific αIIb gene (57,58). These observations have been expanded to show that direct contact is needed between the N-terminal zinc finger of GATA-1 and FOG-1, and that this synergism applies to multiple megakaryocyte-specific genes and also involves a specific Ets-family transcription factor (see below) (58). Further studies suggest that the N-terminal of FOG-1 is involved in this megakaryocyte-specific function (59). The importance of the interaction in megakaryopoiesis of GATA-1 and FOG-1 was the recent description of a number of patients with significant thrombocytopenia and variable anemia who have mutations within or adjacent to the FOG-1 binding domain of GATA-1 (60–62).

Friend-leukemia Integration-1 (Fli-1) and Translocation-Ets-Leukemia (Tel)

At the same time that a number of laboratories were defining the importance of GATA-1 as a *trans*-acting factor in the regulated expression of multiple megakaryocyte-specific genes, it became clear that the proximal promoters for many of these genes had in addition to the consensus GATA-binding sites in their proximal promoters, but also consensus Ets binding sites (48,50,63,64). The Ets family of transcription factors is highly diverse with over 30 family members, which have in common an Ets binding domain that binds to a GGAA consensus sequence (65). Multiple family members have subsequently been described to be present in primary megakaryocytes or megakaryocytic cell lines, especially Ets-1, Ets-2, PU.1, Fli-1, and Tel (63,66–69). While a number of studies have suggested functional importance to Ets-1 (70), the clearest story appears to be that for Fli-1. GATA-1/FOG-1 synergy for many megakaryocyte-specific genes appears to involve Fli-1 (58), and clearly Fli-1 binds to the proximal promoter of these genes in vivo. The molecular basis of this synergy is still not fully known, but clearly Fli-1 is able to specifically bind to GATA-1 (71). Besides the facts that overexpression of Fli-1 can drive hematopoietic cell lines into a megakaryocytic phenotype (67) and that the Fli-1 targeted disruption mice have abnormal megakaryocytes with thrombocytopenia (72), it appears that hemizygous deficiency of Fli-1 expression is sufficient to cause thrombocytopenia associated with abnormal megakaryocytes in patients with Paris-Trousseau syndrome (73).

Whether other Ets family members are also important is unclear at the moment. Tel is part of the pointed domain subfamily to which Fli-1 belongs (74). The pointed domain of Tel is a short N-terminal domain involved in oligomerization of the transcription factor. Like Fli-1 overexpression, Tel overexpression can drive megakaryocytic differentiation of hematopoietic cell lines (68). Targeted disruption of the Tel gene in the hematopoietic lineage results in a specific defect in megakaryopoiesis (75).

NF-E2

NF-E2 is a hematopoietic-specific basic transcription factor consisting of a tissue-specific p45 leucine zipper transcription factor dimerized with a more ubiquitous smaller p18 subunit (76). In vitro studies clearly demonstrated a role in the regulated expression of erythroid-specific genes. Surprisingly, when the p45 gene was disrupted, mice did not develop anemia, but rather had an almost complete absence of circulating platelets with the marrow containing a large number of immature, abnormal megakaryocytes (77). The molecular basis for this effect has yet to be resolved. It may well be that intracellular signaling pathways, perhaps related to Rab27b (78) or cytoskeletal genes (79), are underexpressed in these mice, leading to the inability for proplatelet formation and platelet release (see below).

RUNX1

Runt-related transcription factor1 (RUNX1) or acute myeloid leukemia1 (AML1) is a hematopoietic-specific protein first noted because of its involvement in several chromosomal translocations resulting in leukemia, particularly the translocation resulting in the AML1-ETO chimera protein (80). It became clear that RUNX1 is the core-binding factor α-2 (CBFA2) that bound to DNA and that in turn bound to the β-subunit CBFB that did not directly bind DNA (81). Initially thought to be primarily involved in myeloid differentiation (82), the disruption of the RUNX1 gene demonstrated that the gene was important as well during AGM formation and early hematopoiesis and vasculogenesis (83). A role for RUNX1 in adult megakaryopoiesis became clear when the etiology of a rare, dominantly inherited thrombocytopenia associated with an increased risk of developing acute myeloblastic leukemia was shown to be due to haploinsufficiency for RUNX1 (84,85). Similar studies of the role of RUNX1 in adult megakaryopoiesis in a murine model were shown as well (86). RUNX1 appears to interact with GATA-1 and regulate αIIb expression (87), and overexpression of RUNX1 can drive hematopoietic cell lines into a megakaryocytic phenotype (88).

MORPHOLOGICALLY RECOGNIZABLE MEGAKARYOCYTES

The most recognizable features of a mature megakaryocyte are its size and its polyploidy nucleus, which is secondary to endomitosis, where the nuclear material doubles, but the cell does not divide (89). The details of mitosis have been well studied with many of the involved proteins defined (90). Many of these have been examined for their role in megakaryocytic endomitosis. Thus the mitosis-promoting factor, a multiprotein complex involving cdc2 and cyclin B1, has been proposed as a potential factor in this process (91); however, levels of cdc2 and cyclin B1 are normal in cells undergoing endomitosis (92). On the other hand, Aurora and Ipl-1 like midbody associated protein-1 (AIM-1), a serine/threonine kinase of the Aurora family (93) that may be involved in mitosis, is found at reduced levels at the start of endomitosis (94). Overexpression of AIM-1 inhibits polyploidization (95), and suppression enhances the process (96).

Another feature of developing megakaryocytes is a system of interconnected flattened cisternae and tubules called the demarcation membrane system (97) that was formerly thought to be involved in "platelet territories" (98). This canalicular system is connected to the outside surface and is now thought to represent extra membrane that exvaginates upon platelet activation.

Megakaryocytes also contain two specific sets of granules, the α-granules and δ-granules. Understanding the formation of these granules has been advanced by the fact that defects of megakaryocyte granular formation in humans and animals often result in pigmentary changes in the hair and other parts of the body. This is especially true of the molecular basis of the disorder Hermansky-Pudlak syndrome for which 6 human and 11 mouse genes have been linked and have provided insights into δ-granular synthesis (99). Additional murine pigment mutant mice have provided insights into the biology of neural granular release as well, showing that proteins associated with neural granular release, such as syntaxin-13 and Rab protein activity, are also involved in platelet granular release (100,101).

PLATELET FORMATION AND RELEASE

As mentioned above, megakaryocytes may undergo an orderly progression of maturation as they move from stromal niche toward the marrow sinusoids (35). However, what leads to the release of platelets is unclear. In fact, it is unclear whether megakaryocytes shed their platelets within the bone marrow or within the pulmonary bed (102–105). Studies have shown that one can detect circulating megakaryocytes in the pulmonary arteries relative to the aorta (106). However, megakaryocyte nuclei, which are readily detected in the marrow of TPO-stimulated mice, are difficult to detect in the pulmonary bed (107). To date, there are two reports of platelet formation in vitro from cultured megakaryocytes (108,109). Both show morphologically recognizable platelets, but the biological studies are limited, and the number of isolated platelets have been inadequate for standard functional studies such as platelet aggregation curves. Whether these studies are actually reporting real platelet formation in vitro remains an open issue.

Megakaryocytes in culture clearly form proplatelet processes, which appear to be beads on a string(110). Microtubular polymerization is central to this process. The distal end of each proplatelet stalk contains a microtubule bundle that forms several peripheral loops before re-entering the shaft, forming a teardrop-shaped structure (111). This microtubular organization is much like the marginal band in circulating platelets (112). The process driving this microtubular organization is myosin/actin-based (113). It is interesting that the molecular basis of the giant platelet disorder May Hegglin syndrome is due to mutations in non-muscle myosin heavy-chain chain 9 (MYH9), an ATPase motor that binds to actin filaments and generates force contraction (114). Another protein that appears to be involved in proplatelet and platelet formation is β1-tubulin, a tissue-specific β-tubulin (112). Absence of β1-tubulin in a murine model results in thrombocytopenia and spherocytic platelets (115). Whether this is due to linkage of the microtubular bands to the cytoskeleton is unclear. Certainly, this process may also explain the thrombocytopenia and the presence of spherocytic macrothombocytes in Bernard-Soulier syndrome, which is due to defective GPIb/IX receptors (116). The GPIb/IX complex is bound to the spectrin/actin cytoskeleton directly (117), and this may explain why in Bernard-Soulier syndrome one has a defect in the size and number of platelets as well as in the GPIb/IX receptor function.

REFERENCES

1. Packham MA. Role of platelets in thrombosis and hemostasis. Can J Physiol Pharmacol 1994; 72:278–284.
2. Palis J, Koniski A. Analysis of hematopoietic progenitors in the mouse embryo. Methods Mol Med 2004; 105:289–302.
3. Kanz L, Straub G, Bross KG, Fauser AA. Identification of human megakaryocytes derived from pure megakaryocytic colonies (CFU-M), megakaryocytic-erythroid colonies (CFU-M/E), and mixed hemopoietic colonies (CFU-GEMM) by antibodies against platelet associated antigens. Blut 1982; 45:267–274.
4. Branehog I, Ridell B, Swolin B, Weinfeld A. Megakaryocyte quantifications in relation to thrombokinetics in primary thrombocythaemia and allied diseases. Scand J Haematol 1975; 15:321–332.
5. de Sauvage FJ, Hass PE, Spencer SD, et al. Stimulation of megakaryocytopoiesis and thrombopoiesis by the c-Mpl ligand. Nature 1994; 369:533–538.
6. Cajano A, Polosa P. Contribution to the study of the morphology of megakaryocytes and blood platelets with Feulgen's test. Haematologica 1950; 34:1113–11121.
7. Odell TT, Jr., Jackson CW, Gosslee DG. Maturation of rat megakaryocytes studied by microspectrophotometric measurement of DNA. Proc Soc Exp Biol Med 1965; 119:1194–1199.
8. Ebbe S. Biology of megakaryocytes. Prog Hemost Thromb 1976; 3:211–229.
9. Long MW. Megakaryocyte differentiation events. Semin Hematol 1998; 35:192–199.
10. Cserhati I, Kelemen E. Acute prolonged thrombocytosis in mice induced by thrombocythaemic sera; a possible human thrombopoietin; a preliminary communication. Acta Med Acad Sci Hung 1958; 11:473–475.
11. Gordon MS, Hoffman R. Growth factors affecting human thrombocytopoiesis: potential agents for the treatment of thrombocytopenia. Blood 1992; 80:302–307.
12. Vainchenker W, Debili N, Mouthon MA, Wendling F. Megakaryocytopoiesis:cellular aspects and regulation. Crit Rev Oncol Hematol 1995; 20:165–192.
13. Orazi A, Cooper RJ, Tong J, et al. Effects of recombinant human interleukin-11 (Neumega rhIL-11 growth factor) on megakaryocytopoiesis in human bone marrow. Exp Hematol 1996; 24:1289–1297.
14. Methia N, Louache F, Vainchenker W, Wendling F. Oligodeoxynucleotides antisense to the proto-oncogene c-mpl specifically inhibit in vitro megakaryocytopoiesis. Blood 1993; 82:1395–1401.
15. Bartley TD, Bogenberger J, Hunt P, et al. Identification and cloning of a megakaryocyte growth and development factor that is a ligand for the cytokine receptor Mpl. Cell 1994; 77:1117–1124.
16. Lok S, Kaushansky K, Holly RD, et al. Cloning and expression of murine thrombopoietin cDNA and stimulation of platelet production in vivo. Nature 1994; 369:565–568.
17. Kaushansky K, Lok S, Holly RD, et al. Promotion of megakaryocyte progenitor expansion and differentiation by the c-Mpl ligand thrombopoietin. Nature 1994; 369:568–571.
18. Arnold JT, Daw NC, Stenberg PE, Jayawardene D, Srivastava DK, Jackson CW. A single injection of pegylated murine megakaryocyte growth and development factor (MGDF) into mice is sufficient to produce a profound stimulation of megakaryocyte frequency, size, and ploidization. Blood 1997; 89:823–833.

19. Gurney AL, Carver-Moore K, de Sauvage FJ, Moore MW. Thrombocytopenia in c-mpl-deficient mice. Science 1994; 265:1445–1447.
20. Alexander WS, Roberts AW, Nicola NA, Li R, Metcalf D. Deficiencies in progenitor cells of multiple hematopoietic lineages and defective megakaryocytopoiesis in mice lacking the thrombopoietic receptor c-Mpl. Blood 1996; 87:2162–2170.
21. Murone M, Carpenter DA, de Sauvage FJ. Hematopoietic deficiencies in c-mpl and TPO knockout mice. Stem Cells 1998; 16:1–6.
22. Borge OJ, Ramsfjell V, Veiby OP, Murphy MJ, Jr., Lok S, Jacobsen SE. Thrombopoietin, but not erythropoietin, promotes viability and inhibits apoptosis of multipotent murine hematopoietic progenitor cells in vitro. Blood 1996; 88:2859–2870.
23. Debili N, Wendling F, Katz A, et al. The Mpl-ligand or thrombopoietin or megakaryocyte growth and differentiative factor has both direct proliferative and differentiative activities on human megakaryocyte progenitors. Blood 1995; 86:2516–2525.
24. Jelkmann W. The role of the liver in the production of thrombopoietin compared with erythropoietin. Eur J Gastroenterol Hepatol 2001; 13:791–801.
25. Kaushansky K. Thrombopoietin: understanding and manipulating platelet production. Annu Rev Med 1997; 48:1–11.
26. Ihara K, Ishii E, Eguchi M, et al. Identification of mutations in the c-mpl gene in congenital amegakaryocytic thrombocytopenia. Proc Natl Acad Sci USA 1999; 96:3132–3136.
27. van den Oudenrijn S, Bruin M, Folman CC, et al. Mutations in the thrombopoietin receptor, Mpl, in children with congenital amegakaryocytic thrombocytopenia. Br J Haematol 2000; 110:441–448.
28. Ballmaier M, Germeshausen M, Krukemeier S, Welte K. Thrombopoietin is essential for the maintenance of normal hematopoiesis in humans: development of aplastic anemia in patients with congenital amegakaryocytic thrombocytopenia. Ann N Y Acad Sci 2003; 996:17–25.
29. Kuter DJ, Begley CG. Recombinant human thrombopoietin: basic biology and evaluation of clinical studies. Blood 2002; 100:3457–3469.
30. Oda A, Miyakawa Y, Druker BJ, et al. Thrombopoietin primes human platelet aggregation induced by shear stress and by multiple agonists. Blood 1996; 87:4664–4670.
31. Wang JF, Liu ZY, Groopman JE. The alpha-chemokine receptor CXCR4 is expressed on the megakaryocytic lineage from progenitor to platelets and modulates migration and adhesion. Blood 1998; 92:756–764.
32. Majka M, Janowska-Wieczorek A, Ratajczak J, et al. Stromal-derived factor 1 and thrombopoietin regulate distinct aspects of human megakaryopoiesis. Blood 2000; 96:4142–4151.
33. Kowalska MA, Ratajczak J, Hoxie J, et al. Megakaryocyte precursors, megakaryocytes and platelets express the HIV co-receptor CXCR4 on their surface: determination of response to stromal-derived factor-1 by megakaryocytes and platelets. Br J Haematol 1999; 104:220–229.
34. Hamada T, Mohle R, Hesselgesser J, et al. Transendothelial migration of megakaryocytes in response to stromal cell-derived factor 1 (SDF-1) enhances platelet formation. J Exp Med 1998; 188:539–548.

35. Avecilla ST, Hattori K, Heissig B, et al. Chemokine-mediated interaction of hematopoietic progenitors with the bone marrow vascular niche is required for thrombopoiesis. Nat Med 2004; 10:64–71.
36. Lee B, Ratajczak J, Doms RW, Gewirtz AM, Ratajczak MZ. Coreceptor/chemokine receptor expression on human hematopoietic cells: biological implications for human immunodeficiency virus-type 1 infection. Blood 1999; 93:1145–1156.
37. Gewirtz AM, Calabretta B, Rucinski B, Niewiarowski S, Xu WY. Inhibition of human megakaryocytopoiesis in vitro by platelet factor 4 (PF4) and a synthetic COOH-terminal PF4 peptide. J Clin Invest 1989; 83:1477–1486.
38. Eslin DE, Zhang C, Samuels KJ, et al. Transgenic mice studies demonstrate a role for platelet factor 4 in thrombosis: dissociation between anticoagulant and antithrombotic effect of heparin. Blood 2004; 104:3173–3180.
39. Gewirtz AM, Zhang J, Ratajczak J, et al. Chemokine regulation of human megakaryocytopoiesis. Blood 1995; 86:2559–2567.
40. Kowalska MA, Ratajczak MZ, Majka M, et al. Stromal cell-derived factor-1 and macrophage-derived chemokine: 2 chemokines that activate platelets. Blood 2000; 96:50–57.
41. Clemetson KJ, Clemetson JM, Proudfoot AE, Power CA, Baggiolini M, Wells TN. Functional expression of CCR1, CCR3, CCR4, and CXCR4 chemokine receptors on human platelets. Blood 2000; 96:4046–4054.
42. Gear AR, Camerini D. Platelet chemokines and chemokine receptors: linking hemostasis, inflammation, and host defense. Microcirculation 2003; 10:335–350.
43. Weiss MJ, Orkin SH. GATA transcription factors: key regulators of hematopoiesis. Exp Hematol 1995; 23:99–107.
44. Zon LI, Yamaguchi Y, Yee K, et al. Expression of mRNA for the GATA-binding proteins in human eosinophils and basophils: potential role in gene transcription. Blood 1993; 81:3234–3241.
45. Mouthon MA, Bernard O, Mitjavila MT, Romeo PH, Vainchenker W, Mathieu-Mahul D. Expression of tal-1 and GATA-binding proteins during human hematopoiesis. Blood 1993; 81:647–655.
46. Martin F, Prandini MH, Thevenon D, Marguerie G, Uzan G. The transcription factor GATA-1 regulates the promoter activity of the platelet glycoprotein IIb gene. J Biol Chem 1993; 268:21606–21612.
47. Aird WC, Parvin JD, Sharp PA, Rosenberg RD. The interaction of GATA-binding proteins and basal transcription factors with GATA box-containing core promoters. A model of tissue-specific gene expression. J Biol Chem 1994; 269:883–889.
48. Deveaux S, Filipe A, Lemarchandel V, Ghysdael J, Romeo PH, Mignotte V. Analysis of the thrombopoietin receptor (MPL) promoter implicates GATA and Ets proteins in the coregulation of megakaryocyte-specific genes. Blood 1996; 87:4678–4685.
49. Ludlow LB, Schick BP, Budarf ML, et al. Identification of a mutation in a GATA binding site of the platelet glycoprotein Ibbeta promoter resulting in the Bernard-Soulier syndrome. J Biol Chem 1996; 271:22076–22080.
50. Minami T, Tachibana K, Imanishi T, Doi T. Both Ets-1 and GATA-1 are essential for positive regulation of platelet factor 4 gene expression. Eur J Biochem 1998; 258:879–889.

51. Fujiwara Y, Browne CP, Cunniff K, Goff SC, Orkin SH. Arrested development of embryonic red cell precursors in mouse embryos lacking transcription factor GATA-1. Proc Natl Acad Sci USA 1996; 93:12355–12358.
52. Shivdasani RA, Fujiwara Y, McDevitt MA, Orkin SH. A lineage-selective knockout establishes the critical role of transcription factor GATA-1 in megakaryocyte growth and platelet development. EMBO J 1997; 16:3965–3973.
53. Tsai FY, Keller G, Kuo FC, et al. An early haematopoietic defect in mice lacking the transcription factor GATA-2. Nature 1994; 371:221–226.
54. Fujiwara Y, Chang AN, Williams AM, Orkin SH. Functional overlap of GATA-1 and GATA-2 in primitive hematopoietic development. Blood 2004; 103:583–585.
55. Tsang AP, Visvader JE, Turner CA, et al. FOG, a multitype zinc finger protein, acts as a cofactor for transcription factor GATA-1 in erythroid and megakaryocytic differentiation. Cell 1997; 90:109–119.
56. Zhou M, Ouyang W, Gong Q, et al. Friend of GATA-1 represses GATA-3-dependent activity in CD4+T cells. J Exp Med 2001; 194:1461–1471.
57. Gaines P, Geiger JN, Knudsen G, Seshasayee D, Wojchowski DM. GATA-1- and FOG-dependent activation of megakaryocytic alpha IIB gene expression. J Biol Chem 2000; 275:34114–34121.
58. Wang X, Crispino JD, Letting DL, Nakazawa M, Poncz M, Blobel GA. Control of megakaryocyte-specific gene expression by GATA-1 and FOG-1: role of Ets transcription factors. EMBO J 2002; 21:5225–5234.
59. Cantor AB, Katz SG, Orkin SH. Distinct domains of the GATA-1 cofactor FOG-1 differentially influence erythroid versus megakaryocytic maturation. Mol Cell Biol 2002; 22:4268–4279.
60. Nichols KE, Crispino JD, Poncz M, et al. Familial dyserythropoietic anaemia and thrombocytopenia due to an inherited mutation in GATA1. Nat Genet 2000; 24:266–270.
61. Yu C, Niakan KK, Matsushita M, Stamatoyannopoulos G, Orkin SH, Raskind WH. X-linked thrombocytopenia with thalassemia from a mutation in the amino finger of GATA-1 affecting DNA binding rather than FOG-1 interaction. Blood 2002; 100:2040–2045.
62. Mehaffey MG, Newton AL, Gandhi MJ, Crossley M, Drachman JG. X-linked thrombocytopenia caused by a novel mutation of GATA-1. Blood 2001; 98:2681–2688.
63. Lemarchandel V, Ghysdael J, Mignotte V, Rahuel C, Romeo PH. GATA and Ets cis-acting sequences mediate megakaryocyte-specific expression. Mol Cell Biol 1993; 13:668–676.
64. Uzan G, Prandini MH, Berthier R. Regulation of gene transcription during the differentiation of megakaryocytes. Thromb Haemost 1995; 74:210–212.
65. Oikawa T, Yamada T. Molecular biology of the Ets family of transcription factors. Gene 2003; 303:11–34.
66. Terui K, Takahashi Y, Kitazawa J, Toki T, Yokoyama M, Ito E. Expression of transcription factors during megakaryocytic differentiation of CD34+ cells from human cord blood induced by thrombopoietin. Tohoku J Exp Med 2000; 192:259–273.
67. Athanasiou M, Clausen PA, Mavrothalassitis GJ, Zhang XK, Watson DK, Blair DG. Increased expression of the ETS-related transcription factor FLI-1/ERGB correlates

with and can induce the megakaryocytic phenotype. Cell Growth Differ 1996; 7:1525–1534.
68. Sakurai T, Yamada T, Kihara-Negishi F, et al. Effects of overexpression of the Ets family transcription factor TEL on cell growth and differentiation of K562 cells. Int J Oncol 2003; 22:1327–1333.
69. Zhang C, Gadue P, Scott E, Atchison M, Poncz M. Activation of the megakaryocyte-specific gene platelet basic protein (PBP) by the Ets family factor PU.1. J Biol Chem 1997; 272:26236–42626.
70. Jackers P, Szalai G, Moussa O, Watson DK. Ets-dependent regulation of target gene expression during megakaryopoiesis. J Biol Chem 2004; 279:52183–52190.
71. Eisbacher M, Holmes ML, Newton A, et al. Protein–protein interaction between Fli-1 and GATA-1 mediates synergistic expression of megakaryocyte-specific genes through cooperative DNA binding. Mol Cell Biol 2003; 23:3427–3441.
72. Hart A, Melet F, Grossfeld P, et al. Fli-1 is required for murine vascular and megakaryocytic development and is hemizygously deleted in patients with thrombocytopenia. Immunity 2000; 13:167–177.
73. Raslova H, Komura E, Le Couedic JP, et al. FLI1 monoallelic expression combined with its hemizygous loss underlies Paris–Trousseau/Jacobsen thrombopenia. J Clin Invest 2004; 114:77–84.
74. Mackereth CD, Scharpf M, Gentile LN, MacIntosh SE, Slupsky CM, McIntosh LP. Diversity in structure and function of the Ets family PNT domains. J Mol Biol 2004; 342:1249–1264.
75. Hock H, Meade E, Medeiros S, et al. Tel/Etv6 is an essential and selective regulator of adult hematopoietic stem cell survival. Genes Dev 2004; 18:2336–2341.
76. Andrews NC, Erdjument-Bromage H, Davidson MB, Tempst P, Orkin SH. Erythroid transcription factor NF-E2 is a haematopoietic-specific basic-leucine zipper protein. Nature 1993; 362:722–728.
77. Shivdasani RA, Rosenblatt MF, Zucker-Franklin D, et al. Transcription factor NF-E2 is required for platelet formation independent of the actions of thrombopoietin/MGDF in megakaryocyte development. Cell 1995; 81:695–704.
78. Tiwari S, Italiano JE, Jr., Barral DC, et al. A role for Rab27b in NF-E2-dependent pathways of platelet formation. Blood 2003; 102:3970–3979.
79. Lecine P, Italiano JE, Jr., Kim SW, Villeval JL, Shivdasani RA. Hematopoietic-specific beta 1 tubulin participates in a pathway of platelet biogenesis dependent on the transcription factor NF-E2. Blood 2000; 96:1366–1373.
80. Nucifora G, Rowley JD. AML1 and the 8;21 and 3;21 translocations in acute and chronic myeloid leukemia. Blood 1995; 86:1–14.
81. Speck NA, Stacy T, Wang Q, et al. Core-binding factor: a central player in hematopoiesis and leukemia. Cancer Res 1999; 59:1789s–1793s.
82. Zhang DE, Hohaus S, Voso MT, et al. Function of PU.1 (Spi-1), C/EBP, and AML1 in early myelopoiesis: regulation of multiple myeloid CSF receptor promoters. Curr Top Microbiol Immunol 1996; 211:137–147.
83. Takakura N, Watanabe T, Suenobu S, et al. A role for hematopoietic stem cells in promoting angiogenesis. Cell 2000; 102:199–209.
84. Song WJ, Sullivan MG, Legar RD, et al. Haploinsufficiency of CBFA2 causes familial thrombocytopenia with propensity to develop acute myelogenous leukaemia. Nat Genet 1999; 23:166–175.

85. Michaud J, Wu F, Osato M, et al. In vitro analyses of known and novel RUNX1/AML1 mutations in dominant familial platelet disorder with predisposition to acute myelogenous leukemia: implications for mechanisms of pathogenesis. Blood 2002; 99:1364–1372.
86. Ichikawa M, Asai T, Saito T, et al. AML-1 is required for megakaryocytic maturation and lymphocytic differentiation, but not for maintenance of hematopoietic stem cells in adult hematopoiesis. Nat Med 2004; 10:299–304.
87. Michaud J, Wu F, Osato M, et al. In vitro analyses of known and novel RUNX1/AML1 mutations in dominant familial platelet disorder with predisposition to acute myelogenous leukemia: implications for mechanisms of pathogenesis. Blood 2002; 99:1364–1372.
88. Niitsu N, Yamamoto-Yamaguchi Y, Miyoshi H, et al. AML1a but not AML1b inhibits erythroid differentiation induced by sodium butyrate and enhances the megakaryocytic differentiation of K562 leukemia cells. Cell Growth Differ 1997; 8:319–326.
89. Cramer EM. Megakaryocyte structure and function. Curr Opin Hematol 1999; 6:354–361.
90. Miele L. The biology of cyclins and cyclin-dependent protein kinases: an introduction. Methods Mol Biol 2004; 285:3–21.
91. Wang Zr, Zhang Y, Kamen D, Lees E, Ravid K. Cyclin D3 is essential for megakaryocytopoiesis. Blood 1995; 86:3783–3888.
92. Carow CE, Fox NE, Kaushansky K. Kinetics of endomitosis in primary murine megakaryocytes. J Cell Physiol 2001; 188:291–303.
93. Terada Y, Tatsuka M, Suzuki F, Yasuda Y, Fujita S, Otsu M. AIM-1: a mammalian midbody-associated protein required for cytokinesis. EMBO J 1998; 17:667–676.
94. Zhang Y, Sun S, Chen WC, et al. Repression of AIM-1 kinase mRNA as part of a program of genes regulated by Mpl ligand. Biochem Biophys Res Commun 2001; 282:844–849.
95. Katayama H, Ota T, Morita K, et al. Human AIM-1: cDNA cloning and reduced expression during endomitosis in megakaryocyte-lineage cells. Gene 1998; 224:1–7.
96. Kawasaki A, Matsumura I, Miyagawa J, et al. Downregulation of an AIM-1 kinase couples with megakaryocytic polyploidization of human hematopoietic cells. J Cell Biol 2001; 152:275–287.
97. Mahaut-Smith MP, Thomas D, Higham AB, et al. Properties of the demarcation membrane system in living rat megakaryocytes. Biophys J 2003; 84:2646–2654.
98. Shaklai M, Tavassoli M. Demarcation membrane system in rat megakaryocyte and the mechanism of platelet formation: a membrane reorganization process. J Ultrastruct Res 1978; 62:270–285.
99. Gunay-Aygun M, Huizing M, Gahl WA. Molecular defects that affect platelet dense granules. Semin Thromb Hemost 2004; 30:537–547.
100. Schraw TD, Crawford GL, Ren Q, et al. Platelets from Munc18c heterozygous mice exhibit normal stimulus-induced release. Thromb Haemost 2004; 92:829–837.
101. Shirakawa R, Higashi T, Tabuchi A, et al. Munc13-4 is a GTP-Rab27-binding protein regulating dense core granule secretion in platelets. J Biol Chem 2004; 279:10730–10737.

102. Behnke O, Forer A. From megakaryocytes to platelets: platelet morphogenesis takes place in the bloodstream. Eur J Haematol Suppl 1998; 61:3–23.
103. Melamed MR, Cliffton EE, Mercer C, Koss LG. The megakaryocyte blood count. Am J Med Sci 1966; 252:301–309.
104. Kaufman RM, Airo R, Pollack S, Crosby WH. Circulating megakaryocytes and platelet release in the lung. Blood 1965; 26:720–731.
105. Martin JF, Slater DN, Trowbridge EA. Evidence that platelets are produced in the pulmonary circulation by a physical process. Prog Clin Biol Res 1986; 215:405–416.
106. Levine RF, Eldor A, Shoff PK, Kirwin S, Tenza D, Cramer EM. Circulating megakaryocytes: delivery of large numbers of intact, mature megakaryocytes to the lungs. Eur J Haematol 1993; 51:233–246.
107. Davis RE, Stenberg PE, Levin J, Beckstead JH. Localization of megakaryocytes in normal mice and following administration of platelet antiserum, 5-fluorouracil, or radiostrontium: evidence for the site of platelet production. Exp Hematol 1997; 25:638–648.
108. Choi ES, Nichol JL, Hokom MM, Hornkohl AC, Hunt P. Platelets generated in vitro from proplatelet-displaying human megakaryocytes are functional. Blood 1995; 85:402–413.
109. Fujimoto TT, Kohata S, Suzuki H, Miyazaki H, Fujimura K. Production of functional platelets by differentiated embryonic stem (ES) cells in vitro. Blood 2003; 102:4044–4051.
110. Hartwig J, Italiano J, Jr. The birth of the platelet. J Thromb Haemost 2003; 1:1580–1586.
111. Italiano JE, Jr., Lecine P, Shivdasani RA, Hartwig JH. Blood platelets are assembled principally at the ends of proplatelet processes produced by differentiated megakaryocytes. J Cell Biol 1999; 147:1299–1312.
112. Italiano JE, Jr., Bergmeier W, Tiwari S, et al. Mechanisms and implications of platelet discoid shape. Blood 2003; 101:4789–4796.
113. Barkalow KL, Italiano JE, Jr., Chou DE, Matsuoka Y, Bennett V, Hartwig JH. Alpha-adducin dissociates from F-actin and spectrin during platelet activation. J Cell Biol 2003; 161:557–570.
114. Seri M, Cusano R, Gangarossa S, et al. Mutations in MYH9 result in the May-Hegglin anomaly, and Fechtner and Sebastian syndromes. The May–Hegglin/Fechtner Syndrome Consortium. Nat Genet 2000; 26:103–105.
115. Schwer HD, Lecine P, Tiwari S, Italiano JE, Jr, Hartwig JH, Shivdasani RA. A lineage-restricted and divergent beta-tubulin isoform is essential for the biogenesis, structure and function of blood platelets. Curr Biol 2001; 11:579–586.
116. Kunishima S, Kamiya T, Saito H. Genetic abnormalities of Bernard–Soulier syndrome. Int J Hematol 2002; 76:319–327.
117. Hartwig JH, DeSisto M. The cytoskeleton of the resting human blood platelet: structure of the membrane skeleton and its attachment to actin filaments. J Cell Biol 1991; 112:407–425.

2

Thrombopoietin: Biology and Potential Clinical Applications

David J. Kuter

MGH Cancer Center, Massachusetts General Hospital, Harvard Medical School, Boston, Massachusetts, U.S.A.

INTRODUCTION

Thrombocytopenia is a common problem that affects both oncology and non-oncology patients. Thrombocytopenia is occasionally encountered with conventional chemotherapy regimens used to treat solid tumors, but can be a major clinical problem in the management of patients receiving dose-intensive chemotherapy with stem cell support, bone marrow transplantation, induction and consolidation therapy for leukemia, palliative chemotherapy following multiple previous regimens, and multiple cycles of certain chemotherapeutic regimens (1). Multiagent regimens such as MAID (mesna, adriamycin, ifosfamide, and dacarbazine) and ICE (ifosfamide, carboplatin, and etoposide) used in the treatment of lymphoma, sarcoma, breast, ovarian, and germ-cell tumors often produce thrombocytopenia that requires dose modifications, platelet transfusions, or both to prevent bleeding complications (1,2). Thrombocytopenia associated with the use of newer chemotherapy agents such as gemcitabine and bortezomib may limit their use in patients (3). Additionally, patients with associated bone marrow failure have a higher risk of severe thrombocytopenia and bleeding complications with any chemotherapy regimen.

Thrombocytopenia is also a frequent problem in the management of non-chemotherapy patients with myelodysplastic syndrome (MDS), idiopathic thrombocytopenic purpura (ITP), chronic liver disease, and acquired immunodeficiency syndrome (AIDS) (4–8). The chronic thrombocytopenia observed in these conditions results from defective or diminished platelet production or enhanced immunologic and nonimmunologic platelet destruction and may be associated with abnormal platelet function (4–8).

Patients undergoing liver transplantation, cardiovascular surgery, intraaortic balloon counterpulsation, chronic veno-venous hemofiltration, or receiving supportive intensive care often experience severe, acute thrombocytopenia that is associated with increased mortality (9–11). Thrombocytopenia also complicates the administration of many medications, such as antibiotics, interferon, and IIb/IIIa inhibitors (12–20). Thrombocytopenia is a major dose-limiting toxicity of the treatment of chronic hepatitis C infection with interferon and antiviral medications.

Platelet transfusion therapy is currently the only treatment for severe thrombocytopenia. Although temporarily effective in controlling severe thrombocytopenia, platelet transfusion therapy is associated with several problems, including refractoriness and alloimmunization, transmission of infectious agents, and transfusion reactions (21–27). The limited supply of blood products can also be problematic. The use of dose-intensive chemotherapy regimens and hematopoietic progenitor cell transplantation, as well as intensive support for the medical and surgical patient, has resulted in an increasing demand for platelet products; this demand is likely to escalate in an attempt to improve clinical outcomes for oncology and non-oncology patients. The limitations of platelet transfusions and the increased costs associated with the complications of such transfusions have prompted a search for growth factors that stimulate platelet production, thereby reducing or eliminating the need for platelet transfusions (1,2).

THROMBOPOIETIC GROWTH FACTORS

Over the past two decades, a number of hematopoietic growth factors with thrombopoietic activity have been identified, including recombinant granulocyte-macrophage colony-stimulating factor (GM-CSF); stem cell factor (c-kit ligand or steel factor); interleukin (IL)-1, IL-3, IL-6, and IL11; and thrombopoietin (TPO) (28–38). Early clinical studies of many of these cytokines, including IL-1, IL-3, IL-6, and IL-11, showed their ability to stimulate platelet production directly or indirectly in patients with chemotherapy-induced thrombocytopenia (39–44). In phase I studies, administration of IL-1_{α} before or after carboplatin therapy increased platelet counts and was effective at attenuating thrombocytopenia associated with chemotherapy (39,44). Similarly, both IL-6 and IL-11 have been shown to produce an increase in platelet counts and accelerate platelet recovery after chemotherapy (41,42). Despite its relatively modest effect on megakaryocyte and platelet production, IL-11 has been shown to reduce the need for platelet transfusions in patients with chemotherapy-induced thrombocytopenia (43,45).

Although interleukins stimulate thrombopoiesis, their action on platelets is not their principal physiologic function. Recently, gene-targeting studies have shown that the primary physiologic function of IL-11 is to maintain female fertility; it is not essential for hematopoiesis either in normal physiology or in response to hematopoietic stress (46,47). Furthermore, the pleiotropic effect of interleukins often results in unwanted or unacceptable toxic effects, including hyperbilirubinemia, rapid induction of anemia, fever, fatigue, chills, hypotension, and headache (39,44,48–50). Although administration of IL-11 reduces the need for platelet transfusions by approximately a third in patients with severe chemotherapy-induced thrombocytopenia, it is associated with mild peripheral edema, dyspnea, conjunctival redness, and a low incidence of atrial arrhythmias and syncope (42,45). Thus, despite the ability of interleukins to ameliorate thrombocytopenia in a subset of patients treated with conventional chemotherapy, the moderate toxicity encountered with interleukin treatment may interfere with its therapeutic effect and potential use as a thrombopoietic agent.

In contrast to interleukins, TPO, also known as c-Mpl ligand, is a relatively lineage-specific cytokine that stimulates megakaryocyte growth and maturation in vitro and is a potent in vivo thrombopoietic growth factor. Gene-targeting studies have established that TPO is the most important physiologic regulator of steady-state megakaryocyte and platelet production (51–53). Cloning of the c-Mpl ligand led to the clinical development of various preparations of TPO, including recombinant human thrombopoietin (rhTPO), pegylated recombinant human megakaryocyte growth and development factor (PEG-rHuMGDF), and TPO mimetics. This chapter reviews the biology of the thrombopoietins, the areas of potential clinical use, and the problems encountered in their development.

BIOLOGY OF THROMBOPOIETIN

Isolation of c-Mpl Ligand

The identification of TPO as the ligand for the c-Mpl receptor was heralded with much enthusiasm, as almost 40 years had elapsed since the proposal of the existence of a factor that regulates megakaryocytopoiesis and the generation of platelets (54). As is often the case in research, several independent laboratories simultaneously reported the identification and molecular cloning of TPO (29–33). A sentinel discovery that preceded the purification and molecular cloning of TPO was the cloning of the retroviral oncogene, v-*mpl*, from the murine myeloproliferative leukemia virus (55). Subsequently, the cellular homologue c-*mpl* was cloned and shown to encode a membrane protein that possessed substantial homology with receptors for interleukins and colony-stimulating factors, indicating that it might function as a hematopoietic receptor (56). Additional support for the role of c-Mpl as the putative TPO receptor is provided by the presence of c-Mpl mRNA and protein primarily in platelets, megakaryocytes, and a subpopulation of $CD34^+$ cells, and the absolute requirement for the presence of a functional cMpl to stimulate progenitor cells of the megakaryocyte lineage in bone marrow cultures (57). Several groups were able to isolate, purify, and clone its ligand, which was initially referred to as the c-Mpl ligand, megakaryocyte growth and development factor, megapoietin, or TPO (29–33).

Structure and Biologic Properties of TPO

TPO is synthesized primarily in the human liver as a single 353-amino acid precursor protein. On removal of the 21-amino acid signal peptide, the mature molecule consists of two domains: a receptor-binding domain that shows considerable homology to erythropoietin and a carbohydrate-rich carboxy-terminus of the protein that is highly glycosylated and important in maintaining protein stability (Fig. 1) (30,31,58–60). The crystal structure of TPO has recently been elucidated (61) and reveals an antiparallel four-helix bundle fold. It binds to the TPO receptor with a 1:2 stoichiometry with binding constants of 3.3×10^{-9} M and 1.1×10^{-6} M.

TPO levels usually increase in response to the decline in platelet mass and remain elevated during persistent thrombocytopenia. Although hepatic transcription and translation of the TPO gene appear to be constant (62,63), most studies indicate that the circulating platelet mass directly determines the circulating level of TPO (32,64–69). Transfusion of platelets into thrombocytopenic animals or humans has resulted in a decrease in plasma TPO levels (32,65–67,70), and similar results have been observed when normal platelets are transfused into c-Mpl-deficient mice (64). Upon binding of TPO to its receptor on platelets and probably megakaryocytes, the ligand-receptor complex is internalized (32,65,66). Once internalized, the TPO is degraded (64,71,72) with no recycling of the TPO receptor (68). These findings indicate that TPO is constitutively synthesized in the liver and removed from circulation by binding to the c-Mpl receptor on platelets and possibly bone marrow megakaryocytes (Fig. 2). So far, no endogenous or exogenous modulator has been identified that regulates TPO gene expression.

Some investigators have alternatively suggested that local production of TPO by bone marrow stromal cells is increased during thrombocytopenia and stimulates megakaryocyte growth (73). Direct evidence to support the relative contribution of this mechanism to platelet production is lacking, but in experiments in which livers from $TPO^{-/-}$ mice were transplanted into normal mice, at least 60% of the platelet production could be accounted for by hepatic TPO production (74). Furthermore, in patients with hepatic failure undergoing liver transplantation, the low platelet counts and undetectable TPO levels pre-transplant became normal post-transplant, suggesting that the liver is responsible for virtually all TPO production (75,76).

TPO increases the number of megakaryocyte colony-forming cells (Meg-CFC), increases the size, ploidy, and number of megakaryocytes, and stimulates

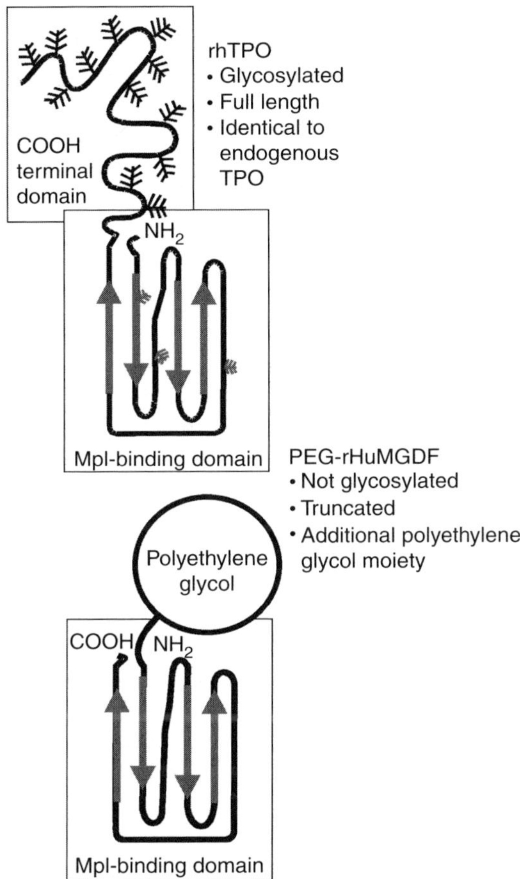

Figure 1 Molecular structures of rhTPO and PEG-rHuMGDF. The receptor-binding domain (Mpl-binding domain) resides in the amino terminus (first 153 amino acids) of TPO and contains 4 conserved cysteine residues and is 17% identical to erythropoietin (~50% identical if neutral substitutions are taken into account). The carboxyl terminus (COOH terminal domain, amino acids 154 to 332) of the molecule appears to be unique to TPO and contains multiple *N*-linked glycosylation sites (indicated by "feathers"). This COOH domain is critical for stabilizing the Mpl binding domain; without it, TPO is rapidly removed from the circulation. rhTPO is a glycosylated full-length TPO molecule, whereas PEG-rHuMGDF is a truncated molecule consisting of the receptor-binding portion of native TPO conjugated to a 20-kD polyethylene glycol moiety; the latter replaces the COOH terminal domain and stabilizes the molecule. *Source*: Courtesy of Amgen Inc., Thousand Oaks, CA.

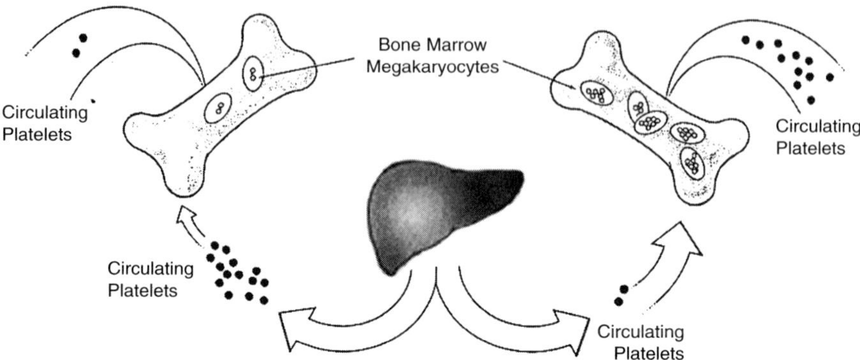

Figure 2 The physiological regulation of thrombopoietin levels. The constitutive hepatic production of thrombopoietin (*center*) is cleared by avid thrombopoietin receptors on platelets resulting in normal levels when the platelet production is normal (*left*) and elevated levels when the platelet production is reduced (*right*). The bone marrow megakaryocytes are stimulated as the circulating thrombopoietin concentration rises.

the expression of platelet-specific markers (32,77,78). The role of TPO as the principal physiologic regulator of platelet production has been confirmed in studies of mutant mice lacking the ability to produce either TPO (TPO$^{-/-}$) or its receptor (c-Mpl$^{-/-}$) (79–83). Genetic elimination of TPO or c-Mpl results in an 85% to 95% reduction in the number of circulating platelets, megakaryocytes, and megakaryocyte progenitor cells (Meg-CFC) (51,82,83). Although TPO-deficient mice are severely thrombocytopenic, they are healthy and show no signs of spontaneous hemorrhage, implying that TPO-independent mechanisms for platelet production exist (82). Recently, "double knock-out" mice that lack the genes for c-Mpl and one other growth factor or its receptor (GM-CSF, IL-3, IL-11, IL-6, or leukemia inhibitory factor) have been created to investigate this observation. The double knockout mice had no additional defect in platelets or their precursors, indicating that GM-CSF, IL-3, IL-11, IL-6, or leukemia inhibitory factor alone are not responsible for the basal platelet production seen in the absence of TPO signaling (52,53,84).

In addition to acting as a potent megakaryocyte colony-stimulating factor, TPO has a major effect on the growth of primitive pluripotent stem cells and progenitor cells from other lineages and synergizes with other hematopoietic growth factors such as erythropoietin or stem cell factor (85–87). Despite normal red and white blood cell numbers, mice deficient in TPO (TPO$^{-/-}$) or c-Mpl (c-Mpl$^{-/-}$) exhibit a 60% to 70% reduction in the number of erythroid and myeloid progenitor cells compared with control animals (51,82). In addition, the ability of hematopoietic cells from these animals to reconstitute the hematopoietic organs of irradiated normal mice is also substantially reduced (88). Administration of TPO to TPO$^{-/-}$ mice expanded the bone marrow and spleen progenitor pools of all hematopoietic lineages and increased the number of circulating platelets (51). Therefore, TPO affects the growth of early precursor cells of all lineages but affects late maturation only of megakaryocytes, thereby increasing only the platelets in the peripheral blood.

Despite its activity on hematopoietic stem cells and early megakaryocytopoiesis, TPO has little direct effect on platelets and on the very late stages of megakaryocyte development (89–92). This contrasts with granulocyte colony-stimulating factor (G-CSF) and GM-CSF, for which an action on late myeloid precursor cells and mature myeloid cells is well established (93,94). Perhaps the most significant consequence of TPO's minimal effect on late-stage megakaryocytes is the inability of TPO to hasten platelet shedding from megakaryocytes. In fact, if anything, TPO inhibits platelet shedding (89).

Although TPO does not directly cause platelet activation, at pharmacologically high doses it does have a modest effect on mature platelets by increasing their reactivity to some aggregation stimuli; TPO-treated platelets require half as much adenosine diphosphate (ADP) for a response (95,96). Other hematopoietic growth factors also reduce the threshold for platelet activation but the clinical relevance of this is unknown. This effect may be mediated by TPO-dependent activation of phosphatidylinositide 3-kinase, which in turn phosphorylates Thr^{306} and Ser^{473} of platelet protein kinase Bα, an important antiapoptotic protein (97). However, TPO does not prevent apoptosis of platelets during ex vivo storage (98–100).

RECOMBINANT THROMBOPOIETINS AND THROMBOPOIETIN MIMETICS

First Generation Recombinant Thrombopoietins—rhTPO and PEG-rHuMGDF

Soon after TPO was first cloned, two recombinant thrombopoietins were rapidly developed for clinical evaluation. Both of these preparations, rhTPO and PEG-rHuMGDF (Fig. 1), have undergone considerable preclinical and clinical evaluation and have taught us much about the clinical behavior of TPO. The amino acid sequence of rhTPO is identical to that of endogenous TPO. rhTPO is produced in mammalian cells and is glycosylated. Nonetheless, its molecular weight is 90 kD, less than the 95 kD of the native molecule (190). PEG-rHuMGDF is produced in *Escherichia coli* and consists of the receptor-binding 163 amino-terminal amino acids of native TPO. It is conjugated on the amino terminus to a 20 kD polyethylene glycol moiety to increase its circulatory half-life and possesses all the biologic activity of native TPO (102). These two recombinant thrombopoietins have similar pharmacologic characteristics (Table 1) and show profound in vitro and in vivo effects on megakaryocyte development and platelet production (103,104).

Table 1 Pharmacologic Characteristics of rhTPO and PEG-rHuMGDF

Characteristic	rhTPO	PEG-rHuMGDF
Terminal $t_{1/2}$ (hr)	24–40	31
K_d for c-Mpl (pM)	150	150
Platelet clearance (mL/h/10^9)	1.28	1.28
Time to onset of effect in mice (d)	3	3
Time to peak effect in mice (d)	4–6	4–6
Truncation	No	Yes
Glycosylation	Yes	No
Pegylation	No	Yes
Human route tested	Intravenous	Subcutaneous

PEG-rHuMGDF, pegylated recombinant human megakaryocyte growth and development factor; rhTPO, recombinant human thrombopoietin.

In healthy animals, these recombinant molecules exert their peripheral blood effects exclusively on platelets, with no increase in white or red blood cells. Administration of either form of recombinant TPO to healthy nonhuman primates results in a dose-dependent increase in megakaryocyte number, size, and ploidy and up to a 5-fold increase in circulating platelet counts (105). There is a requisite lag time of four to five days before the platelet count rises; this reflects the finding that TPO acts primarily on early, not late, precursor cells. Like other hematopoietic growth factors, it takes exponentially greater amounts of TPO to produce linear increases in the platelet count. In murine models of severe chemotherapy—or radiation-induced thrombocytopenia or both, daily administration of recombinant TPO increases megakaryocyte numbers in the bone marrow, ameliorates the depth and duration of thrombocytopenia, but also reduces the severity of leukopenia and anemia (102,106). Similar results have been observed with recombinant TPO in nonhuman primate models of chemotherapy and radiation-induced thrombocytopenia (107–109). However, only platelet responses have been seen in humans (110).

Second Generation Thrombopoietins and Thrombopoietin Mimetics

After the development of rhTPO and PEG-rHuMGDF, a number of other molecules that bind and activate the TPO receptor, cMpl, have been developed (Table 2) in an attempt to eliminate the immunogenicity found with PEG-rHuMGDF (see "Safety of Thrombopoietins" below) or improve efficacy. One of these molecules is a fusion protein of TPO and IL-3. Administration of this molecule has been shown to increase platelet counts in animals, but it has been found to be immunogenic and is no longer under development (111).

Recently, great interest has been focused on the development of TPO peptide (112–114) and non-peptide, small molecule (115) mimetics. These mimetics are designed to bind to the TPO receptor but have no sequence

Table 2 The Thrombopoietins (c-Mpl Ligands)

Endogenous thrombopoietin (TPO)
Recombinant human thrombopoietin (rhTPO)
Pegylated recombinant human growth and development factor (PEG-rHuMGDF)
Promegapoietin (TPO/IL3 fusion protein)
Thrombopoietin peptide mimetics (peptides, pegylated peptides, peptide-immunoglobulin constructs)
Thrombopoietin non-peptide, small molecule mimetics

homology with endogenous TPO. They have been developed by screening peptide and small molecule libraries for the ability to activate the TPO receptor. Many lead compounds have been identified and further modified to increase their efficacy and stability.

Early preclinical work with one of these TPO peptide mimetics (112,113) demonstrated that, to be effective, a TPO peptide mimetic needed to have a long half-life and possess a dimeric structure in order to activate the TPO receptor. Unmodified, monomeric peptides activated the TPO receptor poorly and were rapidly cleared from the circulation.

Although pegylated dimeric TPO peptide mimetics have been developed, a more common approach has been to create TPO mimetics by fusing small peptides containing the receptor-binding region of TPO with another protein sequence such as the IgG heavy chain or Fc region. This provides a dimeric structure with a prolonged half-life. One of these, AMG 531 (formerly AMP 2), consists of four identical peptides that avidly bind c-mpl and are inserted into a dimerized immunoglobulin Fc domain. AMG 531 has a molecular weight of 60,000 Da, a T1/2 in humans of over 100 hr (116) and is cleared and recycled by endothelial FcRn receptors. In vitro it binds the TPO receptor and competes with TPO, activates the JAK2/STAT5 pathway, stimulates the growth of TPO-dependent cell lines, promotes the growth of Meg-CFC, and increases the ploidy and maturation of megakaryocytes (117). When given to healthy human volunteers, it produces a dose-dependent rise in platelet count with no adverse effects (116). It is currently in clinical trials and has been shown to increase the platelet count in some patients with ITP (see below) (118,119). To date no antibody formation has been seen in animals or humans, despite repetitive subcutaneous administration.

Another approach has been to develop small non-peptide TPO mimetics that are potentially orally available. This approach has been surprisingly effective in identifying substances that bind to the TPO receptor, in contrast to the unrewarding search for erythropoietin small molecule mimetics. By using cell lines expressing the TPO receptor, c-mpl, many small molecules that stimulate STAT5 phosphorylation have been identified. Families of hydrazinonaphthalene, azonaphthalene, semicarbazone, and naphtho[1,2-*d*]imidazole TPO mimetics have been described (Fig. 3) (115,120–123). They possess low molecular weights

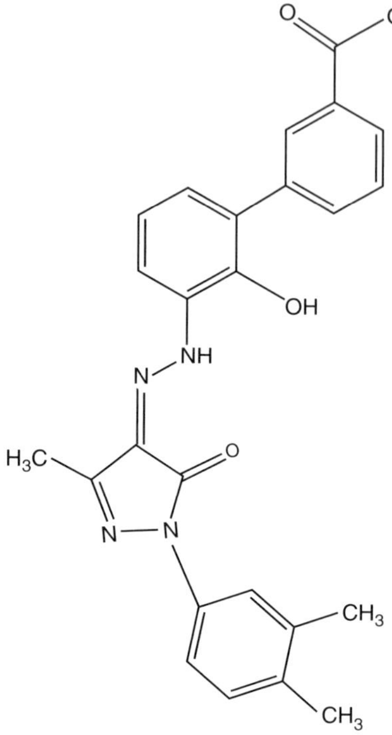

Figure 3 SB-497115, an example of a non-peptide TPO mimetic. The pyrazole-4-ylidenehydrazines have potent thrombopoietic activity. One of these, SB-497115, has a molecular weight of 546 Da, is orally bioavailable, stimulates Meg-CFC growth, increases the platelet count in humans, and does not activate platelets. *Source*: From Refs. 123–125,127.

(MW $<$ 600) and EC_{50} values of 1–20 nM. Preclinical studies have demonstrated stimulation of platelet production identical with TPO. One of these, SB-497115, has a MW of 546 Da, stimulates the growth of TPO-dependent cell lines, promotes the growth of human Meg-CFC and megakaryocytes in culture, and demonstrates striking species-specificity in that it activates human and chimpanzee TPO receptors but not those of any other species (124–126). SB-497115 increases the platelet count in healthy humans (127) and is currently in clinical trials.

Many of these TPO small molecule mimetics possess several striking attributes. One attribute is that they bind the TPO receptor at a site distant from the binding site for TPO and appear to induce signal transduction by a mechanism different from recombinant TPO. It is not yet clear whether they need to dimerize the TPO receptor like the TPO peptide mimetics. By not competing with TPO for binding, they may be active in clinical settings in which TPO failed to act.

A second attribute is that they are highly species-specific (126). For example, non-peptide TPO mimetics developed for the human TPO receptor bind to human and chimpanzee TPO receptor but do not bind the murine or cynomolgus monkey TPO receptor (126). This has been shown to be due to a single amino acid difference in the transmembrane domain of the TPO receptor. Human and chimpanzee TPO receptors have a histidine at residue 499 whereas all of the other species have a leucine. A current model suggests that binding of non-peptide TPO mimetics to His499 and Thr496 in the transmembrane region either induces dimerization of the TPO receptor or directly activates the signal transduction mechanism (126). This species specificity has frustrated preclinical efforts to demonstrate biological effect in vivo and therefore most proof of effect is based on stimulation of human cell lines or growth of Meg-CFC from $CD34^+$ cells (120–122).

Other important aspects of these non-peptide TPO mimetics are that they are orally available and, given their structure, not antigenic. Furthermore, these non-peptide mimetics do not activate platelets. While the recombinant thrombopoietins and the TPO peptide mimetics do not directly activate platelets, they do alter the threshold for other agonists such as ADP. This potentiating effect is not seen with the non-peptide TPO mimetics, probably due to the aforementioned difference in their mechanism of action.

CLINICAL STUDIES OF THE THROMBOPOIETINS

Nonmyeloablative Chemotherapy

The stimulatory effects of PEG-rHuMGDF and rhTPO on megakaryocyte and platelet production have been demonstrated in several clinical trials (128–137). PEG-rHuMGDF, the most widely studied recombinant TPO, has produced dose-dependent increases in platelet counts in patients with advanced malignancies and attenuated chemotherapy-induced thrombocytopenia in randomized, placebo-controlled clinical trials (128,129,135–137). When administered without any chemotherapy as a daily subcutaneous injection, PEG-rHuMGDF produced a dose-dependent increase in peripheral blood platelet counts and a modest increase in megakaryocyte, erythroid, and myeloid progenitor cell levels in patients with advanced cancer (129). No evidence of platelet activation or altered platelet function was observed with PEG-rHuMGDF administration (138).

Subsequent trials evaluated the effects of PEG-rHuMGDF on hematologic recovery after chemotherapy. A randomized, placebo-controlled, dose-escalation study evaluated the effects of PEG-rHuMGDF after carboplatin-paclitaxel chemotherapy in 53 patients with lung cancer (128). Patients treated with PEG-rHuMGDF after chemotherapy had a higher median nadir platelet count (188×10^9/L) than did placebo-treated patients (111×10^9/L) and also showed more rapid recovery of platelet counts (14 days vs. >21 days). The need for platelet transfusions was unaffected because the chemotherapy regimen used did not frequently generate severe thrombocytopenia. In another randomized study in 41 patients with advanced cancer undergoing chemotherapy with carboplatin and cyclophosphamide, treatment with PEG-rHuMGDF enhanced platelet recovery in a dose-related manner (129). Although the platelet nadir occurred earlier in the PEG-rHuMGDF-treated group, its depth was unchanged. Similar results were observed in a dose-scheduling trial of PEG-rHuMGDF with G-CSF carried out in patients with non-small-cell lung cancer treated with carboplatin-paclitaxel (130). PEG-rHuMGDF-treated patients had a higher platelet nadir than did placebo-treated patients (89×10^9/L vs. 27×10^9/L in cycle 1). Moreover, the need for transfusion was lower in the PEG-rHuMGDF group than in the placebo group (17% vs. 64% in the first two cycles). However, in the later cycles, thrombocytopenia became dose-limiting in all treatment groups.

A recent study examined the efficacy of different doses and schedules of PEG-rHuMGDF in 68 patients with advanced cancer (136). Patients received one cycle of carboplatin and cyclophosphamide and were then randomly assigned to receive PEG-rHuMGDF or placebo after the second and subsequent cycles of carboplatin and cyclophosphamide chemotherapy. The platelet nadir was higher and the duration of grade 3 or 4 thrombocytopenia shorter when PEG-rHuMGDF was administered to patients who received the same dose of chemotherapy for at least two cycles. No evidence of an effect on platelet nadir was observed when PEG-rHuMGDF was given before chemotherapy. Unlike in animal chemotherapy models (in which multilineage responses are often seen), no effect of recombinant TPOs on red or white blood cell recovery has been seen in humans.

rhTPO has also produced a dose-dependent increase in platelet counts in patients with sarcomas and gynecologic malignancies (131–134,139). A phase 1 and 2 study examined the effect of rhTPO on megakaryocyte and platelet production before and after chemotherapy with doxorubicin and ifosfamide in patients with sarcomas who were at high risk of developing chemotherapy-induced thrombocytopenia. When given intravenously before chemotherapy, a single dose of rhTPO was associated with a dose-dependent increase in peripheral platelets that began on day 4 and peaked on day 12 in most patients (132). This increase in platelet number was accompanied by a four-fold increase in bone marrow megakaryocytes and a marked expansion and mobilization of erythroid, myeloid, and megakaryocyte progenitor cells. A single dose of rhTPO given intravenously after chemotherapy with doxorubicin and ifosfamide decreased the incidence of thrombocytopenia in some patients (131). A second trial investigated the clinical safety and activity of rhTPO administered subcutaneously to previously treated patients with gynecologic malignancies before and after chemotherapy with carboplatin (134). As observed in the previous study, administration of a single subcutaneous dose of rhTPO before chemotherapy produced a modest dose-dependent rise in circulating platelet counts. Administration of multiple doses of rhTPO after carboplatin chemotherapy produced an earlier platelet count nadir but

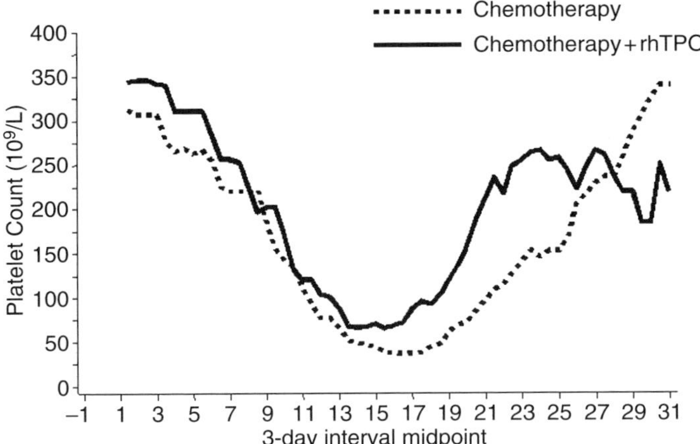

Figure 4 rhTPO increases nadir platelet count. In patients undergoing intensive chemotherapy for gynecologic malignancy, rhTPO (given on days 2, 4, 6, and 8 after chemotherapy) increased the nadir platelet count. The platelet nadir also occurred earlier in patients treated with rhTPO than in untreated patients. *Source*: Courtesy of Pfizer, Inc., from data from Ref. 134.

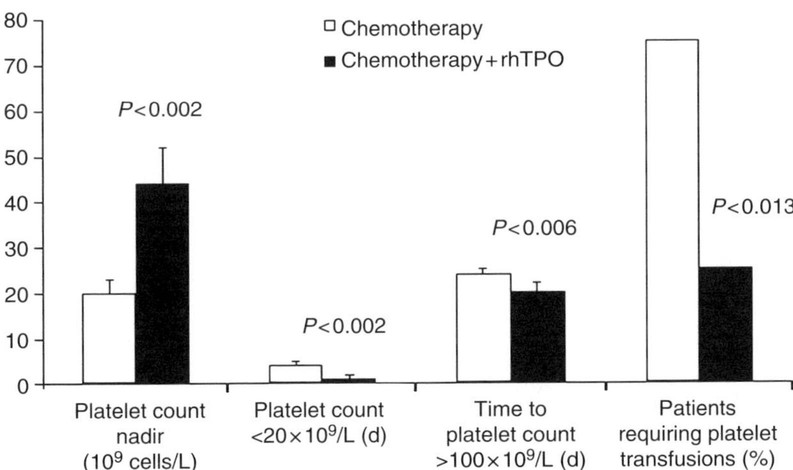

Figure 5 rhTPO decreases the need for platelet transfusions. In patients undergoing intensive chemotherapy for gynecologic malignancy, rhTPO decreased thrombocytopenia and the need for platelet transfusions. *Source*: Courtesy of Pfizer, Inc., from data from Ref. 134.

effectively reduced the depth of the platelet nadir and the duration of severe thrombocytopenia (Fig. 4). The need for platelet transfusions decreased by 75% (Fig. 5) (134).

None of the second generation peptide and non-peptide TPO mimetics have yet been tested in this clinical setting.

Myeloablative Chemotherapy

Prolonged and severe chemotherapy-induced thrombocytopenia is a major cause of morbidity in patients receiving intensive chemotherapy for acute leukemia and those undergoing blood stem cell transplantation (140,141). In recent years, several studies have evaluated the safety and efficacy of PEG-rHuMGDF and rhTPO in the management of thrombocytopenia associated with chemotherapy for acute leukemia and stem cell transplantation (142–155).

In contrast to their effect in the nonmyeloablative setting, PEG-rHuMGDF and rhTPO have not had a clinically significant effect on platelet production when administered to patients receiving dose-intensive therapy for acute leukemia and those undergoing stem cell transplantation after chemotherapy. Moderate increase in peak platelet counts and reduction in time to full platelet recovery were often achieved in patients treated with PEG-rHuMGDF and rhTPO. However, no improvement in time to recovery to a platelet count $\geq 20 \times 10^9$/L and no reduction in the need for platelet transfusions were observed in these studies (142–144,148,149).

In preclinical studies, treatment with TPO before bone marrow harvesting accelerated platelet reconstitution in recipient mice after transplantation, suggesting that this approach may be effective in shortening the time to platelet independence after stem cell transplantation (156). With this approach, one study showed that administration of rhTPO to patients during mobilization of peripheral blood progenitor cells increased $CD34^+$ yield before stem cell transplant. Clinically small, but statistically significant, improvements in neutrophil recovery and platelet and erythrocyte transfusion requirements were noted after transplantation (150).

None of the second generation peptide and non-peptide TPO mimetics have yet been tested in this clinical setting.

Myelodysplastic Syndrome (MDS)

Hematopoietic growth factors have had some success in ameliorating the neutropenia and anemia associated with MDS. The recombinant TPOs may have a similar benefit: some in vitro studies have shown that bone marrow cells of patients with MDS can differentiate into the megakaryocytic lineage when exposed to recombinant TPO (157,158). Because of the underlying heterogeneity of MDS, some individuals might have responsive marrow whereas others might not. Endogenous TPO levels are normal to slightly elevated in MDS (159), so whether they can help predict responsiveness to exogenous TPO requires further investigation. In a preliminary report, various intravenous doses of PEG-rHuMGDF were given daily for 14 days to 21 Japanese patients with MDS (refractory anemia and refractory anemia with ringed sideroblasts) with platelet counts $<30\times10^9$/L. The peak effect of PEG-rHuMGDF occurred 5 to 6 wk later with an average doubling of platelet count; responses were seen in a third of the patients, and a multilineage effect was observed in a few patients (160).

None of the second generation peptide and non-peptide TPO mimetics have yet been tested in this clinical setting.

Human Immunodeficiency Virus (HIV)–Associated Thrombocytopenia

Several studies have examined thrombocytopenia in primates or patients infected with HIV with respect to peripheral platelet mass turnover, marrow megakaryocytopoiesis, and endogenous TPO levels (4,5,161,162). A 10-fold disparity between the reduced platelet production and expanded megakaryocyte mass was observed in the bone marrow of HIV patients with thrombocytopenia (162). This suggests that, despite the expanded megakaryocyte mass, HIV-infected megakaryocytes have a high rate of apoptosis and ineffective thrombopoiesis resulting in thrombocytopenia. Harker and colleagues showed that administration of PEG-rHuMGDF rapidly eliminated thrombocytopenia in thrombocytopenic chimpanzees infected with HIV (161). With normal or slightly elevated endogenous TPO levels in 6 HIV-infected humans, platelet counts in all patients increased 10-fold within 14 days of the start of PEG-rHuMGDF treatment (162). This increase was not associated with change in the megakaryocyte mass, platelet life span, or viral load. What appeared to occur was an increase in the rate of effective platelet production from the bone marrow megakaryocytes of these individuals. These data suggest that, in HIV-related immune thrombocytopenic purpura, TPO can be expected to produce clinically beneficial increases in platelet counts.

Immune Thrombocytopenic Purpura (ITP)

Since recent platelet kinetic studies showed that platelet production was not elevated in up to 75% of patients with ITP (4) and that serum TPO levels were rarely elevated (159), it was hypothesized that TPO might stimulate platelet production and ameliorate thrombocytopenia. Confirmation of this hypothesis has come from several recent studies.

Major increases in platelet count were seen in three of four Japanese patients with non-HIV-related ITP treated with intravenous PEG-rHuMGDF (163). One patient with ITP has been successfully treated twice weekly with

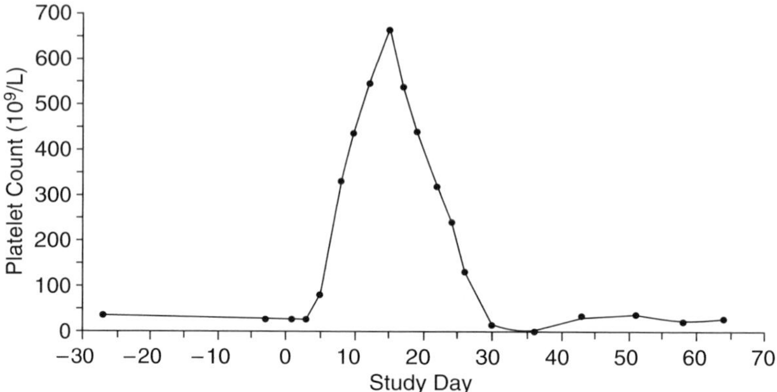

Figure 6 TPO peptide mimetic increases the platelet count in patient with ITP. AMG 531 was administered on day 1 to a patient with chronic ITP, with baseline platelet counts of $\sim 30 \times 10^9$/L for over two years. A peak platelet count rise to 662×10^9/L was observed on day 15. A brief rebound thrombocytopenia to $<5 \times 10^9$/L was noted on day 36. *Source*: From Ref. 118.

subcutaneous PEG-rHuMGDF for over 5 yr (164). In a Phase 1 trial twenty-four patients with chronic ITP were treated in groups of four with six different single doses of the novel TPO mimetic, AMG 531. At AMG 531 concentrations >3 μg/kg, 8/12 (67%) of patients achieved a platelet response (defined as doubling from baseline and an increase above 50×10^9/L) (118). Five of the eight responders (63%) achieved platelet counts $>150 \times 10^9$/L. An illustrative platelet count response to a single injection of AMG 531 is shown in Figure 6. A subsequent Phase 2 randomized, placebo-controlled, double-blind study of weekly injections of AMG 531 vs placebo for 6 weeks showed that 75% of the 16 AMG 531 patients versus 25% of the four placebo-treated patients had their platelet count double from baseline and increase above 50×10^9/L (119). There are several ongoing studies in ITP with AMG 531 as well as with SB-497115.

Liver Disease

Recent understanding of TPO biology suggests that reduced hepatic production of TPO may play a major role in thrombocytopenia associated with liver disease (165,166). TPO is produced primarily in the liver, and thrombocytopenia in animals seems to be proportional to the extent of liver resection (167). In addition, after transplantation of healthy livers into TPO$^{-/-}$ mice, platelet counts returned toward normal, suggesting that the majority of TPO is produced in the liver (74). An association between low platelet counts (median, 84×10^9/L; range, $26–112 \times 10^9$/L) and low levels of TPO (median, <20 pg/mL; range, <20–182 pg/mL) has been reported in patients before orthotopic liver transplantation (75,76). Within four days after orthotopic liver transplantation, TPO levels rose above normal and were accompanied by increased amounts of reticulated platelets, a marker of accelerated platelet production. Fourteen days after transplantation, platelet counts were normal in 14 of 18 patients (median, 254×10^9/L; range, $70–398 \times 10^9$/L) and TPO levels returned to normal in 14 of 18 patients (median, 59 pg/mL; range, $<$20–639 pg/mL). No appreciable change in spleen size was observed. In multivariate analysis, the increase in TPO was the only variable that correlated with the increase in platelet count. Thus, TPO could potentially be used to reduce hemorrhage in patients with thrombocytopenia due to liver disease or to prepare such patients for liver transplantation. Furthermore, TPO might be used to improve platelet counts for patients with chronic hepatitis C infection being treated with interferon and anti-retroviral medications.

Surgery

Approximately 40% of all platelet transfusions are used in surgical settings (168). Pre-operative and post-operative thrombocytopenia complicates surgical procedures and mandates platelet transfusions. No clinical studies have targeted this important area. However, in dogs, the administration of PEG-rHuMGDF 4 days before surgery decreased thrombocytopenia after cardiopulmonary bypass (169). Despite its 5-day lag time before platelet rise, judicial administration of TPO before surgery may ameliorate preoperative and postoperative thrombocytopenia and reduce the need for platelet transfusions. TPO may also be used to maintain an adequate platelet count for surgical or medical procedures in those with religious restrictions on the transfusion of blood products.

Transfusion Medicine

The striking in vivo effect of TPO on the mobilization of $CD34^+$ cells, expansion of multilineage stem cell progenitor pools, and increase in platelet production led to an evaluation of its activity in three areas: mobilization of peripheral blood stem cells before stem cell transplantation, ex vivo expansion of pluripotent stem cells from umbilical cord blood or bone marrow, and increase in the yield of platelet apheresis from healthy platelet donors.

Stem Cell Mobilization

Several pilot studies evaluated the activity of various doses and schedules of rhTPO or PEG-rHuMGDF in combination with G-CSF and chemotherapy as part of a mobilization regimen for stem cell transplantation (129,150–152,170,171). In contrast to peak progenitor cell numbers on days 5–7 usually obtained with G-CSF alone, a peak on days 12–15 was produced by the combination of PEG-rHuMGDF and G-CSF. However, since a full pharmacodynamic response profile to PEG-rHuMGDF was not performed in this study, the exact day of peak stem

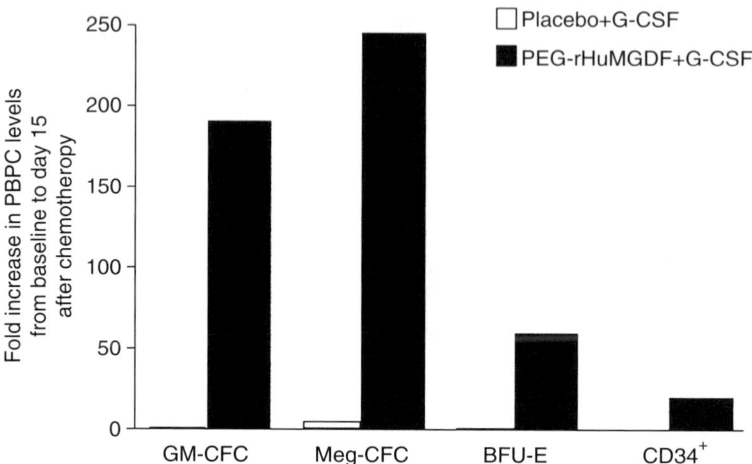

Figure 7 PEG-rHuMGDF increases peripheral blood progenitor cells (PBPCs). Patients undergoing PBPC transplantation underwent stem cell mobilization with chemotherapy and G-CSF with or without PEG-rHuMGDF. Use of PEG-rHuMGDF increased granulocyte-macrophage colony–forming cells (GM-CFC), megakaryocyte colony–forming cells (Meg–CFC), erythroid burst–forming units (BFU-E), and $CD34^+$ cells. *Source*: Adapted from the data of Basser 129.

cell mobilization was not determined. The addition of rhTPO to G-CSF for chemotherapy mobilization regimens substantially increased $CD34^+$ yields (Fig. 7). The promising results observed in these early studies were confirmed in a large randomized phase 2 study of rhTPO in patients undergoing high-dose chemotherapy and transplantation of peripheral blood stem cells (150). Treatment with rhTPO in various doses and schedules reduced the number of aphereses needed to reach a target graft (i.e., $CD34^+ > 5 \times 10^6$/kg) and, compared with placebo treatment, increased the percentage of patients reaching a target graft (from 46% in the placebo group to 79% in the rhTPO group), as well as the percentage of patients reaching the minimum target graft (i.e., $CD34^+ > 2 \times 10^6$/kg) (from 75% in the placebo group to 94% in the rhTPO group). These studies demonstrate the ability of rhTPO to mobilize $CD34^+$ cells safely and effectively and increase the harvest of $CD34^+$ cells used for stem cell transplantation. However, these increased $CD34^+$ harvests have not yet been shown to enhance outcomes in a clinically significant way.

Ex Vivo Expansion of Primitive Stem Cells

The role of TPO in the expansion and prolonged survival of primitive stem cells derived from bone marrow or umbilical cord blood has been the focus of several recent investigations. Yagi demonstrated that administration of TPO alone can sustain ex vivo expansion of hematopoietic stem cells in long-term bone marrow cultures (LTBMCs) from mice (172). The continuous presence of TPO resulted in the generation of long- and short-term colony-forming cells and maintained the relative amount of high-proliferative-potential colony-forming cells. Most importantly, competitive repopulation studies found that the TPO-treated LTBMC cells were as effective as fresh marrow. Subsequent data from this research group suggest that the expanded population of stem cells, when transplanted into recipient mice, is adequate for the long-term repopulation.

Piacibello and colleagues showed that the use of growth factors could expand human cord blood $CD34^+$ cells ex vivo by many million-fold in total number; the $CD34^+$ component and the lineage-specific progenitors increased

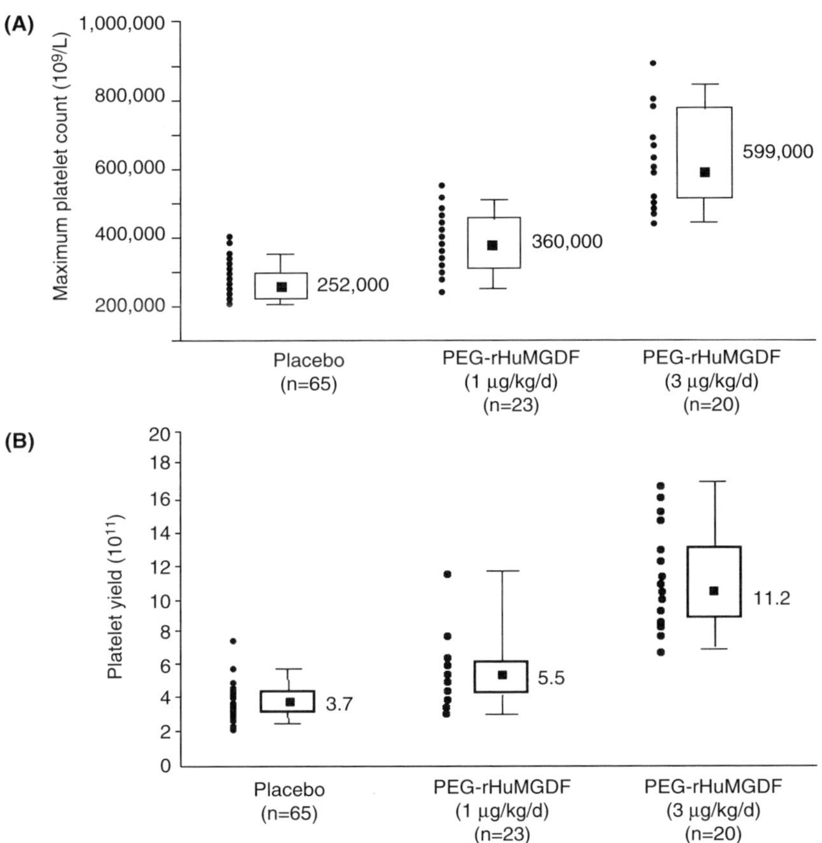

Figure 8 PEG-rHuMGDF increases the yield of platelet apheresis. A single dose of PEG-rHuMGDF was given to routine platelet apheresis donors on day 1. There was a dose-dependent increase in the platelet count (**A**) and platelet yield (**B**) when apheresis was performed 15 days later. *Source*: From Ref. 174.

proportionately (173). Although TPO alone and Flt 3 ligand alone were insufficient in stimulating sustained growth, a combination of the two growth factors accounted for this rapid increase in cell numbers during 24 weeks in culture. However, whether the expanded cell population can be used clinically for transplantation has not been demonstrated.

Platelet Apheresis

Extensive studies have shown that healthy apheresis donors maximally increase their platelet count 10 to 14 days after a single injection of PEG-rHuMGDF (168,174,175). This rise in platelet count is dose-dependent and leads directly to an increase in the apheresis platelet yield (Fig. 8). The platelets collected have normal aggregation responses and normal function on transfusion into thrombocytopenic recipients. Transfusions with the higher platelet doses extended the duration of transfusion independence and possibly reduced bleeding episodes when compared with standard doses. The corrected count increment was also improved when patients were transfused with platelets mobilized by PEG-rHuMGDF rather than with those harvested from control donors.

In a similar study, rhTPO was given to cancer patients about to undergo chemotherapy. Large amounts of platelets were harvested by apheresis, cryopreserved, and successfully transfused back into the donors when they subsequently developed chemotherapy-induced thrombocytopenia. This form of autologous platelet donation may prove to be an important method to support platelet-refractory, allo-immunized patients undergoing dose-intense chemotherapy (176).

Radioprotection

Although there are no studies in humans, the potential for TPO to function as a radioprotectant is another area of clinical interest. In mice, administration of TPO two hours after exposure to sublethal total body irradiation (TBI) dramatically ameliorates the thrombocytopenia that is seen at day 10 in these mice (177). Mice treated with rhTPO before irradiation have a higher platelet count nadir (739×10^9/L) than do those that are untreated before irradiation (144×10^9/L); unirradiated control mice had a platelet count of $1{,}123 \times 10^9$/L. This protective effect was enhanced when rhTPO was administered close to TBI. Stem cells appeared to be highly sensitive to the effects of rhTPO, possibly because it prevented apoptosis when given from two hours before until two hours after TBI. This very narrow window of protection underscores the importance of the timing of the administration of rhTPO vis-à-vis the irradiation. Furthermore, red and white blood cell counts also appeared to be protected somewhat by the administration of rhTPO close to the time of TBI (177). These results suggest a major radioprotective effect of rhTPO on progenitor cells in the bone marrow. This finding is in line with previous data suggesting that pluripotential stem cells are sensitive to the presence of TPO and that TPO can support their survival

(178,179). Similar results have been noted in subsequent studies that investigated the effect of rhTPO in mice exposed to lethal doses of TBI (180). Almost all the mice that received rhTPO close to the time of irradiation survived, whereas all the mice that received placebo died within 30 days of receiving TBI. Furthermore, recovery of blood counts in all lineages improved in those mice that received rhTPO within several hours of TBI.

Whether these results can be expanded to the chemotherapy setting has not been fully explored. Conceivably the antiapoptotic effects of TPO might lessen chemotherapy-induced apoptosis of pluripotential stem cells and thereby ameliorate the pancytopenia of chemotherapy.

SAFETY OF THROMBOPOIETIN

Except for two problems, TPO administration has been remarkably free from adverse effects in the patients studied. Although extensive thrombocytosis may result from TPO treatment, even in cancer patients who are already prone to thromboembolism, no increased rate of thrombosis has been seen (110). TPO did not increase myeloid blast counts in patients with AML, despite the presence of TPO receptors on these cells. Since non-myeloid cells do not contain TPO receptors, stimulation of tumor growth was not expected and was not seen (181). No interactions with other drugs or hematopoietic growth factors have been documented. In most of the studies with TPO in myeloablative and non-myeloablative chemotherapy, patients also received myeloid growth factors. Although interactions of TPO with myeloid growth factors had been seen in one animal model (182), none have been noted in any clinical study.

One problem with recombinant TPO administration to some patients has been increased bone marrow fibrosis. In preclinical studies in animals, long term administration of PEG-rHuMGDF produced reversible bone marrow fibrosis (183). Indeed, overexpression of TPO by transplantation of c-mpl-transfected murine bone marrow cells (184) or by c-mpl retroviral infection in mice (185) creates extensive bone marrow fibrosis, osteosclerosis, and extramedullary hematopoiesis like the human disease agnogenic myelofibrois with myeloid metaplasia (AMM) (186–188). In humans given rhTPO and PEG-rHuMGDF, there has been little clinical evidence for bone marrow fibrosis. But given the brevity of most exposures to recombinant TPO and the lack of bone marrow analysis, this problem has not been fully explored. In the only study where bone marrow analysis was performed, increased bone marrow reticulin was seen in most patients treated with rhTPO. Serial analyses of bone marrow and peripheral blood were conducted in 9 patients who received rhTPO after AML induction therapy and in 8 patients undergoing the same AML induction treatment but without rhTPO treatment (189). Eight of the 9 TPO-treated and 5 of the 8 control patients had increased bone marrow cellularity; 8 of 9 treated and 2 of 6 untreated patients had increased bone marrow reticulin staining. A semi-quantitative measurement of the number of bone marrow megakaryocytes showed that treated patients had 19.5 megakaryocytes per high power field (MHPF) versus 3.7 MHPF for the AML controls and 2.95 MHPF for patients without any bone marrow disease. All of these morphological findings resolved within 42 days of the last dose of rhTPO.

However, a more important complication of TPO treatment has emerged. Administration of multiple doses of one recombinant TPO, PEG-rHuMGDF, to some cancer patients and healthy volunteers was associated with an abrogation of its pharmacologic effect as a result of the development of neutralizing antibodies (130,190–192). These antibodies neutralized both the recombinant and endogenous TPO, resulting in thrombocytopenia. Thrombocytopenia occurred in 4 of 665 cancer/stem cell transplantation/leukemia patients given multiple doses and in 2 of 204 (1.0%) healthy volunteers who received two doses and in 11 of 124 (8.9%) healthy volunteers given three doses of PEG-rHuMGDF (190,191). No subject developed neutralizing antibodies or thrombocytopenia after a single injection. Evaluation of these thrombocytopenic subjects showed that the thrombocytopenia was due to the formation of an IgG antibody to PEG-rHuMGDF that cross-reacted with endogenous TPO and neutralized its biologic activity (190–192). Because endogenous TPO is produced in a constitutive fashion by the liver, megakaryocyte number and ploidy decrease and thrombocytopenia ensues (Fig. 9). In three patients, thrombocytopenia was also

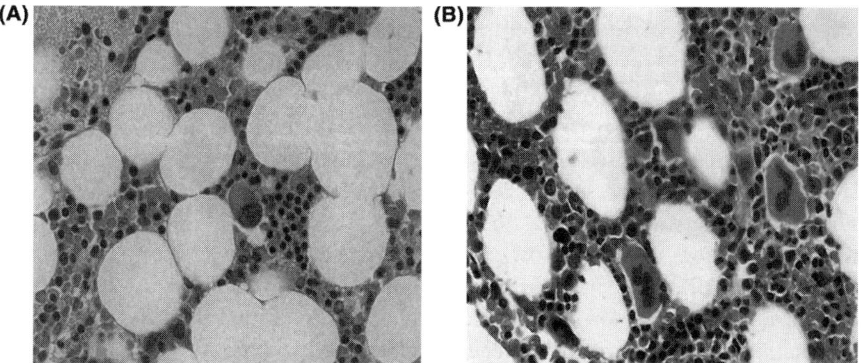

Figure 9 Anti-TPO antibodies may cause amegakaryocytic thrombocytopenia. A normal volunteer received two injections of PEG-rHuMGDF (3 μg/kg) one month apart. She developed profound thrombocytopenia with platelet counts of $10–30 \times 10^9$/L by day 115 and remained at that level for over 700 days. A bone marrow biopsy (**A**) confirmed the virtual absence of megakaryocytes; those present were of low size and ploidy. The patient had a high titer antibody to PEG-rHuMGDF and to endogenous TPO. Her platelet count returned to normal and the antibody disappeared with administration of cyclosporine A (190). Shown in (**B**) is a bone marrow biopsy of a patient with a similar platelet count and ITP; many large, polyploid megakaryocytes are readily seen.

associated with anemia and neutropenia, suggesting an effect on a stem cell population as well (190,192). PEG-rHuMGDF was withdrawn from clinical trials in the United States in September 1998 because of this unexpected effect (193).

To date, the development of neutralizing antibodies in patients treated with intravenous rhTPO has not been reported, although one non-neutralizing antibody was found after subcutaneous injection of rhTPO (132,134).

A possible explanation for the immunogenicity of PEG-rHuMGDF may simply be that this molecule is truncated, nonglycosylated, and pegylated, in contrast to the full-length, glycosylated more "native" rhTPO molecule (Table 1). However, PEG-rHuMGDF has usually been administered subcutaneously, whereas full-length native rhTPO has been injected intravenously. Because TPO is a potent mobilizer of dendritic cells, injection of any form of TPO subcutaneously might enhance its immunogenicity. Support for this latter hypothesis comes from recent experiments in which PEG-ratMGDF was injected into rats once monthly for three months by either a subcutaneous or intravenous route. Most animals treated subcutaneously developed neutralizing antibodies and thrombocytopenia whereas those treated intravenously did not (110).

For AMG 531 and the non-peptide TPO mimetics like SB-497115 there has been no antibody formation seen in the relatively small number of subjects so far treated. The major adverse effect that was seen for AMG 531 was mild headache, a finding seen with many hematopoietic growth factors (118,119).

SUMMARY

The development of recombinant TPO has led to a wide number of discoveries describing the underlying biology of platelet production in normal and pathologic settings. Recombinant TPO has demonstrated a unique pharmacology, unlike other hematopoietic growth factors. Both rhTPO and PEG-rHuMGDF have a prolonged half-life of about 40 hr, and thus continuous dosing with TPO does not seem to be required; one or more appropriately timed doses may even be superior to multiple doses. After a single TPO administration, the platelet count does not increase until day 5 and has its peak effect 10–12 days later. TPO has little effect on mature megakaryocytes and may actually inhibit their shedding of platelets.

TPO is the most specific and effective growth factor identified to date for the prevention and treatment of thrombocytopenia. Preliminary clinical evidence indicates that TPO administration may be a helpful adjunct to the conventional approach of platelet transfusion therapy for some cancer patients with chemotherapy-induced thrombocytopenia. However, the studies with TPO, as with IL-11, mostly involved non-conventional chemotherapy regimens that caused considerable thrombocytopenia. For most routine chemotherapy regimens, clinically significant thrombocytopenia is relatively uncommon. The overall impact of TPO on the need for platelet transfusions will probably not be great, especially with the recent reduction in the threshold "trigger" for platelet transfusions to 10×10^9/L (194–196).

The failure to find any biological effect in myeloablative regimens is still surprising given the success of the myeloid growth factors in these same settings. This is probably not simply due to inadequate dosing schemes; many have been tried. Rather it may reflect aspects of the clinical biology of TPO that are not yet recognized. The elevated endogenous TPO concentration in all of these settings may have already saturated the TPO receptor or, alternatively, may even prevent platelet shedding (197). Since the non-peptide TPO mimetics may act on the TPO receptor by a mechanism different from that of TPO, there remains some optimism that these mimetics may succeed where the recombinant thrombopoietins have failed.

The ultimate clinical indications for recombinant TPO or TPO mimetics will certainly depend on the results of continuing and future studies. Further studies to elucidate their complex and unique biology will help to determine their optimal application in the treatment of thrombocytopenia. While the potential of TPO to reduce the extent of chemotherapy-induced thrombocytopenia and reduce the need for platelet transfusions in the nonmyeloablative chemotherapy setting may be enhanced with innovative dosing schemes, TPO will probably have its greatest impact in non-oncology settings such as the stimulation of platelet apheresis donors, HIV infection, ITP, MDS, and liver disease. A persistent challenge remains for surgical and intensive care patients who account for nearly half of all platelet transfusions (168) and who would benefit from an effective thrombopoietic growth factor. Future efforts will be increasingly focused on developing peptide and non-peptide, orally available TPO mimetics.

ACKNOWLEDGMENTS

Supported in part by grants from the National Institute of Health HL54838, HL61272, HL72299, and HL82889.

REFERENCES

1. Kaushansky K. The thrombocytopenia of cancer. Prospects for effective cytokine therapy. Hematol Oncol Clin North Am 1996; 10:431–455.
2. Prow D, Vadhan-Raj S. Thrombopoietin: biology and potential clinical applications. Oncology (Huntington) 1998; 12:1597–1604.
3. Richardson PG, Barlogie B, Berenson J, et al. A phase 2 study of bortezomib in relapsed, refractory myeloma. N Engl J Med 2003; 348:2609–2617.
4. Ballem PJ, Segal GM, Stratton JR, Gernsheimer T, Adamson JW, Slichter SJ. Mechanisms of thrombocytopenia in chronic autoimmune thrombocytopenic purpura. Evidence of both impaired platelet production and increased platelet clearance. J Clin Invest 1987; 80:33–40.

5. Ballem PJ, Belzberg A, Devine DV, et al. Kinetic studies of the mechanism of thrombocytopenia in patients with human immunodeficiency virus infection. N Engl J Med 1992; 327:1779–1784.
6. Mittelman M, Zeidman A. Platelet function in the myelodysplastic syndromes. Int J Hematol 2000; 71:95–98.
7. Lazarus AH, Ellis J, Semple JW, Mody M, Crow AR, Freedman J. Comparison of platelet immunity in patients with SLE and with ITP. Transfus Sci 2000; 22:19–27.
8. Lawrence SP, Lezotte DC, Durham JD, Kumpe DA, Everson GT, Bilir BM. Course of thrombocytopenia of chronic liver disease after transjugular intrahepatic portosystemic shunts (TIPS). A retrospective analysis. Dig Dis Sci 1995; 40:1575–1580.
9. Alvarez JM, Gates R, Rowe D, Brady PW. Complications from intra-aortic balloon counterpulsation: a review of 303 cardiac surgical patients. Eur J Cardiothorac Surg 1992; 6:530–535.
10. Vonderheide RH, Thadhani R, Kuter DJ. Association of thrombocytopenia with the use of intra-aortic balloon pumps. Am J Med 1998; 105:27–32.
11. Abel G, Kuter DJ. Association of thrombocytopenia with continuous venovenous hemofiltration. Blood 2002; 100:221a.
12. McClure MW, Berkowitz SD, Sparapani R, et al. Clinical significance of thrombocytopenia during a non-ST-elevation acute coronary syndrome. The platelet glycoprotein IIb/IIIa in unstable angina: receptor suppression using integrilin therapy (PURSUIT) trial experience. Circulation 1999; 99:2892–2900.
13. Khaykin Y, Paradiso FL, Madan M. Acute thrombocytopenia associated with eptifibatide therapy. Can J Cardiol 2003; 19:797–801.
14. Nagge J, Jackevicius C, Dzavik V, Ross JR, Seidelin P. Acute profound thrombocytopenia associated with eptifibatide therapy. Pharmacotherapy 2003; 23:374–379.
15. Salengro E, Mulvihill NT, Farah B. Acute profound thrombocytopenia after use of eptifibatide for coronary stenting. Catheter Cardiovasc Interv 2003; 58:73–75.
16. Bougie DW, Wilker PR, Wuitschick ED, et al. Acute thrombocytopenia after treatment with tirofiban or eptifibatide is associated with antibodies specific for ligand-occupied GPIIb/IIIa. Blood 2002; 100:2071–2076.
17. Hongo RH, Brent BN. Association of eptifibatide and acute profound thrombocytopenia. Am J Cardiol 2001; 88:428–431.
18. Dasgupta H, Blankenship JC, Wood GC, Frey CM, Demko SL, Menapace FJ. Thrombocytopenia complicating treatment with intravenous glycoprotein IIb/IIIa receptor inhibitors: a pooled analysis. Am Heart J 2000; 140:206–211.
19. Kuter DJ, Tillotson GS. Hematologic effects of antimicrobials: focus on the oxazolidinone, linezolid. Pharmacotherapy 2001; 21:1010–1013.
20. Gerson SL, Kaplan SL, Bruss JB, et al. Hematologic effects of linezolid: summary of clinical experience. Antimicrob Agents Chemother 2002; 46:2723–2726.
21. Chiu EK, Yuen KY, Lie AK, et al. A prospective study of symptomatic bacteremia following platelet transfusion and of its management. Transfusion 1994; 34:950–954.

22. Davda RK, Collins KA, Kitchens CS. Case report: fatal Staphylococcus aureus sepsis from single-donor platelet transfusion. Am J Med Sci 1994; 307:340–341.
23. Chambers LA, Kruskall MS, Pacini DG, Donovan LM. Febrile reactions after platelet transfusion: the effect of single versus multiple donors. Transfusion 1990; 30:219–221.
24. Contreras M. Diagnosis and treatment of patients refractory to platelet transfusions. Blood Rev 1998; 12:215–221.
25. Engelfriet CP, Reesink HW, Aster RH, et al. Management of alloimmunized, refractory patients in need of platelet transfusions. Vox Sang 1997; 73:191–198.
26. Friedberg RC, Mintz PD. Causes of refractoriness to platelet transfusion. Curr Opin Hematol 1995; 2:493–498.
27. Novotny VM. Prevention and management of platelet transfusion refractoriness. Vox Sang 1999; 76:1–13.
28. Kimura H, Ishibashi T, Shikama Y, et al. Interleukin-1 beta (IL-1 beta) induces thrombocytosis in mice: possible implication of IL-6. Blood 1990; 76:2493–2500.
29. Bartley TD, Bogenberger J, Hunt P, et al. Identification and cloning of a megakaryocyte growth and development factor that is a ligand for the cytokine receptor Mpl. Cell 1994; 77:1117–1124.
30. Lok S, Kaushansky K, Holly RD, et al. Cloning and expression of murine thrombopoietin cDNA and stimulation of platelet production in vivo. Nature 1994; 369:565–568.
31. de Sauvage FJ, Hass PE, Spencer SD, et al. Stimulation of megakaryocytopoiesis and thrombopoiesis by the c-Mpl ligand. Nature 1994; 369:533–538.
32. Kuter DJ, Beeler DL, Rosenberg RD. The purification of megapoietin: a physiological regulator of megakaryocyte growth and platelet production. Proc Natl Acad Sci USA 1994; 91:11104–11108.
33. Kato T, Ogami K, Shimada Y, et al. Purification and characterization of thrombopoietin. J Biochem 1995; 118:229–236.
34. Metcalf D, Burgess AW, Johnson GR, et al. In vitro actions on hemopoietic cells of recombinant murine GM-CSF purified after production in Escherichia coli: comparison with purified native GM-CSF. J Cell Physiol 1986; 128:421–431.
35. Debili N, Masse JM, Katz A, Guichard J, Breton-Gorius J, Vainchenker W. Effects of the recombinant hematopoietic growth factors interleukin-3, interleukin-6, stem cell factor, and leukemia inhibitory factor on the megakaryocytic differentiation of CD34+ cells. Blood 1993; 82:84–95.
36. Leonard JP, Quinto CM, Kozitza MK, Neben TY, Goldman SJ. Recombinant human interleukin-11 stimulates multilineage hematopoietic recovery in mice after a myelosuppressive regimen of sublethal irradiation and carboplatin. Blood 1994; 83:1499–1506.
37. Metcalf D, Begley CG, Williamson DJ, et al. Hemopoietic responses in mice injected with purified recombinant murine GM-CSF. Exp Hematol 1987; 15:1–9.
38. Metcalf D, Begley CG, Johnson GR, Nicola NA, Lopez AF, Williamson DJ. Effects of purified bacterially synthesized murine multi-CSF (IL-3) on hematopoiesis in normal adult mice. Blood 1986; 68:46–57.

39. Vadhan-Raj S, Kudelka AP, Garrison L, et al. Effects of interleukin-1 alpha on carboplatin-induced thrombocytopenia in patients with recurrent ovarian cancer. J Clin Oncol 1994; 12:707–714.
40. Leonardi V, Danova M, Fincato G, Palmeri S. Interleukin 3 in the treatment of chemotherapy induced thrombocytopenia. Oncol Rep 1998; 5:1459–1464.
41. D'Hondt V, Humblet Y, Guillaume T, et al. Thrombopoietic effects and toxicity of interleukin-6 in patients with ovarian cancer before and after chemotherapy: a multicentric placebo-controlled, randomized phase Ib study. Blood 1995; 85:2347–2353.
42. Gordon MS, McCaskill-Stevens WJ, Battiato LA, et al. A phase I trial of recombinant human interleukin-11 (neumega rhIL-11 growth factor) in women with breast cancer receiving chemotherapy. Blood 1996; 87:3615–3624.
43. Tepler I, Elias L, Smith JW, et al. A randomized placebo-controlled trial of recombinant human interleukin-11 in cancer patients with severe thrombocytopenia due to chemotherapy. Blood 1996; 87:3607–3614.
44. Smith JWd, Longo DL, Alvord WG, et al. The effects of treatment with interleukin-1 alpha on platelet recovery after high-dose carboplatin. N Engl J Med 1993; 328:756–761.
45. Vredenburgh JJ, Hussein A, Fisher D, et al. A randomized trial of recombinant human interleukin-11 following autologous bone marrow transplantation with peripheral blood progenitor cell support in patients with breast cancer. Biol Blood Marrow Transplant 1998; 4:134–141.
46. Nandurkar HH, Robb L, Tarlinton D, Barnett L, Kontgen F, Begley GC. Adult mice with targeted mutation of the interleukin-11 receptor (IL11Ra) display normal hematopoiesis. Blood 1997; 90:2148–2159.
47. Robb L, Li R, Hartley L, Nandurkar HH, Koentgen F, Begley CG. Infertility in female mice lacking the receptor for interleukin 11 is due to a defective uterine response to implantation. Nat Med 1998; 4:303–308.
48. Gordon MS, Nemunaitis J, Hoffman R, et al. A phase I trial of recombinant human interleukin-6 in patients with myelodysplastic syndromes and thrombocytopenia. Blood 1995; 85:3066–3076.
49. Lazarus HM, Winton EF, Williams SF, et al. Phase I multicenter trial of interleukin 6 therapy after autologous bone marrow transplantation in advanced breast cancer. Bone Marrow Transplant 1995; 15:935–942.
50. Nieken J, Mulder NH, Buter J, et al. Recombinant human interleukin-6 induces a rapid and reversible anemia in cancer patients. Blood 1995; 86:900–905.
51. Carver-Moore K, Broxmeyer HE, Luoh SM, et al. Low levels of erythroid and myeloid progenitors in thrombopoietin- and c-mpl-deficient mice. Blood 1996; 88:803–808.
52. Gainsford T, Roberts AW, Kimura S, et al. Cytokine production and function in c-mpl-deficient mice: no physiologic role for interleukin-3 in residual megakaryocyte and platelet production. Blood 1998; 91:2745–2752.
53. Gainsford T, Nandurkar H, Metcalf D, Robb L, Begley CG, Alexander WS. The residual megakaryocyte and platelet production in c-mpl-deficient mice is not dependent on the actions of interleukin-6, interleukin-11, or leukemia inhibitory factor. Blood 2000; 95:528–534.
54. Kelemen E, Cserhati I, Tanos B. Demonstration and some properties of human thrombopoietin in thrombocythaemic sera. Acta Haematol 1958; 20:350–355.

55. Wendling F, Tambourin P. The oncogene V-MPL, a putative truncated cytokine receptor which immortalized hemtopoietic progenitors. Nouv Rev Fr Hematol 1991; 33:145–146.
56. Vigon I, Mornon JP, Cocault L, et al. Molecular cloning and characterization of MPL, the human homolog of the v-mpl oncogene: identification of a member of the hematopoietic growth factor receptor superfamily. Proc Natl Acad Sci USA 1992; 89:5640–5644.
57. Methia N, Louache F, Vainchenker W, Wendling F. Oligodeoxynucleotides antisense to the proto-oncogene c-mpl specifically inhibit in vitro megakaryocytopoiesis. Blood 1993; 82:1395–1401.
58. Sohma Y, Akahori H, Seki N, et al. Molecular cloning and chromosomal localization of the human thrombopoietin gene. FEBS Letters 1994; 353:57–61.
59. Foster D, Hunt P. The biological significance of truncated and full-length forms of Mpl ligand. In: Kuter DJ, Hunt P, Sheridan W, Zucker-Franklin D, eds. Thrombopoiesis and Thrombopoietins: Molecular, Cellular, Preclinical, and Clinical Biology. Totowa: Humana Press, 1997:203–214.
60. Foster DC, Sprecher CA, Grant FJ, et al. Human thrombopoietin: gene structure, cDNA sequence, expression, and chromosomal localization. Proc Natl Acad Sci USA 1994; 91:13023–13027.
61. Feese MD, Tamada T, Kato Y, et al. Structure of the receptor-binding domain of human thrombopoietin determined by complexation with a neutralizing antibody fragment. Proc Natl Acad Sci USA 2004; 101:1816–1821.
62. Yang C, Li YC, Kuter DJ. The physiological response of thrombopoietin (c-Mpl ligand) to thrombocytopenia in the rat. Br J Haematol 1999; 105:478–485.
63. Stoffel R, Wiestner A, Skoda RC. Thrombopoietin in thrombocytopenic mice: evidence against regulation at the mRNA level and for a direct regulatory role of platelets. Blood 1996; 87:567–573.
64. Fielder PJ, Gurney AL, Stefanich E, et al. Regulation of thrombopoietin levels by c-mpl-mediated binding to platelets. Blood 1996; 87:2154–2161.
65. Kuter DJ, Rosenberg RD. Appearance of a megakaryocyte growth-promoting activity, megapoietin, during acute thrombocytopenia in the rabbit. Blood 1994; 84:1464–1472.
66. Kuter DJ, Rosenberg RD. The reciprocal relationship of thrombopoietin (c-Mpl ligand) to changes in the platelet mass during busulfan-induced thrombocytopenia in the rabbit. Blood 1995; 85:2720–2730.
67. Kuter DJ. The physiology of platelet production. Stem Cells 1996; 14:88–101.
68. Li J, Xia Y, Kuter DJ. Interaction of thrombopoietin with the platelet c-mpl receptor in plasma: binding, internalization, stability and pharmacokinetics. Br J Haematol 1999; 106:345–356.
69. Broudy VC, Lin NL, Sabath DF, Papayannopoulou T, Kaushansky K. Human platelets display high-affinity receptors for thrombopoietin. Blood 1997; 89:1896–1904.
70. Scheding S, Bergmann M, Shimosaka A, et al. Human plasma thrombopoietin levels are regulated by binding to platelet thrombopoietin receptors in vivo. Transfusion 2002; 42:321–327.
71. Li J, Xia Y, Kuter D. Interaction of thrombopoietin with the platelet c-mpl receptor in plasma: binding, internalization, stability and pharmacodynamics. Br J Haematol 1999; 106:345–356.

72. Fielder PJ, Hass P, Nagel M, et al. Human platelets as a model for the binding and degradation of thrombopoietin. Blood 1997; 89:2782–2788.
73. Sungaran R, Markovic B, Chong BH. Localization and regulation of thrombopoietin mRNa expression in human kidney, liver, bone marrow, and spleen using in situ hybridization. Blood 1997; 89:101–107.
74. Quin S, Fu F, Li W, Chen Q, de Sauvage FJ. Primary role of the liver in thrombopoietin production shown by tissue-specific knockout. Blood 1998; 92:2189–2191.
75. Peck-Radosavljevic M, Zacherl J, Meng YG, et al. Is inadequate thrombopoietin production a major cause of thrombocytopenia in cirrhosis of the liver? J Hepatol 1997; 27:127–131.
76. Peck-Radosavljevic M, Wichlas M, Zacherl J, et al. Thrombopoietin induces rapid resolution of thrombocytopenia after orthotopic liver transplantation through increased platelet production. Blood 2000; 95:795–801.
77. Kaushansky K, Lok S, Holly RD, et al. Promotion of megakaryocyte progenitor expansion and differentiation by the c-Mpl ligand thrombopoietin. Nature 1994; 369:568–571.
78. Broudy VC, Lin NL, Kaushansky K. Thrombopoietin (c-mpl ligand) acts synergistically with erythropoietin, stem cell factor, and interleukin-11 to enhance murine megakaryocyte colony growth and increases megakaryocyte ploidy in vitro. Blood 1995; 85:1719–1726.
79. de Sauvage FJ, Carver-Moore K, Luoh SM, et al. Physiological regulation of early and late stages of megakaryocytopoiesis by thrombopoietin. J Exp Med 1996; 183:651–656.
80. de Sauvage FJ, Villeval JL, Shivdasani RA. Regulation of megakaryocytopoiesis and platelet production: lessons from animal models. J Lab Clin Med 1998; 131:496–501.
81. Alexander WS, Roberts AW, Maurer AB, Nicola NA, Dunn AR, Metcalf D. Studies of the c-Mpl thrombopoietin receptor through gene disruption and activation. Stem Cells 1996; 14:124–132.
82. Alexander WS, Roberts AW, Nicola NA, Li R, Metcalf D. Deficiencies in progenitor cells of multiple hematopoietic lineages and defective megakaryocytopoiesis in mice lacking the thrombopoietic receptor c-Mpl. Blood 1996; 87:2162–2170.
83. Gurney AL, Carver-Moore K, de Sauvage FJ, Moore MW. Thrombocytopenia in c-mpl-deficient mice. Science 1994; 265:1445–1447.
84. Scott CL, Robb L, Mansfield R, Alexander WS, Begley CG. Granulocyte-macrophage colony-stimulating factor is not responsible for residual thrombopoiesis in mpl null mice. Exp Hematol 2000; 28:1001–1007.
85. Rasko JE, O'Flaherty E, Begley CG. Mpl ligand (MGDF) alone and in combination with stem cell factor (SCF) promotes proliferation and survival of human megakaryocyte, erythroid and granulocyte/macrophage progenitors. Stem Cells 1997; 15:33–42.
86. Ku H, Yonemura Y, Kaushansky K, Ogawa M. Thrombopoietin, the ligand for the Mpl receptor, synergizes with steel factor and other early acting cytokines in supporting proliferation of primitive hematopoietic progenitors of mice. Blood 1996; 87:4544–4551.

87. Sitnicka E, Lin N, Priestley GV, et al. The effect of thrombopoietin on the proliferation and differentiation of murine hematopoietic stem cells. Blood 1996; 87:4998–5005.
88. Kimura S, Roberts AW, Metcalf D, Alexander WS. Hematopoietic stem cell deficiencies in mice lacking c-Mpl, the receptor for thrombopoietin. Proc Natl Acad Sci USA 1998; 95:1195–1200.
89. Choi ES, Hokom MM, Chen JL, et al. The role of megakaryocyte growth and development factor in terminal stages of thrombopoiesis. Br J Haematol 1996; 95:227–233.
90. Kojima H, Hamazaki Y, Nagata Y, Todokoro K, Nagasawa T, Abe T. Modulation of platelet activation in vitro by thrombopoietin. Thromb Haemost 1995; 74:1541–1545.
91. Ezumi Y, Takayama H, Okuma M. Thrombopoietin, c-Mpl ligand, induces tyrosine phosphorylation of Tyk2, JAK2, and STAT3, and enhances agonists-induced aggregation in platelets in vitro. FEBS Lett 1995; 374:48–52.
92. Li J, Kuter DJ. The end is just the beginning: megakaryocyte apoptosis and platelet release. Int J Hematol 2001; 74:365–374.
93. Begley CG, Lopez AF, Nicola NA, et al. Purified colony-stimulating factors enhance the survival of human neutrophils and eosinophils in vitro: a rapid and sensitive microassay for colony-stimulating factors. Blood 1986; 68:162–166.
94. Lopez AF, Williamson DJ, Gamble JR, et al. Recombinant human granulocyte-macrophage colony-stimulating factor stimulates in vitro mature human neutrophil and eosinophil function, surface receptor expression, and survival. J Clin Investig 1986; 78:1220–1228.
95. Peng J, Friese P, Wolf RF, et al. Relative reactivity of platelets from thrombopoietin- and interleukin-6-treated dogs. Blood 1996; 87:4158–4163.
96. Harker LA, Hunt P, Marzec UM, et al. Regulation of platelet production and function by megakaryocyte growth and development factor in nonhuman primates. Blood 1996; 87:1833–1844.
97. Kroner C, Eybrechts K, Akkerman JW. Dual regulation of platelet protein kinase B. J Biol Chem 2000; 275:27790–27798.
98. Snyder E, Perrotta P, Rinder H, Baril L, Nichol J, Gilligan D. Effect of recombinant human megakaryocyte growth and development factor coupled with polyethylene glycol on the platelet storage lesion. Transfusion 1999; 39:258–264.
99. Xia Y, Li J, Bertino A, Kuter DJ. Thrombopoietin and the TPO receptor during platelet storage. Transfusion 2000; 40:976–987.
100. Bertino AM, Qi XQ, Li J, Xia Y, Kuter DJ. Apoptotic markers are increased in platelets stored at 37 degrees C. Transfusion 2003; 43:857–866.
101. Allamargot C, Pouplard-Barthelaix A, Fressinaud C. A single intracerebral microinjection of platelet-derived growth factor (PDGF) accelerates the rate of remyelination in vivo. Brain Res 2001; 918:28–39.
102. Hokom MM, Lacey D, Kinstler OB, et al. Pegylated megakaryocyte growth and development factor abrogates the lethal thrombocytopenia associated with carboplatin and irradiation in mice. Blood 1995; 86:4486–4492.
103. Sheridan WP, Kuter DJ. Mechanism of action and clinical trials of Mpl ligand. Curr Opin Hematol 1997; 4:312–316.

104. Begley CG, Basser RL. Biologic and structural differences of thrombopoietic growth factors. Semin Hematol 2000; 37:19–27.
105. Harker LA, Marzec UM, Hunt P, et al. Dose-response effects of pegylated human megakaryocyte growth and development factor on platelet production and function in nonhuman primates. Blood 1996; 88:511–521.
106. Ulich TR, del Castillo J, Yin S, et al. Megakaryocyte growth and development factor ameliorates carboplatin-induced thrombocytopenia in mice. Blood 1995; 86:971–976.
107. Harker LA, Marzec UM, Kelly AB, et al. Prevention of thrombocytopenia and neutropenia in a nonhuman primate model of marrow suppressive chemotherapy by combining pegylated recombinant human megakaryocyte growth and development factor and recombinant human granulocyte colony-stimulating factor. Blood 1997; 89:155–165.
108. Akahori H, Shibuya K, Obuchi M, et al. Effect of recombinant human thrombopoietin in nonhuman primates with chemotherapy-induced thrombocytopenia. Br J Haematol 1996; 94:722–728.
109. Neelis KJ, Hartong SC, Egeland T, Thomas GR, Eaton DL, Wagemaker G. The efficacy of single-dose administration of thrombopoietin with coadministration of either granulocyte/macrophage or granulocyte colony- stimulating factor in myelosuppressed rhesus monkeys. Blood 1997; 90:2565–2573.
110. Kuter DJ, Begley CG. Recombinant human thrombopoietin: basic biology and evaluation of clinical studies. Blood 2002; 100:3457–3469.
111. Giri JG, Smith WG, Kahn LE, et al. Promegapoietin, a chimeric growth factor for megakaryocyte and platelet restoration. Blood 1997; 90:580a.
112. Cwirla SE, Balasubramanian P, Duffin DJ, et al. Peptide agonist of the thrombopoietin receptor as potent as the natural cytokine. Science 1997; 276:1696–1699.
113. de Serres M, Ellis B, Dillberger JE, et al. Immunogenicity of thrombopoietin mimetic peptide GW395058 in BALB/c mice and New Zealand white rabbits: evaluation of the potential for thrombopoietin neutralizing antibody production in man. Stem Cells 1999; 17:203–209.
114. Case BC, Hauck ML, Yeager RL, et al. The pharmacokinetics and pharmacodynamics of GW395058, a peptide agonist of the thrombopoietin receptor, in the dog, a large-animal model of chemotherapy-induced thrombocytopenia. Stem Cells 2000; 18:360–365.
115. Erickson-Miller CL, Delorme E, Tian SS, et al. Discovery and characterization of a selective, non-peptidyl thrombopoietin receptor agonist. Blood 2000; 96:675a.
116. Wang B, Nichol JL, Sullivan JT. Pharmacodynamics and pharmacokinetics of AMG 531, a novel thrombopoietin receptor ligand. Clin Pharmacol Ther 2004; 76:628–638.
117. Broudy VC, Lin NL. AMG531 stimulates megakaryopoiesis in vitro by binding to Mpl. Cytokine 2004; 25:52–60.
118. Bussell JB, George JN, Kuter DJ, et al. An open-label, dose-finding study evaluating the safety and platelet response of a novel thrombopoietic protein (AMG 531) in thrombocytopenic adult patients with immune thrombocytopenic purpura (ITP). Blood 2003; 102:234b.

119. Kuter DJ, Bussel J, Aledort L, et al. A phase 2 placebo controlled study evaluating the platelet response and safety of weekly dosing with a novel thrombopoietic protein (AMG 531) in thrombocytopenic adult patients with immune thrombocytopenic purpura. Blood 2004; 104:148a.
120. Duffy KJ, Darcy MG, Delorme E, et al. Hydrazinonaphthalene and azonaphthalene thrombopoietin mimics are nonpeptidyl promoters of megakaryocytopoiesis. J Med Chem 2001; 44:3730–3745.
121. Duffy KJ, Shaw AN, Delorme E, et al. Identification of a pharmacophore for thrombopoietic activity of small, non-peptidyl molecules. 1. Discovery and optimization of salicylaldehyde thiosemicarbazone thrombopoietin mimics. J Med Chem 2002; 45:3573–3575.
122. Duffy KJ, Price AT, Delorme E, et al. Identification of a pharmacophore for thrombopoietic activity of small, non-peptidyl molecules. 2. Rational design of naphtho[1,2-d]imidazole thrombopoietin mimics. J Med Chem 2002; 45:3576–3578.
123. Erickson-Miller CL, DeLorme E, Tian SS, et al. Discovery and characterization of a selective, nonpeptidyl thrombopoietin receptor agonist. Exp Hematol 2005; 33:85–93.
124. Luengo JI, Duffy KJ, Shaw AN, et al. Discovery of SB-497115, a small-molecule thrombopoietin (TPO) receptor agonist for the treatment of thrombocytopenia. Blood 2004; 104:795a.
125. Erickson-Miller C, Delorme E, Giampa L. Biological activity and selectivity for Tpo receptor of the orally bioavailable, small molecule Tpo receptor agonist, SB-497115. Blood 2004; 104:796a.
126. Erickson-Miller C, Delorme E, Iskander M, et al. Species specificity and receptor domain interaction of a small molecule TPO receptor agonist. Blood 2004; 104:795a.
127. Jenkins J, Nicholl R, Williams D, et al. An oral, non-peptide, small molecule thrombopoietin receptor agonist increases platelet counts in healthy subjects. Blood 2004; 104:797a.
128. Fanucchi M, Glaspy J, Crawford J, et al. Effects of polyethylene glycol-conjugated recombinant human megakaryocyte growth and development factor on platelet counts after chemotherapy for lung cancer. N Engl J Med 1997; 336:404–409.
129. Basser RL, Rasko JE, Clarke K, et al. Randomized, blinded, placebo-controlled phase I trial of pegylated recombinant human megakaryocyte growth and development factor with filgrastim after dose-intensive chemotherapy in patients with advanced cancer. Blood 1997; 89:3118–3128.
130. Crawford J, Glaspy J, Belani C, et al. A randomized, placebo-controlled, blinded, dose scheduling trial of pegylated recombinant human megakaryocyte growth and development factor (PEG-HUMGDF) with filgrastim support in non-small cell lung cancer (NSCLC) patients treated with paclitaxel and carboplatin during multiple cycles of chemotherapy. Proc ASCO 1998; 17:73a.
131. Vadhan-Raj S, Patel S, Broxmeyer HE, et al. Phase I-II investigtion of recombinant human thrombopoietin (rhTPO) in patients with sarcoma receiving high dose chemotherapy (CT) with adriamycin (A) and ifosfamide (I). Blood 1996; 88:448a.

132. Vadhan-Raj S, Murray LJ, Bueso-Ramos C, et al. Stimulation of megakaryocyte and platelet production by a single dose of recombinant human thrombopoietin in patients with cancer. Ann Intern Med 1997; 126:673–681.
133. Vadhan-Raj S, Verschraegen C, McGarry L, et al. Recombinant human thrombopoietin (rhTPO) attenuates high-dose carboplatin (C)-induced thrombocytopenia in patients with gynecological malignancy. Blood 1997; 90:580a.
134. Vadhan-Raj S, Verschraegen CF, Bueso-Ramos C, et al. Recombinant human thrombopoietin attenuates carboplatin-induced severe thrombocytopenia and the need for platelet transfusions in patients with gynecologic cancer. Ann Intern Med 2000; 132:364–368.
135. Basser RL, Rasko JE, Clarke K, et al. Thrombopoietic effects of pegylated recombinant human megakaryocyte growth and development factor (PEG-rHuMGDF) in patients with advanced cancer. Lancet 1996; 348:1279–1281.
136. Basser RL, Underhill C, Davis I, et al. Enhancement of platelet recovery after myelosuppressive chemotherapy by recombinant human megakaryocyte growth and development factor in patients with advanced cancer. J Clin Oncol 2000; 18:2852–2861.
137. Moskowitz C, Nimer S, Gabrilove J, et al. A randomized, double blind, placebo-controlled, dose finding, efficacy and safety study of PEG-rHuMGDF (M) in non-Hodgkin's lymphoma (NHL) patients (pts) treated with ICE (ifosfamide, carboplatin and etoposide). J Clin Oncol 1998; 17:76a.
138. O'Malley CJ, Rasko JE, Basser RL, et al. Administration of pegylated recombinant human megakaryocyte growth and development factor to humans stimulates the production of functional platelets that show no evidence of in vivo activation. Blood 1996; 88:3288–3298.
139. Vadhan-Raj S, Patel S, Broxmeyer H. Schedule-dependent reduction in thrombocytopenia by recombinant human thrombopoietin (rhTPO) in patients with sarcoma receiving high dose chemotherapy (CT) with adriamycin (A) and ifosfamide (I). J Clin Oncol 1999; 18:52A.
140. Tornebohm E, Lockner D, Paul C. A retrospective analysis of bleeding complications in 438 patients with acute leukaemia during the years 1972–1991. Eur J Haematol 1993; 50:160–167.
141. Anderlini P, Luna M, Kantarjian HM. Causes of initial remission induction failure in patients with acute myeloid leukemia and myelodysplastic syndromes. Leukemia 1996; 10:600–608.
142. Archimbaud E, Ottmann OG, Yin JA, et al. A randomized, double-blind, placebo-controlled study with pegylated recombinant human megakaryocyte growth and development factor (PEG-rHuMGDF) as an adjunct to chemotherapy for adults with de novo acute myeloid leukemia. Blood 1999; 94:3694–3701.
143. Archimbaud E, Ottmann O, Lin J, et al. A randomized, double-blind, placebo-controlled study using PEG-rHuMGDF as an adjunct to chemotherapy for adults with de-novo acute myeloid leukemia (AML): Early results. Blood 1996; 99:447a.
144. Schiffer CA, Miller K, Larson RA, et al. A double-blind, placebo-controlled trial of pegylated recombinant human megakaryocyte growth and development factor as an adjunct to induction and consolidation therapy for patients with acute myeloid leukemia. Blood 2000; 95:2530–2535.

145. Cripe L, Neuberg D, Tallman M, et al. A pilot study of recombinant human thrombopoietin (rh-TPO) and GM-CSF following induction therapy in patients older than 55 years with acute myeloid leukemia (AML). Blood 1998; 92:616A.
146. Glaspy J, Vredenburgh J, Demetri GD, et al. Effects of PEGylated recombinant human megakaryocyte growth and development factor (PEG-rHuMGDF) before high dose chemotherapy (HDC) with peripheral blood progenitor cell (PBPC) support. Blood 1997; 90:580a.
147. Bolwell B, Vredenburgh J, Overmoyer B, et al. Safety and biological effect of pegylated recombinant megakaryocyte growth and development factor (PEG-rHuMGDF) in breast cancer patients following autologous peripheral blood progenitor cell transplantation (PBPC). Blood 1997; 90:171a.
148. Nash R, Kurzrock R, DiPersio J, et al. Safety and activity of recombinant human thrombopoietin (rhTPO) in patients (pts) with delayed platelet recovery (DPR). Blood 1997; 90:262a.
149. Nash RA, Kurzrock R, DiPersio J, et al. A phase I trial of recombinant human thrombopoietin in patients with delayed platelet recovery after hematopoietic stem cell transplantation. Biol Blood Marrow Transplant 2000; 6:25–34.
150. Somlo G, Sniecinski I, ter Veer A, et al. Recombinant human thrombopoietin in combination with granulocyte colony-stimulating factor enhances mobilization of peripheral blood progenitor cells, increases peripheral blood platelet concentration, and accelerates hematopoietic recovery following high-dose chemotherapy. Blood 1999; 93:2798–2806.
151. Gajewski J, Korbling M, Donato M, et al. Recombinant human thrombopoietin (rhTPO) for mobilization of peripheral blood progenitor cells (PBPC) for autologous transplantation in breast cancer: preliminary results of a phase I trial. Blood 1997; 90:97A.
152. Linker C, Anderlini P, Herzig R, et al. A randomized, placebo-controlled, phase II trial of recombinant human thrombopoietin (rhTPO) in subjects undergoing high dose chemotherapy (HDC) and PBPC transplant. Blood 1998;92.
153. Linker C. Thrombopoietin in the treatment of acute myeloid leukemia and in stem-cell transplantation. Semin Hematol 2000; 37:35–40.
154. Bolwell B, Vredenburgh J, Overmoyer B, et al. Phase 1 study of pegylated recombinant human megakaryocyte growth and development factor (PEG-rHuMGDF) in breast cancer patients after autologous peripheral blood progenitor cell (PBPC) transplantation. Bone Marrow Transplant 2000; 26:141–145.
155. Schuster MW, Beveridge R, Frei-Lahr D, et al. The effects of pegylated recombinant human megakaryocyte growth and development factor (PEG-rHuMGDF) on platelet recovery in breast cancer patients undergoing autologous bone marrow transplantation. Exp Hematol 2002; 30:1044–1050.
156. Fibbe WE, Heemskerk DP, Laterveer L, et al. Accelerated reconstitution of platelets and erythrocytes after syngeneic transplantation of bone marrow cells derived from thrombopoietin pretreated donor mice. Blood 1995; 86:3308–3313.
157. Liu Yin JA, Adams JA, Brereton ML, Hann A, Harrison BD, Briggs M. Megakaryopoiesis in vitro in myelodysplastic syndromes and acute myeloid leukaemia: effect of pegylated recombinant human megakaryocyte growth and development factor in combination with other growth factors. Br J Haematol 2000; 108:743–746.

158. Fontenay-Roupie M, Dupont JM, Picard F, et al. Analysis of megakaryocyte growth and development factor (thrombopoietin) effects on blast cell and megakaryocyte growth in myelodysplasia. Leuk Res 1998; 22:527–535.
159. Nichol JL. Thrombopoietin levels after chemotherapy and in naturally occurring human diseases. Curr Opin Hematol 1998; 5:203–208.
160. Komatsu N, Okamoto T, Yoshida T, et al. Pegylated recombinant human megakaryocyte growth and development factor (PEG-rHuMGDF) increased platelet counts (plt) in patients with aplastic anemia (AA) and myelodysplastic syndrome (MDS). Blood 2000; 96:296a.
161. Harker LA, Marzec UM, Novembre F, et al. Treatment of thrombocytopenia in chimpanzees infected with human immunodeficiency virus by pegylated recombinant human megakaryocyte growth and development factor. Blood 1998; 91:4427–4433.
162. Harker LA, Carter RA, Marzec UM, et al. Correction of thrombocytopenia and ineffective platelet production in patients infected with human immunodeficiency virus (HIV) by PEG-rHuMGDF therapy. Blood 1998; 92:707a.
163. Nomura S, Dan K, Hotta T, Fujimura K, Ikeda Y. Effects of pegylated recombinant human megakaryocyte growth and development factor in patients with idiopathic thrombocytopenic purpura. Blood 2002; 100:728–730.
164. Rice L, Nichol JL, Delavari M, Roskos L, Bacille MH, McMillan R. Cyclic thrombocytopenia with platelet auto-antibodies: response to PEG-rHu megakaryocyte growth and development factor. Blood 1998; 92:180b.
165. Aref S, Mabed M, Selim T, Goda T, Khafagy N. Thrombopoietin (TPO) levels in hepatic patients with thrombocytopenia. Hematology 2004; 9:351–356.
166. Giannini E, Borro P, Botta F, et al. Serum thrombopoietin levels are linked to liver function in untreated patients with hepatitis C virus-related chronic hepatitis. J Hepatol 2002; 37:572–577.
167. Siemensma NP, Bathal PS, Penington DG. The effect of massive liver resection on platelet kinetics in the rat. J Lab Clin Med 1975; 86:817–833.
168. Kuter DJ. The use of PEG-rhuMGDF in platelet apheresis. Stem Cells 1998; 16:231–242.
169. Nakamura M, Toombs CF, Duarte IG, et al. Recombinant human megakaryocyte growth and development factor attenuates postbypass thrombocytopenia. Ann Thorac Surg 1998; 66:1216–1223.
170. Rasko JE, Basser RL, Boyd J, et al. Multilineage mobilization of peripheral blood progenitor cells in humans following administration of PEG-rHuMGDF. Br J Haematol 1997; 97:871–880.
171. Murray LJ, Luens KM, Estrada MF, et al. Thrombopoietin mobilizes CD34+ cell subsets into peripheral blood and expands multilineage progenitors in bone marrow of cancer patients with normal hematopoiesis. Exp Hematol 1998; 26:207–216.
172. Yagi M, Ritchie KA, Sitnicka E, Storey C, Roth GJ, Bartelmez S. Sustained ex vivo expansion of hematopoietic stem cells mediated by thrombopoietin. Proc Natl Acad Sci USA 1999; 96:8126–8131.
173. Piacibello W, Sanavio F, Garetto L, et al. Extensive amplification and self-renewal of human primitive hematopoietic stem cells from cord blood. Blood 1997; 89:2644–2653.

174. Kuter DJ, Goodnough LT, Romo J, et al. Thrombopoietin therapy increases platelet yields in healthy platelet donors. Blood 2001; 98:1339–1345.
175. Goodnough LT, Kuter DJ, McCullough J, et al. Prophylactic platelet transfusions from healthy apheresis platelet donors undergoing treatment with thrombopoietin. Blood 2001; 98:1346–1351.
176. Vadhan-Raj S, Kavanagh JJ, Freedman RS, et al. Safety and efficacy of transfusions of autologous cryopreserved platelets derived from recombinant human thrombopoietin to support chemotherapy-associated severe thrombocytopenia: a randomised cross-over study. Lancet 2002; 359:2145–2152.
177. Neelis KJ, Visser TP, Dimjati W, et al. A single dose of thrombopoietin shortly after myelosuppressive total body irradiation prevents pancytopenia in mice by promoting short-term multilineage spleen-repopulating cells at the transient expense of bone marrow-repopulating cells. Blood 1998; 92:1586–1597.
178. Kaushansky K, Lin N, Grossmann A, Humes J, Sprugel KH, Broudy VC. Thrombopoietin expands erythroid, granulocyte-macrophage, and megakaryocytic progenitor cells in normal and myelosuppressed mice. Exp Hematol 1996; 24:265–269.
179. Kaushansky K. Thrombopoietin: more than a lineage-specific megakaryocyte growth factor. Stem Cells 1997; 15:97–103.
180. Mouthon MA, Van der Meeren A, Gaugler MH, et al. Thrombopoietin promotes hematopoietic recovery and survival after high- dose whole body irradiation. Int J Radiat Oncol Biol Phys 1999; 43:867–875.
181. Columbyova L, Loda M, Scadden DT. Thrombopoietin receptor expression in human cancer cell lines and primary tissues. Cancer Res 1995; 55:3509–3512.
182. Molineux G, Hartley C, McElroy P, McCrea C, Kerzic P, McNiece I. An analysis of the effects of combined treatment with rmGM-CSF and PEG- rHuMGDF in murine bone marrow transplant recipients. Stem Cells 1997; 15:43–49.
183. Ulich TR, del Castillo J, Senaldi G, et al. Systemic hematologic effects of PEG-rHuMGDF-induced megakaryocyte hyperplasia in mice. Blood 1996; 87:5006–5015.
184. Villeval JL, Cohen-Solal K, Tulliez M, et al. High thrombopoietin production by hematopoietic cells induces a fatal myeloproliferative syndrome in mice. Blood 1997; 90:4369–4383.
185. Frey BM, Rafii S, Teterson M, Eaton D, Crystal RG, Moore MA. Adenovector-mediated expression of human thrombopoietin cDNA in immune- compromised mice: insights into the pathophysiology of osteomyelofibrosis. J Immunol 1998; 160:691–699.
186. Abina MA, Tulliez M, Lacout C, et al. Major effects of TPO delivered by a single injection of a recombinant adenovirus on prevention of septicemia and anemia associated with myelosuppression in mice: risk of sustained expression inducing myelofibrosis due to immunosuppression. Gene Ther 1998; 5:497–506.
187. Yan XQ, Lacey D, Fletcher F, et al. Chronic exposure to retroviral vector encoded MGDF (mpl-ligand) induces lineage-specific growth and differentiation of megakaryocytes in mice. Blood 1995; 86:4025–4033.
188. Yan XQ, Lacey D, Hill D, et al. A model of myelofibrosis and osteosclerosis in mice induced by overexpressing thrombopoietin (mpl ligand): reversal of disease by bone marrow transplantation. Blood 1996; 88:402–409.

189. Douglas VK, Tallman MS, Cripe LD, Peterson LC. Thrombopoietin administered during induction chemotherapy to patients with acute myeloid leukemia induces transient morphologic changes that may resemble chronic myeloproliferative disorders. Am J Clin Pathol 2002; 117:844–850.
190. Li J, Yang C, Xia Y, et al. Thrombocytopenia caused by the development of antibodies to thrombopoietin. Blood 2001; 98:3241–3248.
191. Yang C, Xia Y, Li J, Kuter DJ. The appearance of anti-thrombopoietin antibody and circulating thrombopoietin-IgG complexes in a patient developing thrombocytopenia after the injection of PEG-rHuMGDF. Blood 1999; 94:681a.
192. Basser RL, O'Flaherty E, Green M, et al. Development of pancytopenia with neutralizing antibodies to thrombopoietin after multicycle chemotherapy supported by megakaryocyte growth and development factor. Blood 2002; 99:2599–2602.
193. F-D-C- Reports. In Brief: Amgen Megagen. The Pink Sheet. 1998; 60:27.
194. Rebulla P, Finazzi G, Marangoni F, et al. The threshold for prophylactic platelet transfusions in adults with acute myeloid leukemia. N Engl J Med 1997; 337:1870–1875.
195. Rebulla P. Trigger for platelet transfusion. Vox Sang 2000; 78:179–182.
196. Wandt H, Frank M, Ehninger G, et al. Safety and cost effectiveness of a 1010(9)/L trigger for prophylactic platelet transfusions compared with the traditional 2010(9)/L trigger: a prospective comparative trial in 105 patients with acute myeloid leukemia. Blood 1998; 91:3601–3606.
197. Kuter DJ. Whatever happened to thrombopoietin? Transfusion 2002; 42:279–283.

3

Congenital (Inherited, Familial) Thrombocytopenias (CTPs)

James B. Bussel

Platelet Disorders Center, Division of Pediatric Hematology-Oncology, Department of Pediatrics, Weill Medical College of Cornell University, New York, New York, U.S.A.

Congenital (inherited, familial) thrombocytopenias (CTPs) are relatively infrequent compared to acquired causes of low platelets, such as immune thrombocytopenic purpura (ITP) (Table 1). The absolute percentage of each among all cases of thrombocytopenia is not known and likely varies considerably depending upon the population being assessed. Common experience would suggest, however, that all nonimmune causes of thrombocytopenia, both acquired and congenital, represent at most 5–10 percent of the cases of thrombocytopenia seen by hematologists. Even if known infections complicated by mild or moderate thrombocytopenia are excluded and only isolated thrombocytopenia considered, approximately 90–95% of thrombocytopenia in both children and adults results from ITP or drug-induced thrombocytopenia.

DIAGNOSING CONGENITAL THROMBOCYTOPENIA

An important factor in considering the diagnosis of thrombocytopenia is that routine platelet counts are performed in otherwise healthy patients with increasing frequency. Unless thrombocytopenia is severe, or the platelets dysfunctional, most individuals with thrombocytopenia have few symptoms or signs of bleeding and thus escape detection until a platelet count is performed for another purpose.

Table 1 Causes of Acquired Thrombocytopenia

Immune causes	
	Immune thrombocytopenic purpura (ITP)
	Neonatal alloimmune thrombocytopenia
	Posttransfusion purpura (PTP)
	Drug-induced thrombocytopenia
Nonimmune causes	
	Shortened circulation
	Disseminated intravascular coagulopathy (DIC)
	Thrombotic thrombocytopenic purpura (TTP)[a]
	Heparin-induced thrombocytopenia (HIT)[a]
	Splenomegaly/splenic sequestration
	Turbulent blood flow (hemangiomas, abnormal cardiac valves, intra-aortic balloon pumps)
	Decreased production
	Drug-induced marrow suppression
	Chemotherapy
	Viral infection (hepatitis C virus, HIV, cytomegalovirus)
	Bacterial infection (sepsis)
	Alcoholism/bone marrow suppression
	Myelodysplastic syndrome (MDS)
	Myelofibrosis/myelophthisis
	Aplastic anemia
	Hematologic malignancy (leukemias, lymphomas, myeloma)
	Solid tumor infiltrating bone marrow

[a] These disorders may have an immune component to their pathogenesis, but are not associated with auto antiplatelet antibodies.

Thus, unsuspected thrombocytopenia is often noted incidentally when complete blood counts are obtained using modern autoanalyzers that routinely measure the platelet count (1). The detection of unsuspected thrombocytopenia is augmented by an increasing emphasis on preventative care, including not only annual evaluations, but also relatively frequent blood tests in settings such as prior to surgery, or as part of work, camp, or school "physicals." Considerations such as these explain the occasional identification of CTP not only in mildly or asymptomatic children, but also adults, and in turn increases the number of cases of "isolated" thrombocytopenia referred to specialists.

Concern has been raised about the importance of correctly diagnosing CTP, or misdiagnosing it as ITP. Two recent studies have highlighted the fact that a number of cases of CTP have been misdiagnosed as ITP, and that affected patients have been subjected to inappropriate therapy such as corticosteroids, splenectomy and/or cyclophosphamide, among others (2,3). Reports such as these highlight the importance of correct diagnosis of congenital thrombocytopenias. An additional concern is that in emergent situations in which the platelet count must be increased acutely, the management of thrombocytopenia in patients with ITP (steroids, IVIG, etc) is markedly different than that in patients with congenital thrombocytopenias (platelet transfusions).

The diagnosis of CTP may be difficult, given that cases are both relatively infrequent and heterogeneous; indeed, CTP is not a single entity, but rather a group of approximately 20 separate clinical syndromes. Several clinical and historical findings should lead one to suspect CTP. The most obvious of these is the family history. While ITP is thought to result from the effects of antiplatelet autoantibodies, the lack of a family history in most cases argues against a simple genetic predisposition to the disease process. Though occasional patients with ITP may have affected family members with similar disorders, these individuals are often first or second cousins at the closest and it is uncommon in the author's personal and others' reported experiences to have immediate family members affected. Reports of "ITP" in close relatives may instead represent autoimmune disorders in which the family history is more consistent with systemic lupus (SLE). While the presence of immediate family members with thrombocytopenia is consistent with CTP, it is important to realize that some types of CTP may also result from autosomal recessive inheritance. Thus any family history of thrombocytopenia needs to be considered from the perspective of CTP, with the caveat that the affected individual may be the propositus/index case (Table 2).

Another important point to consider is that there is no diagnostic laboratory testing available for ITP. Therefore, ITP is a "diagnosis of exclusion" and prone to misdiagnosis. Thus, a family member diagnosed with "ITP" may or may not have autoimmune thrombocytopenia. While current antigen-specific platelet antibody testing for ITP has greater predictive value and specificity than tests utilizing the intact platelet as a target, it remains to be demonstrated whether this testing will indeed distinguish ITP from CTP. Moreover, certain syndromes of CTP may also have an autoimmune component (see below).

Thrombocytopenia that is either stable over a long period of time and/or has an apparent onset at birth also suggests the diagnosis of CTP. In fact, the most efficient way to eliminate CTP as a consideration is documentation of a normal platelet count in the past, as it it is much more likely that a platelet count will be falsely low than falsely normal. Therefore, it is important to obtain the results of any previous blood work, even if these studies had been performed years ago. In the absence of a previously normal platelet count, the timing of onset of the thrombocytopenia (as best as it is known) may also be important. The probability of CTP would be increased if the thrombocytopenias existed for many years, especially if first documented in early childhood. In the author's experience, adults are remarkably poor historians regarding their childhood blood counts, and query of their parents may be worthwhile.

A stable platelet count over time is another marker of CTP, though a recent evaluation of platelet counts spanning months to years in 30 patients with chronic ITP also suggested surprising stability (unpublished data). Therefore, while this criterion may not be highly specific, it should suggest CTP in certain ambiguous cases of thrombocytopenia.

Table 2 Classification of Congenital Thrombocytopenia based on Inheritance Pattern

Autosomal dominant	Autosomal recessive	X-linked
May-Hegglin anomaly	Congenital amegakaryocytic thrombocytopenia (CAMT)	Wiskott-Aldrich syndrome (WAS)
Fechtner syndrome		
Epstein syndrome	Thrombocytopenia and absent radii (TAR)	X-linked thrombocytopenia (WAS)
Sebastian syndrome		
Mediterranean thrombocytopenia/Bernard-Soulier carrier	Bernard-Soulier syndrome	*GATA1* mutation (1) XLTT (2) X-linked thrombocytopenia and dyserythropoiesis with or without anemia
Velocardiofacial / DiGeorge syndrome		
Platelet-type or pseudo von Willebrand's disease		
Familial platelet disorder/acute myeloid leukemia		
Amegakaryocytic thrombocytopenia with radio-ulnar synostosis		
Chromosome 10/THC2		
Paris-Trousseau thrombocytopenia/Jacobsen syndrome		
Gray platelet syndrome		
Montreal platelet syndrome		
Macrothrombocytopenia with platelet expression of glycophorin A		
Thrombocytopenia and radial synostosus		

Perhaps the most important initial diagnostic step in evaluating a patient with possible CTP is review of the peripheral blood smear. Newer automated blood cell analyzers have been significantly improved in terms of their ability to recognize large platelets, and thus estimate platelet size (i.e., the mean platelet volume, MPV). However, there is no substitute for a visual examination of the patient's platelets, since for very small or very large platelets, and at very low platelet counts, the accuracy of measurement of both the platelet count itself and the MPV obtained in standard laboratories is uncertain. Hence, visual inspection of the peripheral smear remains the gold standard for evaluating platelets of abnormal size and morphology. The presence of megathrombocytes, defined as very large platelets that are equal in size or larger than red blood cells, is compatible with a number of syndromes that comprise CTP (Table 3). Indeed, it appears that producing excessively large platelets is a common feature of many disorders in which the pathogenesis involves a disturbance in the development of megakaryocytes or platelets. Acquisition of normal platelet size requires that the megakaryocyte demarcatory membrane system delineates platelets by subdivision of megakaryocyte cytoplasm. Any significant interruption of this process may result in larger platelets. Examples of syndromes associated with large platelets include Bernard-Soulier syndrome (4) and the MYH9 defects (5), e.g., May-Hegglin, Sebastian, Fechtner, Epstein, and Alport syndromes. The gray platelet syndrome (6) and von Willebrand disease (vWD) type IIB are also associated with large platelets. A critical distinction to make on the peripheral blood film is that in CTP one may routinely see many megathrombocytes, while in ITP, large platelets also occur, but they are less common and not as large.

The presence of very small platelets is consistent with the Wiskott-Aldrich syndrome (WAS), either the complete syndrome or the less symptomatic XLT (X-linked thrombocytopenia) form (7,8). The reason that small platelets occur in these individuals is uncertain, but may reflect deficiencies in thrombopoiesis or more avid removal of larger platelets by the spleen. Small platelets may be difficult to recognize without very careful examination of the peripheral blood

Table 3 Inherited Thrombocytopenias Classified by Platelet Size

Small platelets, MPV less than 7 fL	Normal platelets, MPV 7–11 fL	Large/giant platelets, MPV greater than 11 fL
Wiskott-Aldrich syndrome (WAS)	Familial platelet disorder/ acute myeloid leukemia	May-Hegglin anomaly
		Fechtner syndrome
X-linked thrombocytopenia (WAS)		Epstein syndrome
	Chromosome 10/THC2	Sebastian syndrome
		Mediterranean thrombocytopenia
	Congenital amegakaryocytic thrombocytopenia	Bernard-Soulier syndrome
		Velocardiofacial / DiGeorge syndrome
		GATA1 mutation
	Thrombocytopenia and absent radii	Gray platelet syndrome
	von Willebrand type IIB	Paris-Trousseau thrombocytopenia / Jacobsen syndrome

film, and their presence in the newborn may depend upon sufficient maturation of the mononuclear phagocyte system. Other entities that may result in thrombocytopenia with small platelets include congenital CMV or rubella infections, though these are usually diagnosed by other features such as the "blueberry muffin" rash, hepatosplenomegaly and/or presence of high fever.

Pseudothrombocytopenia (9) is artifactual thrombocytopenia caused by platelet clumping in the presence of Ethylenediaminetetraacetic Acid. In the absence of free calcium, certain platelet glycoproteins may undergo conformational change with resultant exposure of a neoepitope that is recognized by latent antibodies in the patient plasma. These clumped (agglutinated) platelets are not recognized as such by automated counters, leading to artifactual thrombocytopenia, though they are evident on the peripheral blood film. Platelet clumping on the peripheral blood film may also suggest type IIb vWD, though this is much less common than pseudothrombocytopenia. Pseudothrombocytopenia may be excluded either by using citrate as the anticoagulant prior to automated platelet counting, or making peripheral blood films from a drop of blood placed directly on a glass slide.

The gray platelet syndrome (6) results from the absence of platelet alpha granule contents. Therefore, the small, purple granules normally seen in platelets on the blood film are absent, and the platelets appear uniformly gray. Döhle-like bodies in neutrophils, in conjunction with very large platelets, suggests the May-Hegglin anomaly (MYH9-RD) (5). Microcytosis and thrombocytopenia suggest the XLT-T form of CTP involving a mutation in the DNA binding face of GATA-1 (4). Dyserythropoiesis is also consistent with the XLT form of CTP, involving a mutation of GATA-1 that disrupts its interaction with FOG (10–13). These manifestations may sometimes be difficult to differentiate from those occurring in myelodysplastic syndromes (MDS).

CLINICAL FINDINGS THAT SUGGEST CONGENITAL THROMBOCYTOPENIC DISORDERS

Bleeding out of proportion to the platelet count is actually less common in CTP than once thought, but may be a feature of several entities, such as the familial thrombocytopenia-leukemia syndrome (14), both variants of the Wiskott Aldrich syndrome, and type IIB vWD. Patients with these disorders may develop petechiae and/or ecchymoses at platelet counts $>50{,}000$/ul, suggesting intrinsic platelet dysfunction in addition to thrombocytopenia. The differential diagnosis of this presentation may also include ITP due to a platelet autoantibody that inhibits platelet function by binding to critical functional epitopes on specific platelet glycoproteins, such as GPIIbIIIa, causing an "acquired" Glanzmann's thrombasthenia. While routine testing for such antibodies is generally not available, all of the CTP syndromes noted above that are associated with platelet dysfunction have other diagnostic features that allow their identification.

A lack of response to ITP therapies is another observation that should suggest the possibility of CTP. Since definitions of "response" to such therapy, and the rate of responses to various agents vary among reports, deciding what constitutes a treatment failure may be subjective. Moreover, cases initially considered to be ITP in which the patients do not respond to therapy are more likely to represent MDS or impending aplastic anemia than CTP, and the relationship between the absolute value of any observed platelet count increment and a diagnosis of ITP vs CTP remains uncertain. Most experts believe, however, that a failure to increase the platelet count, even transiently, following ITP therapy, is consistent with CTP. In particular, a lack of any response to IVIG or to IV anti-D (in an Rh(D)+patient) seems to be unequivocal evidence against ITP and, by inference, for CTP. Likewise, the platelet increment and survival following a platelet transfusion may facilitate the distinction between ITP and CTP, though again there are no strict guidelines as to what constitutes a "normal" response to platelet transfusion in a patient with ITP versus CTP. The concept is that patients with CTP should respond to platelet transfusion, while the response of those with ITP is likely to be blunted both in terms of the observed platelet increment and survival.

These comments must be tempered by the realization that some cases of CTP are indeed associated with autoimmune thrombocytopenia. The most well described of these is the velocardiofacial syndrome (VCF) (14), which may be associated with immune mediated thrombocytopenia and autoimmune hemolytic anemia (Evan's syndrome). Patients with WAS may also have an ITP-like component to their thrombocytopenia, which often responds to splenectomy.

Associated clinical features of congenital thrombocytopenic disorders may also provide important clues to the diagnosis. These may occur either in the patient or in family members. Table 4 lists many of these, which although helpful may be difficult to interpret due to their variable presence and heterogeneity among specific individuals affected by CTP. While there should not be a high threshold to *suspect* CTP, being certain of the diagnosis, especially using only associated features, is challenging unless the presentation is both unique and classic. For example, a constellation of associated features in patients with CTP includes high tone hearing loss, renal disease, and cataracts, along with leukocyte inclusions (Döhle-like bodies) and large platelets. Having all or most of these features in more than one family member is highly consistent with MYH9-RD. Another example is the abnormality of the radius associated with congenital amegakaryocytopenia (TAR (15–16); thrombocytopenia with absent radii). However, even the diagnosis of TAR, which is now so well known and easily recognized that it is often diagnosed by prenatal ultrasound (17) or in the neonatal nursery prior to measurement of a platelet count, has become more complex following the description of another syndrome called CTRUS (18) (congenital thrombocytopenia and radio-ulnar synostosis). In contrast, some features associated with CTP are not well appreciated, for example the mental retardation that may be observed in association with the Jacobson and Paris-Trousseau (19)

Table 4 Inherited Thrombocytopenias Classified by Associated Findings

Syndrome	Associated findings
MYH9-related thrombocytopenia	
May-Hegglin anomaly	Neutrophil inclusions, sensorineural hearing loss, nephritis, cataracts
Fechtner syndrome	
Epstein syndrome	
Sebastian syndrome	
Mediterranean thrombocytopenia/ Bernard-Soulier carrier	None
Bernard-Soulier syndrome	None
Velocardiofacial/DiGeorge syndrome (CATCH 22)	Cardiac, facial, parathyroid, and thymus anomalies, cognitive/learning impairment, reduced expression of GPIb in a subpopulation of large platelets
Familial platelet disorder/acute myeloid leukemia	Myelodysplasia, acute myeloid leukemia, solid tumors
Chromosome 10/THC2	None
Paris-Trousseau thrombocytopenia/ Jacobsen syndrome	Psychomotor retardation, facial anomalies (Jacobsen syndrome)
Gray platelet syndrome	None
Congenital amegakaryocytic thrombocytopenia	Marrow failure during first and second decades
Thrombocytopenia and absent radii	Shortened/absent radii bilaterally
Thrombocytopenia and radial synostosis	Fused radius, incomplete range of motion especially supination/ pronation
Wiskott-Adrich syndrome (WAS)	Immunodeficiency, eczema, lymphoma
X-linked thrombocytopenia (WAS)	None
GATA-1 mutation	
Dyserythropoietic anemia with thrombocytopenia	Anemia (mild to severe), red cell anisopoikilocytosis, dysmegakaryocytopoiesis. Large platelets.
X-linked thrombocytopenia with thalassemia (XLTT)	Anemia (mild to nil), unbalanced globin chain synthesis resembling ß-thalassemia, peripheral red cell hemolysis, dysmegakaryocytopoiesis, splenomegaly. Large platelets.
Thrombocytopenia 2	Dysmegakaryocytopoiesis. Normal platelet size.
Platelet-type or pseudo von Willebrand disease	Spontaneous platelet aggregation in vitro and/or increased platelet agglutination to low-dose ristocetin.
Montreal platelet syndrome	Spontaneous platelet aggregation in vitro. Large platelets.

syndromes. Finally, some associated features may be subtle, for example the "heart disease" of the DiGeorge/VCF may be only a right-sided aortic arch (14), while the immune deficiency may not be clinically apparent; thus, the presence of immune thrombocytopenia may complicate the diagnosis by making the case appear as only a slightly atypical ITP.

SYNTHESIZING THE FINDINGS TO REACH A DIAGNOSIS

The various clinical and laboratory findings described above may lead one to suspect a clinical diagnosis of CTP; however, reaching a definitive diagnosis by either accepting or rejecting this suspicion may be difficult. Characteristics which lead one to suspect such a disorder, such as a failure to respond to ITP therapy, are often not useful in reaching a specific diagnosis. Indeed, the difficulty of making such a diagnosis depends considerably upon the individual diseases and their characteristics, specifically those considered essential for diagnosis. On one end of the spectrum are certain disorders that can be diagnosed clinically without special testing or molecular analysis (20). On the other end of the spectrum are diagnoses in which the molecular lesion has not been well characterized, or in which the specific diagnostic laboratory studies are difficult to perform and not generally available. In general, associated clinical features, such as platelet dysfunction, may be useful in pinpointing the specific syndrome when present. Similar considerations apply to specific findings observed when examining the peripheral blood film, although certain findings, such as large platelets, may narrow the differential diagnosis yet be consistent with several CTP syndromes (Table 5). Suggested classification schemes for CTP which are based on either genetic studies, mechanisms of thrombocytopenia, or other findings in affected patients are suggested in Table 6. Specific molecular defects associated with syndromes of congenital thrombocytopenia are listed in Table 7 (20), and key growth and transcription factors implicated in pathogenesis of several CTP syndromes are listed in Table 8.

Below, we summarize several CTP syndromes, attempting to highlight their distinguishing features and molecular characteristics, when known.

Table 5 Confirmation of a Specific Congenital Thrombocytopenia in a Thrombocytopenic Patient[a]

(A)	Detection of the specific molecular defect
(B)	Identification of one or more laboratory findings considered to be diagnostic
(C)	Assembly of clinical and laboratory features which, while not individually diagnostic, together strongly suggest a specific diagnosis

[a] Ideally a diagnosis would first be made by "C" and then followed by "A" and/or "B".

Table 6 Classification Schemes for Congenital Thrombocytopenias

(A)	Specific genetic/molecular defect
(B)	Mechanism whereby thrombocytopenia results
(C)	Mode of inheritance
(D)	Size of the platelet on smear including other abnormal findings on the smear
(E)	Presence of diagnostic clinical features either in the proband or in family members

SPECIFIC INHERITED THROMBOCYTOPENIAS

Amegakaryocytic Thrombocytopenia

Congenital amegakaryocytic thrombocytopenia (CAMT) (15,21,22) typically presents as severe neonatal thrombocytopenia that is often recognized on the first day of life, or at least within the first month. It may initially be confused with fetal and neonatal alloimmune thrombocytopenia, but the platelet count does not improve with time (weeks) and responds only to platelet transfusion rather than to IVIG and corticosteroids. Eventually a diagnostic bone marrow examination including a biopsy is performed leading to the correct diagnosis. Ten to 30% of cases of CAMT are associated with orthopedic or neurologic abnormalities. Intracranial hemorrhage (ICH) is common, occurring in 5 of 24 cases in the largest series (5), and treatment other than platelet transfusions is largely ineffective although responses to IL-3 and IL-11 may occur in a limited number of cases.

Fifty percent of the 24 cases in the same large survey progressed to aplastic pancytopenia within the first five years of life; one case of leukemia was seen (5). The underlying defect in the majority of cases has been found to be a mutation in the thrombopoietin (TPO) receptor, c-mpl (22). Recently, Ballmaier has suggested that the specific type of mutation within c-mpl determines the severity of the disease (21). In the absence of a signal from TPO, megakaryocytes do not proliferate. The prevailing hypothesis to account for the later onset of aplastic pancytopenia is that c-mpl is also required for stem cell maturation. Therefore, in the absence of the anti-apoptotic influences of TPO, stem cell depletion may lead to aplasia.

While certain cytokines may have limited efficacy in individual patients, none are consistently effective and their use may result in substantial toxicity. TPO, or a thrombopoietic agent dependent on c-mpl seems unlikely to be of use because the underlying defect is a mutation in the receptor, and only a limited number of patients have sufficiently functional c-mpl to transmit TPO initiated signaling responses.

Platelet transfusions are administered for very low platelet counts (usually $<10{,}000/\mu l$) and as prophylaxis in patients who have had major bleeds. Specific transfusion strategies have not been well-defined, thus the schedule must be individualized by the treating hematologist. Matching strategies for compatible

Table 7 Inherited Thrombocytopenias Classified by Genetic Mutations

Syndrome	Gene mutation	Chromosomal location
MYH9-related thrombocytopenia		
May-Hegglin anomaly	MYH9	22q12-13
Fechtner syndrome	MYH9	22q12-13
Epstein syndrome	MYH9	22q12-13
Sebastian syndrome	MYH9	22q12-13
Mediterranean thrombocytopenia/Bernard-Soulier carrier	GP1Bβ, possibly others	17pter-p12
Bernard-Soulier syndrome	GP1Bα GP1Bβ, GPIX	17p13 22q11 3q21
Velocardiofacial/DiGeorge syndrome (CATCH 22)	?GP1Bβ	22q11
Familial platelet disorder/ acute myeloid leukemia	AML1	21q22.2
Chromosome 10/THC2	?FLJ14813	10p12-11.2
Paris-Trousseau thrombocytopenia/Jacobsen syndrome	FLI1, Ets-1	11q23
Gray platelet syndrome	Unknown	Unknown
Congenital amegakaryocytic thrombocytopenia	MPL	1p34
Thrombocytopenia and absent radii (TAR)	Unknown	Unknown
Thrombocytopenia and radial synostosus	HOXA11	7p15-p14.2
Wiskott-Adrich syndrome	WAS	Xp11.23-p11.22
X-linked thrombocytopenia	WAS	Xp11.23-p11.22
GATA-1 mutation	GATA1	Xp11.23
Amegakaryocytic thrombocytopenia with radio-ulnar synostosis (CTRUS, 605432)	HOX11A	7p15-14
Dyserythropoietic anemia with thrombocytopenia	GATA-1	Xp11
X-linked thrombocytopenia with thalassemia	GATA-1	Xp11
Mediterranean macrothrombocytopenia	Unknown	Unknown
Thrombocytopenia 2	Unknown	10p2
Platelet-type or pseudo von Willebrand disease	GPIbα	17p13
Montreal platelet syndrome	Unknown	Unknown

Table 8 Stem Cells to Platelets: Platelet Production

	Commitment	Differentiation	Maturation
HoxA11	X	X	
CBFA2	X	X	
FOG1/GATA1	X	X	X
FOG1/GATA2	X	X	
TPO	X	X	X
FLI1 (ETS1)			X

platelets are generally pursued only in the context of refractoriness to leukocyte-reduced random donor units.

The only definitive treatment thus far has been allogeneic stem cell transplant (HSCT) from a matched sibling donor. An approach to gene therapy is being pursued in which a dimerized c-mpl is utilized to convey a growth advantage to stem cells that express the construct, allowing them to eventually repopulate the marrow with cells that are TPO responsive.

Thrombocytopenia and Absent Radii (TAR)

The diagnosis of TAR (15,16) is suggested by the finding of isolated, severe neonatal thrombocytopenia (similar to CAMT) accompanied by characteristic physical anomalies (associated features) as indicated above. These features are not limited to absent radii but also include other orthopedic abnormalities (18). For example, one survey identified an isolated abnormality of the radii in only 4 of 54 cases of TAR, whereas abnormalities of the ulna and knees occurred in well over 50% of the patients (15). Patients with TAR have a high incidence of serious bleeding including ICH and gastrointestinal (GI) bleeding. However, in contrast to patients with CAMT, patients with TAR tend to improve and their platelet counts increase with time. The general impression has always been that patients with TAR will achieve normal platelet counts within one year of birth (16). However, milder thrombocytopenia often persists and the platelets, after initially increasing, may decrease again during early adulthood (15). Signaling via the TPO receptor is abnormal, but the defect in the signaling pathway has not been defined. Because of the findings of abnormalities in HOX11a in patients with CTRUS (see below), a parallel study of cases of TAR was performed but did not identify mutations in this or other Hox genes.

Amegakaryocytic Thrombocytopenia (AMT) with Radial-Ulnar Synostosis (CTRUS)

CTRUS (18) is a rare entity (three cases reported) that presents in a manner similar to TAR, with initially severe thrombocytopenia and subsequent improvement (8). In the newborn, the forearm initially appears normal or only subtle abnormalities may be detected. The diagnosis of CTRUS is made later when pronation and supination of the forearm is discovered to be very restricted. Hox 11a was reported to be abnormal in the initial cases, but not all cases have this abnormality.

Microcytosis and X-Linked Inheritance

These familial thrombocytopenias are of two primary varieties—those accompanied by microcytic anemia, i.e., the XLT-T syndrome (X-linked thrombocytopenia—thalassemia), and those accompanied by dyserythropoiesis (XLT) (10–13).

Patients with both types of familial thrombocytopenia have large platelets that, in combination with the microcytic erythrocytes, distinguish them from XLT/WAS. XLT with dyserythropoiesis may be considered to be a form of myelodysplasia (MDS). These cases reflect the importance of GATA-1 in both thrombopoiesis and erythropoiesis. The recent evaluation of a second family with the XLT-beta thalassemia mutation suggests that anemia derived from mutations of GATA-1 that affect its binding site for FOG (Friend of GATA) is more severe than that derived from a previously described mutation that leads to deficient binding of GATA-1 to DNA.

Some cases of Fanconi's anemia may also present with thrombocytopenia with mild microcytic anemia. Other anomalies characteristic of Fanconi's anemia (abnormal thumbs, failure to thrive, renal anomalies, etc.), may not be initially apparent.

XLT-WAS

Patients with either WAS or the XLT form of WAS (8–9) classically have severe thrombocytopenia and smaller than normal platelets. The only other entity in which such distinctly small platelets are found is in patients with TORCH (Toxoplasma-Rubella-Cytomegalovirus-Herpes) infections, particularly with cytomegalovirus (CMV). In addition to severe thrombocytopenia, WAS is an important congenital immunodeficiency syndrome characterized by an inability to make anti-polysaccharide antibodies, resulting in a predilection to pneumococcal sepsis. Eczema is common, although its relationship to the underlying defect is unclear. Very young infants may present with thrombocytopenia, milk allergy and hematochezia, the latter apparently resulting from the combination of the prominent milk allergy and low platelets. The platelets may not appear small at birth, possibly because of a lack of splenic maturity. The XLT form of WAS seems to involve defects primarily in exon 2 of the WAS gene; these patients have minimal immunodeficiency. WAS/XLT is unusual for syndromes of CTP, in that the thrombocytopenia usually responds to splenectomy (9), which may remove a site of clearance of platelets with defective membrane. The possibility that patients with WAS make anti-platelet antibodies as part of the immunodeficiency state is unlikely in other than exceptional cases.

Even when thrombocytopenia is only moderately severe, the risk of hemorrhage may be high because the platelet mass is low relative to the platelet count, and the platelets may also be dysfunctional. WAS and XLT patients with severe thrombocytopenia have an especially high risk of ICH because of this triad of low counts, small and possibly dysfunctional platelets. Treatment focused on increasing the platelet count beyond what can be accomplished by repeated platelet transfusions involves either splenectomy or stem cell transplantation (HSCT). In XLT or in patients with WAS for whom a HSCT cannot be performed, splenectomy is appropriate (9). However, in WAS, and even in XLT, there is an increased risk of overwhelming post splenectomy sepsis. Determining an adequate response to pneumococcal vaccine, either Pneumovax or Prevnar®, is important, and careful antibiotic prophylaxis as well as monitoring antibody levels is mandatory. IVIG may need to be given monthly. There is approximately a 10% cumulative incidence of lymphoma in either WAS or XLT in those who have not undergone transplantation, which is very close to the mortality from allogeneic HSCT. Mutational analysis of the WAS gene to confirm the diagnosis is commercially available. While the clinical features of the syndrome are often self evident, the distinction of WAS from XLT can be suggested by the site of the mutation and is an important reason to proceed with this type of confirmatory testing.

Velocardiofacial Syndrome (DiGeorge Syndrome or VCF)

Another form of thrombocytopenia, with similarities to XLT, and the first of the large platelet syndromes to be discussed, is *VCF* (14). VCF, like WAS/XLT, also involves a variable clinical immunodeficiency but the thrombocytopenia is generally mild. Right-sided heart disease, neonatal hypocalcemia, cleft lip-palate, neuropsychologic issues, autoimmune thrombocytopenia and autoimmune hemolytic anemia (Evans syndrome) suggest the possibility of VCF. VCF is associated with mutations in chromosome 1q22 and 10p4 and molecular diagnosis of at least the former mutation is available on a routine basis. Although gene defects have been identified, patients with nearly identical clinical features have not had a mutation identified.

In VCF, two forms of thrombocytopenia may be seen—one autoimmune and one hereditary. The autoimmune thrombocytopenia in VCF may respond to ITP therapy, but is often severe, likely to be chronic, and can be associated with Evans syndrome (autoimmune hemolytic anemia). Milder forms of VCF without prominent heart disease or hypocalcemia may not be identified until adolescence or adulthood for the following reasons:

(1) The immunodeficiency may be subtle.
(2) The thrombocytopenia may be asymptomatic.
(3) The "heart disease" may be clinically silent, i.e., a right-sided aortic arch.
(4) Either the oropharyngeal findings are subtle, such as a bifid uvula, or a cleft palate was repaired in the first year of life and subsequently forgotten.

The presence of Evans syndrome and immunodeficiency in patients with VCF is typically associated with poor prognosis immune thrombocytopenia. This indicates that the disease will be chronic, persistent, and either not responsive to treatment, or that tachyphylaxis to treatment will develop. Underlying behavioral abnormalities associated with VCF may be initiated or worsened by corticosteroids administered to treat presumed autoimmune thrombocytopenia or autoimmune hemolytic anemia.

The non-immune hereditary component of the thrombocytopenia may be linked to the gene for platelet glycoprotein Ib which is also located in the 1q22 region. This gene, when mutated or deleted, results in the Bernard-Soulier syndrome with typically mild macrothrombocytopenia.

MYH9-Related Diseases

The most common forms of CTP are accompanied by macrothrombocytopenia, and among these the most frequent are a group now known collectively as the MYH9-RD (myosin heavy chain 9 related diseases) (5). What had been previously considered separate but overlapping syndromes (May-Hegglin, Fechtner, Sebastian, and Epstein syndromes) have now been shown to involve mutations of the gene that codes for non-muscle myosin IIA. Platelets and neutrophils only express myosin IIA, while myosin IIB is normally expressed in other cell types. Some of the findings common to these disorders, such as leukocyte inclusions, are a result of abnormal precipitated myosin in these cells. Other associated features of these disorders include renal failure, hearing loss, and cataracts. In the commonest form of MYH9 disorders, the May-Hegglin anomaly, Dohle-like bodies may be seen in neutrophils in addition to the very large (giant) platelets identified on peripheral smear. The platelet count varies and may be <20,000/uL; however, the very large platelets often lead to reporting of falsely low platelet counts. Platelet function is generally preserved, and cases of these syndromes are often identified in asymptomatic patients.

While not yet conclusively defined, the current consensus is that the associated features of these overlapping syndromes are not dependent upon the site of the mutation within the MYH9 gene. Mutational analysis of the MYH9 gene can be obtained through commercial laboratories.

Familial Thrombocytopenia-Leukemia (Tel-AML1)

The familial thrombocytopenia-leukemia (Tel-AML1) syndrome (14) is important to identify, since it is the form of congenital thrombocytopenia most closely linked to malignancy. Fortunately, it has a somewhat unique presentation. Tel-AML1 displays autosomal dominant inheritance. The thrombocytopenia is usually mild, approximately 80–100,000/uL. However, signs and symptoms of bleeding, such as ecchymoses, are common; this immediately sets it apart from other causes of CTP. Platelet function testing reveals evidence of a storage pool disorder. Approximately half of the thrombocytopenic family members may go on to develop a malignancy, 2/3 of which are myeloid leukemias and 1/3 solid tumors. Mutations in the transcription factor CBFA2 have been identified in at least two families with this syndrome, and the defects in this molecule appear responsible for the development of malignancy. The inheritance pattern has been shown to be such that a single mutation in 1 of 2 genes is responsible and sufficient for the thrombocytopenia via a dominant negative platelet effect. If a second mutation occurs knocking out the wild type allele, then malignancy will ensue. Specialists in bone marrow transplantation believe that the Tel-AML gene defect is the most common type of familial thrombocytopenia, whereas hematologists who treat benign disease consider it quite rare. It is difficult to determine point mutations in the tel-AML gene, and these analyses are not widely available.

Bernard-Soulier Syndrome

The Bernard-Soulier syndrome should be considered when a patient presents with macrothrombocytopenia and bleeding out of proportion to the platelet count in the absence of other clinical or hematologic abnormalities (4). Bernard-Soulier syndrome results from the absence of the GPIb-IX-V complex on the platelet surface, and homozygous and heterozygous forms of the disease that overlap in their clinical manifestations have been described. In homozygotes and certain heterozygotes, the platelets are comparable in size to those seen in the MYH9 syndromes. Automated platelet counts are often inaccurate because of the large platelets, but typically the thrombocytopenia is not severe. Epistaxis is relatively common.

Diagnosis in the routine laboratory can be strongly suspected by lack of or diminished aggregation (agglutination) of platelets by ristocetin, a result which may also occur in patients with vWD; the latter, however, may be essentially ruled out by documentation of normal levels of von Willebrand factor antigen and a normal von Willebrand factor multimer pattern. Heterozygotes have a less profound platelet deficiency in ristocetin induced agglutination, and may be more difficult to identify. Flow cytometry may be used to quantify platelet glycoproteins; this approach may be diagnostic for heterozygotes as well if GPIb-IX-V is absent or present but reduced in its expression. Milder variants, e.g., "Bolzano," have been described in which dysfunctional platelet glycoproteins are expressed on the platelet surface. Since the genes for these proteins have been sequenced, the Bernard-Soulier syndrome can also be identified by molecular testing on a research basis.

von Willebrand Disease 2B (vWD2B)

vWD type 2B (vWD 2B) is an autosomal dominant disorder caused by the production of an abnormal vWF molecule with a propensity to form ultra-large multimers that bind more avidly to platelets than normal vWF. These large multimers promote platelet clumping, and thus this disorder represents a classic gain of function mutation. Platelets in these patients are normal to large in size and platelet counts tend to fluctuate, especially with stress and hormonal changes such as those associated with pregnancy. Postpartum hemorrhage may occur as the levels of vWF fall rapidly after delivery. Menstrual bleeding may be heavy, and bleeding of other mucous membranes may occur as well. Desmopressin acetate (DDAVP®) may cause more severe thrombocytopenia by stimulating the release of abnormal vWF from storage sites, and exacerbating platelet agglutination. vWF multimer analysis may distinguish Type IIB vWD from the much less common "platelet type" vWD in which mutations in GPIb are responsible for the enhanced interaction of platelets with normal von Willebrand factor.

Gray Platelet Syndrome

On the peripheral blood film, platelets from patients with this disorder appear uniformly gray due to the absence of purple staining alpha granule constituents (6). The gene defect underlying this disorder is not yet known, nor is the explanation for the large platelets that are often present. Current thought concerning this unusual disorder suggests that alpha granules may be normally formed in megakaryocytes, but that the granule contents are not properly stored. Release of mitogenic growth factors such as platelet derived growth factor and transforming growth factor β are thought to account for the myelofibrosis that may accompany the gray platelet syndrome.

Mediterranean Macrothrombocytopenia

Mediterranean macrothrombocytopenia is a confusing and apparently heterogeneous disorder. Some use this term to denote the differences in platelet count and size among Europeans of Northern and Mediterranean origin (23). However, the most common cause of autosomal dominant macrothrombocytopenia in Italy is probably, heterozygous Bernard-Soulier syndrome. Reports describe thrombocytopenia and large platelets, sometimes associated with a mild bleeding predisposition, but not attributable to either the May-Hegglin anomaly or Bernard-Soulier syndrome (23). Mediterranean macrothrombocytopenia may also describe a disorder featuring large platelets, but without other associated clinical features, possibly related to a defect in the demarcatory membrane system by which megakaryocytes divide their cytoplasm into platelets. As a consequence, fewer larger platelets are released, but the overall platelet mass is thought to remain approximately normal.

Miscellaneous Causes of Congenital Thrombocytopenia

Several additional causes of congenital thrombocytopenia are rare and will only be mentioned briefly. The Paris-Trousseau syndrome and Jacobsen syndrome (19) appear to share the same genetic defect, a deletion at 11q23.3, leading to absence of the FLI1 transcription factor. This observation suggests an important role for FLI1 in megakaryopoiesis, and FLI1 corrects in vitro megakaryopoiesis in cells from these patients. These syndromes are characterized by micromegakaryocytes, large platelets containing giant α granules, and a moderate bleeding diathesis. They may also be accompanied by mental retardation and facial and other dysmorphic features. THC2 is a syndrome of autosomal dominant thrombocytopenia associated with a mutation in the FLJ14813 gene. Patients are variably affected by generally mild clinical manifestations including mild thrombocytopenia, normal platelet function, and normal appearance of the bone marrow despite evidence of increased megakaryocyte precursors in hematopoietic colony assays. Finally, the Montreal platelet syndrome is characterized by abnormal platelet size and shape following exposure to agents such as ADP and thrombin known to induce platelet shape change. Individuals with this disorder may have prolonged bleeding times but normal platelet aggregation studies; platelets appear deficient in calcium-activated neutral proteinase (calpain). Further information on these disorders is available in reviews by Balduini (3,20) or at OMIM-online Mendelian Inheritance in Man http://www.ncbi.nlm.nih.gov/entrez/query.fcgi?db=OMIM.

MANAGEMENT OF PATIENTS WITH CONGENITAL THROMBOCYTOPENIAS

There is no uniform approach to the treatment of patients with CTP who are bleeding or are to undergo surgery. Potentially useful agents include DDAVP and/or antifibrinolytic agents such as Amicar (epsilon-aminocaproic acid), especially for mouth or nose bleeding, as well as hormonal therapy for excessive menstrual bleeding.

Platelet transfusion remains the mainstay of therapy for most patients with CTP, though this should be reserved only for the management of severe bleeding episodes in order to reduce the probability of platelet alloimmunization. Leukocyte-reduced platelets should be used routinely in these individuals, as these preparations dramatically lessen sensitization to platelets and the development of refractoriness to platelet transfusion.

Finally, for life threatening bleeds refractory to the interventions noted above, recombinant factor VIIa (rVIIa) has been used successfully, most often in patients with Glanzmann thrombasthenia. The optimum dose of rVIIa remains to be defined, as its use has been anecdotal. Doses in the range of 20–40 units/kg instead of the more standard 90 units/kg used for hemophiliacs with inhibitors have been reported to be effective in some patients.

Hematopoietic stem cell transplantation is used occasionally for severe cases of CTP such as CAMT or the homozygous Bernard-Soulier syndrome.

Whether the emerging family of thrombopoietic agents will have a future role in the management of at least some of these entities seems probable, but remains unexplored.

CONCLUSIONS

A considerable amount has been learned about the hereditary thrombocytopenias in the past 10 years, yet much remains to be discovered. Classification schemes for these disorders continue to evolve as more information concerning their pathogenesis and molecular basis accumulates. Above all else, suspicion that a congenital thrombocytopenia exists remains the key element in reaching an accurate diagnosis; this suspicion may then be followed by confirmatory studies, if available. However, even in experienced hands, at least 40% of suspected cases of CTP are ultimately classified as unknown. While sobering, this observation suggests that continued study of these rare diseases is likely to uncover additional key molecules that play central roles in megakaryo- and thrombopoiesis.

REFERENCES

1. Aledort LM, Hayward C, Chen MG, Nichol J, Bussel JB. Prospective screening of 205 patients with ITP including diagnosis, serological markers, and the relationship of platelet counts, endogenous thrombopoietin, and circulating anti-thrombopoietin antibodies. Am J Hematol 2004; 76:205–213.
2. Bader-Meunier B, Proulle V, Trichet C, et al. Misdiagnosis of chronic thrombocytopenia in childhood. J Pediatr Hematol Oncol 2003; 25:548–552.
3. Balduini CL, Iolascon A, Savoia A. Inherited thrombocytopenias: from genes to therapy. Haematologica 2002; 87:860–880.
4. Budarf ML, Konkle BA, Ludlow LB, et al. Identification of a patient with Bernard-Soulier syndrome and a deletion in the DiGeorge/velo-cardio-facial chromosomal region in 22q11.2. Hum Mol Genet 1995; 4:763–766.
5. Seri M, Cusano R, Gangarossa S, et al. Mutations in MYH9 result in the May-Heglin anomaly, and Fechtner and Sebastian syndromes. The May-Heggllin/Fechtner syndrome consortium. Nat Genet 2000; 26:103–105.
6. White JG. Ultrastructural studies of gray platelet syndrome. Am J Pathol 1979; 95:445–462.
7. Mullen CA, Anderson KD, Blaese RM. Splenectomy and/or bone marrow transplantation in the management of the Wiskott-Aldrich syndrome: long-term follow-up of 62 cases. Blood 1993; 82:2961–2966.
8. Ochs HD. The Wiskott-Aldrich syndrome. Clin Rev Allergy Immunol 2001; 20:61–86.
9. Mant MJ, Doery JC, Gauldie J, Sims H. Pseudo-thrombocytopenia due to platelet aggregation and degranulation in blood collected in EDTA. Scand J Haematol 1975; 15:161–170.
10. Yu C, Niakan KK, Matsushita M, Stamatoyannopoulos G, Orkin SH, Raskind WH. X-linked thrombocytopenia with thalassemia from a mutation in the amino finger of GATA-1 affecting DNA binding rather than FOG-1 interaction. Blood 2002; 100:2040–2045.
11. Balduini CL, Pecci A, Loffredo G, et al. Effects of the R216Q mutation of GATA-1 on erythropoiesis and megakaryocytopoiesis. Thromb Haemost 2004; 91:129–140.

12. Mehaffrey MG, Newton AL, Gandhi MJ, Crossley M, Drachman JG. X-linked thrombocytopenia caused by a novel mutation of GATA-1. Blood 2001; 98:2681–2688.
13. Nichols KE, Crispino JD, Poncz M, et al. Familial dyserythropoietic anaemia and thrombocytopenia due to an inherited mutation in GATA1. Nat Genet 2000; 24:266–270.
14. Song WJ, Sullivan MG, Legare RD, et al. Haplo-insufficiency of CBFA2 causes familial thrombocytopenia with propensity to develop acute myelogenous leukemia [see comments]. Nat Genet 1999; 23:166–175.
15. Merola PR, Guinan E, Blanchette V, Novoa M, Bussel JB, Thrombocytopenia Absent Radii (TAR) and Congenital Amegakaryocytic Thrombocytopenia (CAMT), in preparation.
16. Hedberg VA, Lipton JM. Thrombocytopenia with absent radii. A review of 100 cases. Am J Pediatr Hematol Oncol 1988; 10:51–64.
17. Hohlfeld P, Forestier F, Kaplan C, Tissot JD, Daffos F. Fetal thrombocytopenia: a retrospective survey of 5, 194 fetal blood samplings. Blood 1994; 84:1851–1856.
18. Thompson AA, Woodruff K, Feig SA, Nguyen LT, Schanen NC. Congenital thrombocytopenia and radio-ulnar synostosis: a new familial syndrome. Br J Haematol 2001; 113:866–870.
19. Breton-Gorius J, Favier R, Guichard J, et al. A new congenital dysmegakaryopoietic thrombocytopenia (Paris-Trousseau) associated with giant platelet alpha-granules and chromosome 11 deletion at 11q23. Blood 1995; 85:1805–1814.
20. Balduini CL, Savoia A, Inherited thrombocytopenias: molecular mechanisms. Seminars in thrombosis and hemostasis 2004; 30(5): 513–523. Review.
21. Ballmaier M, Germeshausen M, Schulze H, et al. c-mpl mutations are the cause of congenital amegakaryocytic thrombocytopenia. Blood 2001; 97:139–146.
22. Van den Oudenrijn S, Bruin M, Folman CC, et al. Mutations in the thrombopoietin receptor, Mpl, in children with congenital amegakaryocytic thrombocytopenia. Br J Haematol 2000; 110:441–448.
23. Behrens WE. Mediterranean macrothrombocytopenia. Blood 1975; 46:199–208.

4

Thrombocytopenia Due to Deficient Platelet Production

Marc J. Kahn
Section of Hematology/Medical Oncology, Department of Medicine, School of Medicine, Tulane University Health Sciences Center, New Orleans, Louisiana, U.S.A.

Cindy Leissinger
Section of Hematology/Medical Oncology, Department of Medicine, School of Medicine, Louisiana Comprehensive Hemophilia Care Center, Tulane University Health Sciences Center, New Orleans, Louisiana, U.S.A.

INTRODUCTION

The regulation of megakaryocyte proliferation and differentiation in the marrow and the subsequent production of platelets from megakaryocytes is a complicated process that, until recently, has not been well understood. In 1958, the existence of a humoral substance, termed "thrombopoietin," was surmised to provide for platelet production during thrombocytopenic states (1). However, it took another 36 years for human thrombopoietin (TPO) to be cloned and characterized. TPO, in concert with a number of other cytokines including steel factor, interleukins 3, 6, and 11, leukemia inhibitor factor, and erthropoietin (2,3,4), stimulates megakaryocyte development, expression of platelet-specific markers, and colony formation, though it does not promote platelet budding from megakaryocytes and may actually inhibit this process (5). As with other stimulating factors, plasma concentrations of TPO are typically inversely related to circulating platelet counts in patients with marrow suppression (6). TPO is synthesized primarily by the liver (7), and as demonstrated in mice lacking its receptor, c-Mpl, is subsequently removed from the circulation by binding to c-Mpl on platelets and megakaryocytes (8). Therefore, most patients with thrombocytopenia from diminished marrow production display increased TPO levels because of a reduced platelet/megakaryocyte mass. Exceptions to this rule include some instances of liver disease and states in which autoantibodies to TPO are present. In these situations, despite a low platelet count, TPO is either decreased or not functional.

In this chapter, thrombocytopenia secondary to deficient platelet production will be discussed. The differential diagnosis of hypoproliferative thrombocytopenia is shown in Table 1.

LOW TPO STATES AND CONDITIONS OF TPO HYPORESPONSIVENESS

Liver Disease

Studies showing normalization of platelet counts in TPO-deficient mice transplanted with normal livers strongly suggest that the liver is the primary site of TPO production (9). Additional studies in humans awaiting orthotopic liver transplantation have shown an association between low TPO levels and the degree of thrombocytopenia (7,10) Hepatectomy represents the classic TPO deficient state. Similarly, patients infected with hepatitis C have low TPO levels,

Table 1 Thrombocytopenias Secondary to Diminished Platelet Production

Hereditary disorders
Fanconi's anemia
Thromboytopenia absent radii syndrome
May-Hegglin abnormality
Alport's syndrome
Wiskott-Aldrich
Liver disease
Autoantibodies to TPO or c-Mpl
Megakaryocytic aplasia
Cyclic thrombocytopenia
Myelodysplasia
Paroxysmal nocturnal hemoglobinuria
Marrow infiltration
Infections
Drugs and toxins
Nutritional deficiencies
Cobalamin
Folate
Iron

with the degree of TPO reduction related to the degree of liver fibrosis (11). In contrast, patients with either acute liver failure or chronic cirrhosis unrelated to hepatitis C have not been shown to display the same inverse relationship between circulating TPO levels and platelet counts (12,13) However, patients with cirrhosis may have decreased expression of platelet TPO receptor, c-Mpl (14). The relationship between thrombocytopenia and hepatitis C will be discussed in more detail later in this chapter.

Autoantibodies

Following the successful cloning and development of human TPO as a therapeutic agent, animal studies suggested that the protein could be immunogenic and lead to the development of neutralizing antibodies (15). Thrombocytopenia secondary to the development of autoantibodies to TPO has been described in patients treated with pegylated recombinant human megakaryocyte growth and development factor (16). Measured TPO levels were variable in this small series but the antibodies were found to neutralize the biologic activity of endogenous TPO in all subjects, leading to severe thrombocytopenia. Interestingly, antibodies to c-Mpl have also been described in thrombocytopenic patients with lupus and megakaryocytic hypoplasia (17). TPO levels were variable in these patients.

NORMAL AND ELEVATED TPO STATES

Congenital Disorders

Fanconi's anemia, the thrombocytopenia-absent radii (TAR) syndrome, May-Hegglin abnormality, Alport's syndrome, and the Wiskott-Aldrich syndrome all represent congenital disorders of marrow thrombocyte hypoproduction, with elevated or normal TPO levels. They have been discussed in detail in Chapter 3 and will not be discussed further in this chapter.

Acute Amegakaryocytic Thrombocytopenic Purpura (AATP)

AATP is a rare disorder characterized by megakaryocytic hypoplasia in an otherwise normal marrow. This disorder may precede the diagnosis of aplastic anemia (18) and has also been seen in a patient with lymphoma (19). Patients typically present with varying degrees of thrombocytopenia related to the degree of megakaryocyte aplasia, and may also display erythrocyte macrocytosis. Early studies speculated that the disorder was due to either a defect in the megakaryocyte colony-forming unit itself, or to antibodies that inhibit colony formation (20). Subsequent studies confirmed the presence of a serologic inhibitory factor (21). Additionally, cell-mediated suppression of megakaryopoiesis has been demonstrated in AATP (22). As expected, TPO levels in AATP are elevated (23). Treatment of AATP involves immunosuppression with cytotoxic therapy, cyclosporin A (24), danazol (25), antithymocyte globulin (26), or intravenous immunoglobulin. Unfortunately, most patients do not respond to such immunosuppressive therapy and progress to frank aplastic anemia (27).

Cyclic Thrombocytopenia (CT)

A disorder in megakaryopoiesis related to AATP, CT is a syndrome of unknown etiology. Unlike AATP, where megakaryocytes are absent from the marrow, CT is characterized by periodic fluctuations in megakaryocyte mass. In canines, CT may be acute and is often related to infection with Ehrlichia species (28). CT has been described in patients following classic immune thrombocytopenic purpura (29). In this scenario, megakaryocyte ploidy is inversely related to circulating platelet count number. Cases of CT in which the platelet count varies as a function of the menstrual cycle have also been described in females (30). In this setting, platelet nadirs often occur at the onset of menses and maximum platelet counts are seen 5–14 days later. One hypothesis that has been suggested to explain this observation is that estrogens increase Fc gamma receptor expression on monocytes, which facilitates platelet clearance. Another report of a patient with menses-associated CT has demonstrated fluctuations in IgM anti-GPIIb/IIIa antibody levels which were inversely related to platelet counts (31). In contrast, in males, CT is characterized by periodic alterations in megakaryocyte mass rather than variations in peripheral platelet destruction (32). In one case, CT has been shown to be associated with a clonal T-cell disorder (33), with platelet counts being inversely related to TPO levels—suggesting production failure as the cause of thrombocytopenia. Cyclic changes in platelet counts corresponding to changes in the levels of IL-7, stem cell factor, and transforming growth factor beta with reciprocal changes in macrophage colony-stimulating factor, TPO, and erythropoietin have been described in a patient with CT, suggesting changes in both megakaryopoieis and platelet destruction as etiologies of the disease (34).

The treatment of CT is similar to the treatment of AATP, with variable responses to therapy.

Myelodysplasia

A small percentage of patients with myelodysplasia present with isolated thrombocytopenia. Examination of the bone marrow in these patients reveals dysmorphic megakaryocytes with one or two nuclei and prominent cytoplasmic vacuoles (35). Many of these patients have complex cytogenetic abnormalities (36). Refractory thrombocytopenia, as this is termed, frequently progresses to acute myelogenous leukemia (37). Treatment of this disorder is usually not successful, but thrombocytopenias have been shown to respond to androgen therapy (38). This condition can be confused with immune thrombocytopenic purpura despite its refractoriness to therapy and propensity to progress to acute leukemia.

Paroxysmal Nocturnal Hemoglobinuria (PNH)

PNH is a clonal disorder related to mutations in the X-linked *PIG-A* gene that encodes an enzyme critical in the synthesis of glycophosphotidylinositol (GPI) anchors. Erythrocytes from patients with PNH display increased sensitivity to complement. Hematopoiesis in these individuals is diminished, and may lead to aplastic anemia. The cause of the hematopoietic defect is not clear. A majority of patients with PNH have thrombocytopenia due to diminished platelet production, (39) with this being a poor prognostic feature (40). Interestingly, mutations in PIG-A have been found retrospectively in patients diagnosed with aplastic anemia (41) or myelodysplasia (42), suggesting that there may be some overlap in these three conditions. PNH can be definitively treated by bone marrow or stem cell transplantation. Alternatively, immunosuppression with glucocortocoids, cyclosporine A (43), or antithymocyte globulin (44) has been used to alleviate cytopenias in these patients.

Marrow Infiltration

It should not be surprising that patients with infiltrative disorders of the marrow can have thrombocytopenia. This may result from either "crowding out" of megakaryocyte precursors in the marrow, or from humoral suppression of thrombopoiesis. Such disorders include metastatic neoplasms, leukemia, lymphoma, myelofibrosis, Gaucher's disease, and infectious and histiocytic disorders, among others. Treatment is directed at the underlying disorder.

Infections

Thrombocytopenia, either alone or in combination with other hematologic abnormalities, is commonly associated with infectious diseases. The mechanisms of thrombocytopenia associated with infection vary widely depending on the specific infectious agent, the severity of disease, the pathophysiologic impact of the infectious agent, and in some cases, factors unique to the infected individual. Often, particularly in patients with severe or protracted infections, there may be multiple causes of thrombocytopenia. While direct suppression of thrombopoiesis is clearly associated with some infections, this does not appear to be the most common cause of infection associated with thrombocytopenia. Other etiologies may include platelet destruction due to immunologic mechanisms, or direct damage to platelets. Microangiopathic processes such as disseminated intravascular coagulation (DIC) or thrombotic thrombocytopenic purpura/hemolytic uremic syndrome (TTP/HUS) may also occur in the setting of infection. DIC may be associated with acute or severe infections and must always be considered when evaluating causes of thrombocytopenia in these individuals. Other causes of thrombocytopenia in infected patients include marrow suppression due to medications, nutritional deficiencies, and drug or alcohol exposure.

Viruses

Thrombocytopenia is a manifestation of many viral illnesses. Although suppression or alteration of platelet production can occur in viral infections, enhanced clearance of platelets due to direct viral damage or antibody binding are far more common mechanisms (45,46). Limited experimental data suggest that "early" thrombocytopenias occurring during the active viremic stage of infection are more likely due to direct viral effects on platelets and megakaryocytes, whereas thrombocytopenias that occur after the viremic phase are more likely to be immunologic in nature, often leading to an ITP-like picture. Establishing that suppression of megakaryopoiesis plays a role in thrombocytopenia is difficult without thrombokinetic studies to assess platelet production. Such studies are technically difficult and are generally restricted to research laboratories.

Human Immunodeficiency Virus Type 1 Infection

Thrombocytopenia is a common finding in patients with HIV infection, affecting as many as 50% of patients at some time during the course of their disease. Approximately 10% of patients will develop a thrombocytopenic syndrome that is indistinguishable from classic ITP on the basis of clinical features, bone marrow findings, and response to therapy (47,48). In the remaining 40% of HIV patients, low platelet counts will be the result of a host of problems and complications that are associated with progressive HIV infection or its management. HIV-associated thrombocytopenia is the best studied model of virus-induced thrombocytopenia. Studies have revealed some intriguing and unexpected findings concerning the mechanisms by which viruses can affect megakaryocytes and platelets.

Early electron microscopy studies of megakaryocytes from HIV-infected patients demonstrated ultrastructural abnormalities and denuded megakaryocyte nuclei even in patients with normal platelet counts (49). Further investigation demonstrated the presence of HIV-mRNA in megakaryocytes from infected patients, supporting the likelihood of direct HIV-1 infection of megakaryocytes (50). More recently, several investigators have demonstrated the presence of CD4 receptors as well as the HIV co-receptor CXCR4 on megakaryocytes and platelets, (51,52) and in vitro studies have confirmed that purified megakaryocytic progenitors and maturing megakaryocytes can be productively infected with HIV via these receptors (53). It now seems likely that most if not all patients with HIV have productive infection of megakaryocytes and platelets in vivo. Interestingly, such infection does not always result in low platelet counts. Recently, some investigators have found that patients who develop thrombocytopenia are more likely to have syncytium-inducing HIV strains infecting their megakaryocytes, (54) and that megakaryocytes from thrombocytopenic patients display increased apoptosis and impaired survival in vitro (55). These results suggest that in some cases thrombocytopenia may be related to specific properties of the infecting virus itself.

Studies of TPO levels have shown that non-thrombocytopenic HIV patients have TPO levels nearly twice as high as healthy, non-HIV-infected controls, further supporting the concept that HIV infection likely results in a diminished megakaryocyte/platelet receptor mass (56,57). These are interesting observations since platelet counts remain normal, but perhaps help to explain why HIV patients may have particular susceptibility to thrombocytopenia in the face of additional insults.

Two studies have examined platelet kinetics in healthy HIV-infected patients with normal platelet counts (58,59). Results of these studies demonstrate that mean platelet survival was reduced by about 25% in these individuals. The greatest discrepancy in the two studies was in the measurement of platelet production. In the first study (58), performed prior to the era of highly active antiretroviral therapy (HAART), half the patients were on zidovudine (AZT) and the other half were on no antiretroviral therapy. The healthy HIV patients on no antiretroviral therapy showed platelet production rates essentially the same as in normal controls, despite having shortened survival times. By contrast, the group on AZT demonstrated an increased rate of platelet production compared to the non-AZT group. In the second study (59), half of the patients had shortened platelet survival with a life span of 4–5 days, while the other half had normal survival. All patients with normal platelet survival had normal platelet production, though platelet production was increased in the group with shortened platelet survival. Which of these HIV-infected patients were on antiretroviral therapy was not stated, though it is likely that most of these individuals were. Thus, slightly shortened platelet survival may be common in non-thrombocytopenic patients infected with HIV, possibly related to direct effects of HIV on platelets or low grade autoimmune processes. Platelet production appears to be adequate in patients with normal platelet counts despite the megakaryocytic changes noted earlier. AZT, which is known to improve HIV-associated thrombocytopenia (60,61), appears to exert this effect by enhancing platelet production.

Several studies have evaluated platelet kinetics in HIV patients who present with thrombocytopenia (58,59,62–64). The difficulty in evaluating these results is ascertaining whether the subjects may have had other HIV or medication-related effects that could affect platelet kinetics. In the largest study, 85 patients with thrombocytopenia were studied without regard to the etiology of thrombocytopenia (64). Platelet survival was decreased to a greater extent in asymptomatic patients compared to those with AIDS, while platelet production rates were more likely to be decreased in patients with AIDS. The other studies selected patients with a clinical diagnosis of HIV-associated immune thrombocytopenia. While all patients had thrombocytopenia that appeared consistent with immune thrombocytopenic purpura, most of the studies did not require bone marrow examination and included patients with relatively advanced HIV disease, high HIV viral load measurements, and/or mild thrombocytopenia (59). These studies also did not comment on concurrent antiretroviral therapy. The results demonstrated that platelet survival times in patients with a clinical diagnosis of HIV-associated immune thrombocytopenic purpura were decreased, though they did not appear to be as short as those previously reported for patients with classic ITP and similar platelet counts (58,65). Most of these reports also found that platelet production was likely to be lower in HIV-associated versus classic ITP, and that although platelet production was quite low in patients not on AZT, it was increased in those on AZT, consistent with the observations described above in non-thrombocytopenic HIV patients.

In summary, it appears that most patients infected with HIV show evidence of direct infection of megakaryocytes by the virus. In most patients with normal platelet counts, platelet survival is slightly diminished (probably on the basis of direct effects of the virus on platelets), but platelet production is adequate to maintain normal platelet counts. When platelet survival times shorten even further (such as with immune-mediated destruction), platelet production is not adequate to compensate. At least one effective therapy for HIV-associated thrombocytopenia, AZT, appears to increase platelet production.

Hepatitis C Virus (HCV)

Thrombocytopenia is a relatively common finding in patients with HCV infection, even in those without advanced liver disease or hypersplenism. As many as 40% of patients with HCV infection will have thrombocytopenia during the course of their disease (66). Numerous investigators have shown that HCV-associated thrombocytopenia may be autoimmune in nature, based on characteristic bone marrow findings and responsiveness therapies such as prednisone and intravenous immunoglobulin (IVIg) directed at the treatment of ITP (66–71). However, a study of platelet kinetics in six thrombocytopenic HCV patients found a nearly normal platelet life span with depressed platelet production (perhaps related to low TPO levels), and evidence of direct infection of megakaryocytes by HCV (72). Several other groups of investigators have reported finding HCV mRNA in platelets from thrombocytopenic HCV-infected patients, and have demonstrated the ability of HCV to infect megakaryocytic cell lines (73–75). In a study of 13 patients with HCV-associated thrombocytopenia, eight of eight patients treated with low dose interferon alpha showed good platelet responses irrespective of HCV response, prompting the authors to speculate that the therapeutic effect of interferon may have resulted from direct inhibition of infection of platelets and megakaryocytes by HCV (76). Taken together, these findings suggest some similarities to studies in HIV-infected patients which have demonstrated increased platelet destruction accompanied by platelet underproduction. It may be possible to explain both by the direct effects of the virus and/or virus-induced antibodies on megakaryocytes and platelets.

Epstein-Barr Virus (EBV)

Over 50% of patients with EBV infection develop mild to moderate thrombocytopenia; severe thrombocytopenia develops in approximately 1%. While one study has reported the detection of EBV in megakaryocytes from infected patients, there is little other experimental work to link thrombocytopenia with inhibition of thrombopoiesis (77). Numerous studies have noted that most cases of thrombocytopenia are clinically indistinguishable from classic ITP on the basis of increased megakaryocytes in the marrow and response to therapies such as steroids and IVIg (78–81). Survival of infused platelets is short, further supporting the likelihood that the major mechanism of thrombocytopenia in these patients is due to immunologic platelet destruction (82,83).

Cytomegalovirus (CMV)

Clinically significant thrombocytopenia rarely occurs in patients infected with CMV. In the majority of cases, thrombocytopenia is moderate, although there have been numerous reports of severe thrombocytopenia associated with acute CMV infection. Bone marrow examination from one child with congenital CMV and persistent mild thrombocytopenia revealed increased numbers of megakaryocytes with abnormal vacuolization and inclusions, (84) and one adult with severe thrombocytopenia and myelodysplasia developed in association with CMV infection has been reported (85). Early studies in animal models and in vitro assay systems also demonstrated that CMV can directly infect megakaryocytes and other pluripotent stem cells, (86,87) though the majority of cases of CMV-associated thrombocytopenia, as with EBV, appear to be immune-mediated based on clinical responses to steroids, IVIG, and splenectomy (88).

Varicella Zoster Virus

Thrombocytopenia is an infrequent, but occasionally severe manifestation of Varicella zoster infection. One early study using electron microscopy demonstrated direct viral infection of megakaryocytes in a child who presented with fatal purpura fulminans (89). More commonly, thrombocytopenia occurs several days to a week after the eruption of varicella skin lesions, following the acute viremic stage. Several studies, including one study of platelet survival, suggest that these cases are secondary to platelet destruction, most likely by cross reactive antibodies (90,91).

Parvovirus B19

Parvovirus B19 is the etiologic agent responsible for the common childhood illness, fifth disease, generally a mild illness of young children. Because of its association with cases of pure red cell aplasia, the marrow-suppressing effects of parvovirus B19 have been extensively studied, and its ability to infect red cell precursors in the marrow has been shown (92,93). A single case report of thrombocytopenia and amegakaryocytosis that resolved following the acute infection (94) has led to the suggestion that thrombocytopenia may also be associated with parvovirus B19 infection. One in vitro study demonstrated that megakaryocytic colony formation could be suppressed by infection of normal marrow cultures with parvovirus B19, though the clinical relevance of this observation is uncertain (95). Moreover, several studies have reported increased megakaryocytes in marrows of patients with parvovirus-associated thrombocytopenia, suggesting that these result from immune-mediated platelet destruction (96,97). Finally, it appears that significant numbers of newly diagnosed cases of childhood may be associated with recent parvovirus B19 infection (98,99).

Hantavirus

Infection by different members of hantavirus genus may lead to a variety of clinical presentations. A recently identified hantavirus in the United States has been associated with a severe pulmonary syndrome and high fatality rate due to respiratory failure. Patients often present with mild to moderate thrombocytopenia and coagulopathy, but do not experience symptomatic hemorrhage (100). In Asia, the prototypical hantavirus presentation is characterized by a hemorrhagic fever associated with severe thrombocytopenia and renal disease. Recent experimental work suggests that the virus closely interacts with cellular β3-integrins. β3 integrins are part of the GP IIbIIIa (integrin αIIbβ3) complex of platelets and megakaryocytes. Binding of the virus to related receptors mediates its entry into endothelial cells. Although the mechanism of viral-induced thrombocytopenia has not been clearly defined, it has been suggested that viral binding to αIIbβ3 may allow entry into megakaryocytes, and interfere with platelet and megakaryocytic activation and function (101,102).

Other Viruses

Several common viruses such as rubella, rubeola, and mumps can rarely be associated with thrombocytopenia. Thrombocytopenia occurs approximately one week after the onset of the presenting rash. Early studies revealed findings consistent with platelet destruction at the time of thrombocytopenia, including increased bone marrow megakaryocytes and short survival of transfused platelets, (103–107) due to either cross-reacting antibodies, a direct toxic effect, or immune complex deposition (108–110). While megakaryocytes may be affected by these same processes, more data are needed on megakaryopoiesis and thrombokinetics in these disorders.

More severe hemorrhagic viral infections, known as "hemorrhagic fevers," are characterized by thrombocytopenia in association with other coagulopathies. Viruses responsible for hemorrhagic fevers include Ebola, Marburg, Dengue, Lassa and Rift Valley fever, among others. It appears that the severe bleeding diathesis and thrombocytopenias associated with these disorders are primarily related to the inexorable, progessive microangiopathy of DIC and shock, and result in relatively high mortality rates (111). However, it is worth noting that mild degrees of thrombocytopenia are often seen in early infection prior to the development of DIC and are postulated to be due to direct cytotoxic effects on platelets or megakaryocytes. In the case of dengue fever, there is experimental data that shows evidence of bone marrow suppression beginning 3–4 days after infection. Experimental work has shown that, in vitro, both stromal and hematopoietic progenitor cells become infected with the dengue virus and then undergo phagocytosis by marrow dendritic cells. Infected stromal cells also demonstrate alterations in cytokine production, which may inhibit normal hematopoiesis (112).

A recent severe infectious outbreak due to a new virus thus far designated as severe acute respiratory syndrome or SARS results in thrombocytopenia in 55% of patients (113). Many of those cases were followed by rebound thrombocytosis. Only 2.5% of cases were diagnosed with concomitant DIC, making this an unlikely explanation for most cases of thrombocytopenia. The mechanism of thrombocytopenia awaits further study.

Other Infections

Malaria

Of all parasitic infections, malaria is most frequently associated with thrombocytopenia. Over 50% of patients with Plasmodium falciparum will have low platelet counts and many will have severe thrombocytopenia. Recent studies have identified thrombocytopenia as predictive for a poor prognosis for disease outcome in children (114,115). Early studies demonstrated that abnormally large platelets may be present in association with malarial infection, and that malarial parasites could be found within platelets (116,117). Thrombokinetic studies demonstrated poor platelet recovery suggestive of splenic pooling and decreased platelet life-span, with normal or increased platelet production (118,119), suggesting that the major mechanism of thrombocytopenia is platelet destruction.

Babesiosis

Babesiosis is a tick borne illness caused by Babesia microti, a parasite that infects red blood cells. In a recent case control study of 34 patients with babesiosis, platelet counts were the only hematologic parameter significantly lower than in case controls (120). Thrombocytopenia tended to be moderate although severe cases were noted. The mechanism of thrombocytopenia in these patients is unknown.

Bacterial and Fungal Infections

Few specific bacterial or fungal infections are associated with thrombocytopenia as a presenting feature except in the presence of advanced sepsis, DIC, or bone marrow infiltration by organisms or granulomata. In addition, certain bacterial infections (particularly brucellosis and mycobacterial infections) can rarely be associated with a hemophagocytic syndrome (HPS) that results in severe thrombocytopenia, generally in association with pancytopenia and evidence of hemophagocytic histiocytes in the bone marrow (121,122). Any organism associated with sepsis may be associated with thrombocytopenia. It was recently shown that thrombocytopenia in sepsis may be related to platelet phagocytosis mediated by monocytic activation due to an increase in macrocyte colony-stimulating factor (M-CSF) (123,124). In animal studies, administration of macrophage colony-stimulating factor resulted in transient dose-dependent thrombocytopenia associated with shortened platelet survival but normal platelet production (124). In a study of patients with sepsis and thrombocytopenia, hemophagocytosis was associated with overproduction of M-CSF (123).

Human Granulocyte Ehrlichiosis (HGE)

HGE is an obligate intracellular bacterium that infects human granulocytes. Thrombocytopenia and neutropenia are characteristic of the acute phase of the disease; both tend to normalize by the second week of infection, even without specific therapy (125). A recent cross-sectional case study of 144 cases showed that thrombocytopenia was more prevalent than leukopenia, with nearly 100% of infected patients having mild to moderate thrombocytopenia by day 6 of the acute illness (126). Bone marrow examination has been reported to show normal or hypercellular marrow (127); however, studies in a murine model have suggested that the rapid thrombocytopenia after infection is not due to immune platelet destruction or splenic sequestration (128). Although these results suggest that thrombocytopenia may be related to direct effects of HGE on platelets or megakaryocytes, additional thrombokinetic studies are needed to assess platelet production.

Spirochetal Infections

Thrombocytopenia has been reported in 54–90% of patients infected with leptospirosis and a significant percentage of patients infected with some borrelia species (129–131). In leptospirosis, thrombocytopenia appears to be associated with sepsis and renal failure, but not necessarily DIC (130). At least one report demonstrated that megakaryocyte morphology is normal in the face of severe thrombocytopenia, and suggested a direct effect of leptospirosis on platelets (132). Early studies in patients infected with Borrelia hermsii (relapsing fever) demonstrated thrombocytopenia associated with normal numbers of bone marrow megakaryocytes, and platelet-associated spirochetes were present on patients' blood smears (133). Recent studies have shown that both Borrelia hermsii and Borrelia burgdorferi (Lyme disease agent), can bind to activated platelets through the platelet integrin αIIb-β3 (131,134). This mechanism seems likely to contribute to early removal of affected platelets from the circulation. Since megakaryocytes also express these integrins, further studies are needed to determine if such interactions also affect megakaryopoiesis.

Drugs and Toxins

Numerous drugs have been implicated in thrombocytopenia (see Chap. 7). Although most are thought to exert their effect via a drug-dependent immune mechanism, studies confirming immune-mediated destruction are lacking in the majority of cases. In a recent review, George et al. have developed evidence-based criteria for assessing the relationship between suspect drugs and drug-dependent immune thrombocytopenia (135).

While it seems obvious that given the large number and variety of pharmacologic agents available today, some may have the ability to interfere with megakaryopoiesis and platelet production, few have been clearly shown to do so. The difficulty in defining a marrow-suppressing mechanism for many of these reports reflects a lack of available tests to measure platelet production and survival. The following is a discussion of drugs known or suspected to be associated with suppression of thrombopoiesis. It is important to note that other drugs may cause thrombocytopenia through this mechanism; however, experimental data is lacking.

Drugs that Suppress Platelet Production

Anagrelide

Anagrelide is used to treat essential thrombocythemia and thrombocytosis associated with other myeloproliferative disorders, and is the only drug known that exerts selective depression of megakaryocyte maturation in a non-idiosyncratic manner. Anagrelide inhibits platelet production in a dose-dependent fashion, but has no effect on other hematopoietic elements (136). Studies in normal controls and in patients with essential thrombocythemia have shown that anagrelide inhibits both megakaryocytic maturation and platelet production (137).

Interferons

Thrombocytopenia is a common side effect of interferon therapy. With interferon-alpha (IFN), thrombocytopenia is dose-dependent and may be dose-limiting in some individuals. There appear to be at least two mechanisms by which IFN causes thrombocytopenia. Several studies have reported the development of an ITP-like syndrome, especially in patients being treated for hepatitis C (138,139). However, the most common mechanism for falling platelet counts associated with IFN therapy is direct suppression of platelet production. IFN receptors have been demonstrated on megakaryocytic cell lines (140), and in vitro studies demonstrate that IFN may inhibit both megakaryocytic colony formation and growth (141). More recent studies have shown that IFN-alpha inhibits TPO-dependent megakaryopoiesis in culture, possibly through the induction of a protein that interferes with TPO signaling (142).

Cytotoxic Chemotherapeutic Agents

Cytotoxic chemotherapeutic agents are designed to disrupt replication, growth, and/or maturation of rapidly dividing malignant cells. A nearly universal and accepted effect of these agents is suppression of normal cells that have a high mitotic rate. Hematopoietic progenitor cells, including megakaryocytes, are thus frequently affected by administration of these agents. These effects are dose-dependent and normally reversible following the discontinuation of the causative agent(s). It is not understood why some chemotherapeutic agents affect platelet production to a greater or lesser degree than other hematopoietic elements.

Idiosyncratic Reactions to Drugs

Drugs with Selective Megakaryocytic Suppression

Mild to moderate thrombocytopenia has rarely been reported in association with chlorothiazide diuretic use. Some early reports suggested that megakaryocytes were decreased or absent in these patients, while other reports noted normal marrow megakaryocytes (143,144). Definitive studies on the etiology of thrombocytopenia are lacking, but the weight of evidence suggests that most cases of thiazide-associated thrombocytopenia are secondary to immune platelet destruction.

Drugs that Lead to Aplastic Anemia

There are numerous reports of drugs associated with marrow aplasia with consequent pancytopenia—the most well established examples of aplastic anemia have occurred with chloramphenicol and quinacrine (145). The risk of developing aplastic anemia has been estimated to be 1 in 20,000 for patients treated with chloramphenicol, (146) and between 1 in 10,000 to 1 in 40,000 for patients treated with quinacrine (147). Other drugs that have been associated with sporadic cases of aplastic anemia include non-steroidal anti-inflammatory drugs, sulfonamides, phenylbutazone, hydantoins, phenothiazines, penicillamine, and anti-thyroid drugs.

Toxins

As many as 80% of patients hospitalized for ethanol withdrawal have thrombocytopenia, often in addition to other hematologic and coagulation abnormalities. For most patients the cause is multifactorial and often related to nutritional deficiencies. However, several studies have demonstrated that ethanol alone directly and specifically suppresses the platelet count in a dose-dependent manner when used daily for at least 5–10 days. Upon cessation of ethanol ingestion, platelet counts begin to rise within 3–5 days and may reach abnormally high (rebound) levels before returning to normal by 3–4 weeks (148–150). Early thrombokinetic studies showed a direct association between ethanol ingestion and a decrease in platelet survival (of approximately 50%) and production in patients who develop thrombocytopenia (150). Studies in both humans and animals have demonstrated that ethanol disrupts megakaryocytic differentiation (151,152). At levels usually achieved in vivo, ethanol does not directly suppress early megakaryocytic progenitors, but rather targets maturing megakaryocytes, leading to ineffective thrombopoiesis.

Benzene and Other Environmental Toxins

Several organic solvents and pesticides have been causally linked to the development of severe bone marrow disorders such as aplastic anemia, myelodysplasia or acute leukemia (153–155). Thrombocytopenia almost always occurs in conjunction with other cytopenias. Benzene, the prototype for such an effect, was first noted to cause hematologic abnormalities over 90 years ago. In workers regularly exposed to benzene, the incidence of aplastic anemia was reported to be six times higher than in the general population (156). Although benzene and its multiple toxic metabolites have been shown to have a wide variety of effects in hematopoietic cell culture systems, precise mechanisms leading to its varied clinical effects remain unclear. Unlike patients with myelodysplasia and acute leukemia, patients with aplastic anemia rarely display chromosomal abnormalities, suggesting that more than one mechanism is responsible for bone marrow toxicity (154). In addition, certain individuals may be predisposed to benzene toxicity due to genetic polymorphisms leading to a decreased ability to enzymatically detoxify harmful benzene metabolites (157). Other organic compounds, most notably pesticides, have also been associated with an increased risk of aplastic anemia (155,158). Recent epidemiologic studies further suggest that occupational exposure to some organic solvents, pesticides, semi-metals, metals, and inorganic dusts are associated with myelodysplasia and chromosomal abnormalities (159,160).

Radiation

Ionizing radiation causes marrow aplasia involving all hematopoietic cell lines in a dose-dependent manner. Following acute, sub-lethal exposures, these changes are reversible; however, exposure to radiation results in a long term risk of development of aplastic anemia, myelodysplasia or leukemia (161,162). Radiation induces DNA strand breaks as well as mutations of DNA repair genes that may lead to deregulated growth of hematopoietic stem cells, ultimately resulting in myelodysplasia or aplastic anemia.

Nutritional Deficiencies

Iron Deficiency

Although the association of thrombocytosis with blood loss and iron deficiency has been recognized for the past 100 years (163), thrombocytopenia which responds rapidly to iron replacement has also been reported in children with iron deficiency (164). Megakaryocytic hypoplasia and severe thrombocytopenia have also been reported in an adult female with severe anemia secondary to menorrhagia (165). Thrombocytopenia has also been reported as a complication of iron replacement (166). The mechanisms underlying disordered platelet kinetics in patients with iron deficiency have not been well studied. However, it has been suggested that iron enhances platelet production in some patients and inhibits thrombopoiesis in others (167). The precise reason for this dichotomy has not been elucidated.

B12 and Folate Deficiency

Approximately one-fifth of patients with B12 deficiency have concurrent thrombocytopenia (168). Thrombocytopenia from B12 deficiency is usually due to ineffective platelet production, since both megakaryocyte mass and platelet survival are usually normal in these individuals (169,170). However, some patients with B12 or folate deficiency can have marrow aplasia or even amegakaryocytic thrombocytopenic purpura (171). Severe hemorrhage has been described in thrombocytopenic patients with folate deficiency (172,173). Although microangiopathy has been reported in association with B12 deficiency (174), the typical blood smear in B12 or folate deficiency reveals macrocytosis with hypersegmentated neutrophils, and the marrow reveals megaloblastic changes. Thrombocytopenia usually resolves rapidly with vitamin replacement.

REFERENCES

1. Keleman E, Scerhati I, Tanos B. Demonstration and some properties of human thrombopoietin in thrombocythaemic sera. Acta Hematologica 1958; 20:350–355.
2. Kaushansky K. Thrombopoietin. N Engl J Med 1998; 339:746–754.
3. de Sauvage FJ, Hass PE, Spencer SD, et al. Stimulation of megakaryocytopoiesis and thrombopoiesis by the c-Mpl ligand. Nature 1994; 369:533–538.
4. Lok S, Kaushansky K, Holly RD, et al. Cloning and expression of murine thrombopoietin cDNA and stimulation of platelet production in vivo. Nature 1994; 369:565–568.
5. Choi ES, Hokom MM, Chen JL, et al. The role of megakaryocyte growth and development factor in terminal stages of thrombopoiesis. Br J Haematol 1996; 95:227–233.
6. Nichol JL, Hokom MM, Hornkohl A, et al. Megakaryocyte growth and development factor. Analyses of in vitro effects on human megakaryopoiesis and endogenous serum levels during chemotherapy-induced thrombocytopenia. J Clin Invest 1995; 95:2973–2978.
7. Peck-Radosavljevic M, Wichlas M, Zacherl J, et al. Thrombopoietin induces rapid resolution of thrombocytopenia after orthotopic liver transplantation through increased platelet production. Blood 2000; 95:795–801.
8. Fielder PJ, Gurney AL, Stefanich E, et al. Regulation of thrombopoietin levels by c-mpl-mediated binding to platelets. Blood 1996; 87:2154–2161.
9. Qian S, Fu F, Li W, Chen Q, de Sauvage FJ. Primary role of the liver in thrombopoietin production shown by tissue-specific knockout. Blood 1998; 92:2189–2191.
10. Peck-Radosavljevic M, Zacherl J, Meng YG, et al. Is inadequate thrombopoietin production a major cause of thrombocytopenia in cirrhosis of the liver? J Hepatol 1997; 27:127–131.

11. Giannini E, Borro P, Botta F, et al. Serum thrombopoietin levels are linked to liver function in untreated patients with hepatitis C virus-related chronic hepatitis. J Hepatol 2002; 37:572–577.
12. Schiodt FV, Balko J, Schilsky M, Harrison ME, Thornton A, Lee WM. Thrombopoietin in acute liver failure. Hepatology 2003; 37:558–561.
13. Stockelberg D, Andersson P, Bjornsson E, Bjork S, Wadenvik H. Plasma thrombopoietin levels in liver cirrhosis and kidney failure. J Intern Med 1999; 246:471–475.
14. Ishikawa T, Ichida T, Sugahara S, et al. Thrombopoietin receptor (c-Mpl) is constitutively expressed on platelets of patients with liver cirrhosis, and correlates with its disease progression. Hepatol Res 2002; 23:115–121.
15. de Serres MEB, Dillberger JE, et al. Immunogenicity of thrombopoietin mimetic peptide GW395058 in Balb/c mice and New Zealand white rabbits: evaluation of the potential for thrombopoietin neutralizing antibody production in man. Stem Cells 1999; 17:203–209.
16. Li J, Yang C, Xia Y, et al. Thrombocytopenia caused by the development of antibodies to thrombopoietin. Blood 2001; 98:3241–3248.
17. Kuwana M, Okazaki Y, Kajihara M, et al. Autoantibody to c-Mpl (thrombopoietin receptor) in systemic lupus erythematosus: relationship to thrombocytopenia with megakaryocytic hypoplasia. Arthritis Rheum 2002; 46:2148–2159.
18. King JA, Elkhalifa MY, Latour LF. Rapid progression of acquired amegakaryocytic thrombocytopenia to aplastic anemia. South Med J 1997; 90:91–94.
19. Lugassy G. Non-Hodgkin's lymphoma presenting with amegakaryocytic thrombocytopenic purpura. Ann Hematol 1996; 73:41–42.
20. Hoffman R, Bruno E, Elwell J, et al. Acquired amegakaryocytic thrombocytopenic purpura: a syndrome of diverse etiologies. Blood 1982; 60:1173–1178.
21. Katai M, Aizawa T, Ohara N, et al. Acquired amegakaryocytic thrombocytopenic purpura with humoral inhibitory factor for megakaryocyte colony formation. Intern Med 1994; 33:147–149.
22. Gewirtz AM, Sacchetti MK, Bien R, Barry WE. Cell-mediated suppression of megakaryocytopoiesis in acquired amegakaryocytic thrombocytopenic purpura. Blood 1986; 68:619–626.
23. Mukai HY, Kojima H, Todokoro K, et al. Serum thrombopoietin (TPO) levels in patients with amegakaryocytic thrombocytopenia are much higher than those with immune thrombocytopenic purpura. Thromb Haemost 1996; 76:675–678.
24. Azuno Y, Yaga K. Successful cyclosporin A therapy for acquired amegakaryocytic thrombocytopenic purpura. Am J Hematol 2002; 69:298–299.
25. Kashyap R, Choudhry VP, Pati HP. Danazol therapy in cyclic acquired amegakaryocytic thrombocytopenic purpura: a case report. Am J Hematol 1999; 60:225–228.
26. Trimble MS, Glynn MF, Brain MC. Amegakaryocytic thrombocytopenia of 4 years duration: successful treatment with antithymocyte globulin. Am J Hematol 1991; 37:126–127.
27. Manoharan A, Williams NT, Sparrow R. Acquired amegakaryocytic thrombocytopenia: report of a case and review of literature. Q J Med 1989; 70:243–252.
28. Harrus S, Aroch I, Lavy E, Bark H. Clinical manifestations of infectious canine cyclic thrombocytopenia. Vet Rec 1997; 141:247–250.

29. Shirota T, Yamamoto H, Fujimoto H, et al. Cyclic thrombocytopenia in a patient treated with cyclosporine for refractory idiopathic thrombocytopenic purpura. Am J Hematol 1997; 56:272–276.
30. Tomer A, Schreiber AD, McMillan R, et al. Menstrual cyclic thrombocytopenia. Br J Haematol 1989; 71:519–524.
31. Kosugi S, Tomiyama Y, Shiraga M, et al. Cyclic thrombocytopenia associated with IgM anti-GPIIb-IIIa autoantibodies. Br J Haematol 1994; 88:809–815.
32. Nagasawa T, Hasegawa Y, Kamoshita M, et al. Megakaryopoiesis in patients with cyclic thrombocytopenia. Br J Haematol 1995; 91:185–190.
33. Fureder W, Mitterbauer G, Thalhammer R, et al. Clonal T cell-mediated cyclic thrombocytopenia. Br J Haematol 2002; 119:1059–1061.
34. Kimura F, Nakamura Y, Sato K. Cyclic change of cytokines in a patient with cyclic thrombocytopenia. Br J Haematol 1996; 94:171–174.
35. Tricot G, Criel A, Verwilghen RL. Thrombocytopenia as presenting symptom of preleukaemia in 3 patients. Scand J Haematol 1982; 28:243–250.
36. Ridell B, Kutti J, Swolin B, Wadenvik H. Dysplastic megakaryopoiesis with thrombocytopenia and chromosomal aberration. Am J Clin Pathol 1992; 98:227–230.
37. Menke DM, Colon-Otero G, Cockerill KJ, Jenkins RB, Noel P, Pierre RV. Refractory thrombocytopenia. A myelodysplastic syndrome that may mimic immune thrombocytopenic purpura. Am J Clin Pathol 1992; 98:502–510.
38. Wattel E, Cambier N, Caulier MT, Sautiere D, Bauters F, Fenaux P. Androgen therapy in myelodysplastic syndromes with thrombocytopenia: a report on 20 cases. Br J Haematol 1994; 87:205–208.
39. Dacie JV, Lewis SM. Paroxysmal nocturnal haemoglobinuria: clinical manifestations, haematology, and nature of the disease. Ser Haematol 1972; 5:3–23.
40. Socie G, Mary JY, de Gramont A. Paroxysmal nocturnal haemoglobinuria: long-term follow-up and prognostic factors. French Society of Haematology. Lancet 1996; 348:573–577.
41. Lin LI, Liu CH, Chen YC. PIG-A gene mutations in four Taiwanese patients with paroxysmal nocturnal haemoglobinuria following aplastic anaemia. Br J Haematol 1997; 97:286–292.
42. Wang H, Chuhjo T, Yasue S, Omine M, Nakao S. Clinical significance of a minor population of paroxysmal nocturnal hemoglobinuria-type cells in bone marrow failure syndrome. Blood 2002; 100:3897–3902.
43. Schubert J, Scholz C, Geissler RG, Ganser A, Schmidt RE. G-CSF and cyclosporin induce an increase of normal cells in hypoplastic paroxysmal nocturnal hemoglobinuria. Ann Hematol 1997; 74:225–230.
44. Paquette RL, Yoshimura R, Veiseh C, Kunkel L, Gajewski J, Rosen PJ. Clinical characteristics predict response to antithymocyte globulin in paroxysmal nocturnal haemoglobinuria. Br J Haematol 1997; 96:92–97.
45. Rand ML, Wright JF. Virus-associated idiopathic thrombocytopenic purpura. Transfus Sci 1998; 19:253–259.
46. Baranski B, Young N. Hematologic consequences of viral infections. Hematol Oncol Clin North Am 1987; 1:167–183.
47. Ratner L. Human immunodeficiency virus-associated autoimmune thrombocytopenic purpura: a review. Am J Med 1989; 86:194–198.

48. Sloand EM, Klein HG, Banks SM, Vareldzis B, Merritt S, Pierce P. Epidemiology of thrombocytopenia in HIV infection. Eur J Haematol 1992; 48:168–172.
49. Zucker-Franklin D, Termin CS, Cooper MC. Structural changes in the megakaryocytes of patients infected with the human immune deficiency virus (HIV-1). Am J Pathol 1989; 134:1295–1303.
50. Zucker-Franklin D, Cao YZ. Megakaryocytes of human immunodeficiency virus-infected individuals express viral RNA. Proc Natl Acad Sci USA 1989; 86:5595–5599.
51. Kouri YH, Borkowsky W, Nardi M, Karpatkin S, Basch RS. Human megakaryocytes have a CD4 molecule capable of binding human immunodeficiency virus-1. Blood 1993; 81:2664–2670.
52. Kowalska MA, Ratajczak J, Hoxie J, et al. Megakaryocyte precursors, megakaryocytes and platelets express the HIV co-receptor CXCR4 on their surface: determination of response to stromal-derived factor-1 by megakaryocytes and platelets. Br J Haematol 1999; 104:220–229.
53. Chelucci C, Federico M, Guerriero R, et al. Productive human immunodeficiency virus-1 infection of purified megakaryocytic progenitors/precursors and maturing megakaryocytes. Blood 1998; 91:1225–1234.
54. Voulgaropoulou F, Tan B, Soares M, Hahn B, Ratner L. Distinct human immunodeficiency virus strains in the bone marrow are associated with the development of thrombocytopenia. J Virol 1999; 73:3497–3504.
55. Zauli G, Catani L, Gibellini D, et al. Impaired survival of bone marrow GPIIb/IIa+ megakaryocytic cells as an additional pathogenetic mechanism of HIV-1-related thrombocytopenia. Br J Haematol 1996; 92:711–717.
56. Harker LA. Physiology and clinical applications of platelet growth factors. Curr Opin Hematol 1999; 6:127–134.
57. Espanol I, Muniz-Diaz E, Margall N, et al. Serum thrombopoietin levels in thrombocytopenic and non-thrombocytopenic patients with human immunodeficiency virus (HIV-1) infection. Eur J Haematol 1999; 63:245–250.
58. Ballem PJ, Belzberg A, Devine DV, et al. Kinetic studies of the mechanism of thrombocytopenia in patients with human immunodeficiency virus infection. N Engl J Med 1992; 327:1779–1784.
59. Van Wyk V, Kotze HF, Heyns AP. Kinetics of indium-111-labelled platelets in HIV-infected patients with and without associated thrombocytopaenia. Eur J Haematol 1999; 62:332–335.
60. Hymes KB, Greene JB, Karpatkin S. The effect of azidothymidine on HIV-related thrombocytopenia. N Engl J Med 1988; 318:516–517.
61. Zidovudine for the treatment of thrombocytopenia associated with human immunodeficiency virus (HIV). A prospective study. The Swiss Group for Clinical Studies on the Acquired Immunodeficiency Syndrome (AIDS). Ann Intern Med, 1988;109:718–721.
62. Cole JL, Marzec UM, Gunthel CJ, et al. Ineffective platelet production in thrombocytopenic human immunodeficiency virus-infected patients. Blood 1998; 91:3239–3246.
63. Tomer A, Hanson SR, Harker LA. Autologous platelet kinetics in patients with severe thrombocytopenia: discrimination between disorders of production and destruction. J Lab Clin Med 1991; 118:546–554.

64. Najean Y, Rain JD. The mechanism of thrombocytopenia in patients with HIV infection. J Lab Clin Med 1994; 123:415–420.
65. Leissinger CA. Platelet kinetics in immune thrombocytopenic purpura and human immunodeficiency virus thrombocytopenia. Curr Opin Hematol 2001; 8:299–305.
66. Nagamine T, Ohtuka T, Takehara K, Arai T, Takagi H, Mori M. Thrombocytopenia associated with hepatitis C viral infection. J Hepatol 1996; 24:135–140.
67. Ramos-Casals M, Garcia-Carrasco M, Lopez-Medrano F, et al. Severe autoimmune cytopenias in treatment-naive hepatitis C virus infection: clinical description of 35 cases. Medicine (Baltimore) 2003; 87:87–96.
68. Pawlotsky JM, Bouvier M, Fromont P, et al. Hepatitis C virus infection and autoimmune thrombocytopenic purpura. J Hepatol 1995; 23:635–639.
69. Blanche P, Bouscary D. Ribavirin therapy for cryoglobulinemia and thrombocytopenia associated with hepatitis C virus infection. Clin Infect Dis 1997; 25:1472–1473.
70. Jaccard A, Loustaud V, Turlure P, Rogez S, Bordessoule D. Ribavirin and immune thrombocytopenic purpura. Lancet 1998; 351:1660–1661.
71. Hernandez F, Blanquer A, Linares M, Lopez A, Tarin F, Cervero A. Autoimmune thrombocytopenia associated with hepatitis C virus infection. Acta Haematol 1998; 99:217–220.
72. Bordin G, Ballare M, Zigrossi P, et al. A laboratory and thrombokinetic study of HCV-associated thrombocytopenia: a direct role of HCV in bone marrow exhaustion? Clin Exp Rheumatol 1995; 13:S39–S43.
73. Pawlotsky JM, Ben Yahia M, Andre C, et al. Immunological disorders in C virus chronic active hepatitis: a prospective case-control study. Hepatology 1994; 19:841–848.
74. Jimenez-Saenz M, Rojas M, Pinar A, et al. Sustained response to combination therapy in a patient with chronic hepatitis C and thrombocytopenia secondary to alpha-interferon. J Gastroenterol Hepatol 2000; 15:567–569.
75. Li X, Jeffers LJ, Garon C, et al. Persistence of hepatitis C virus in a human megakaryoblastic leukaemia cell line. J Viral Hepat 1999; 6:107–114.
76. Garcia-Suarez J, Burgaleta C, Hernanz N, Albarran F, Tobaruela P, Alvarez-Mon M. HCV-associated thrombocytopenia: clinical characteristics and platelet response after recombinant alpha2b-interferon therapy. Br J Haematol 2000; 110:98–103.
77. Morgan D, Ablashi DV. Detection of EBNA and rescue of transformine EBV in megakaryocyte cells established in culture. In: Levine PH, Abashi DV, Pearson GR, Kotardis, eds. Epstein-Barr Virus Malignant Associated Disease, International symposium on Epstein-Barr Virus Malignant Associated Diseases. Boston: Martinus Nijhoff Publishing, 1985:402–407.
78. Pipp ML, Means ND, Sixbey JW, Morris KL, Gue CL, Baddour LM. Acute Epstein-Barr virus infection complicated by severe thrombocytopenia. Clin Infect Dis 1997; 25:1237–1239.
79. Flanagan NG, Rowlands AJ, Sloan ME, Ridway JC. Infectious mononucleosis with acute thrombocytopenia. J Infect 1989; 61:61–63.
80. Duncombe AS, Amos RJ, Metcalfe P, Pearson TC. Intravenous immunoglobulin therapy in thrombocytopenic infectious mononucleosis. Clin Lab Haematol 1989; 11:11–15.

81. Cyran EM, Rowe JM, Bloom RE. Intravenous gammaglobulin treatment for immune thrombocytopenia associated with infectious mononucleosis. Am J Hematol 1991; 38:124–129.
82. Casey TP, Matthews JR. Thrombocytopenic purpura in infectious mononucleosis. N Z Med J 1973; 77:318–320.
83. Steeper TA, Horwitz CA, Moore SB. Severe thrombocytopenia in Epstein-Barr virus-induced mononucleosis. West J Med 1989; 150:170–173.
84. Modlin JF, Grant PE, Makar RS, Roberts DJ, Krishnamoorthy KS. Case records of the Massachusetts General Hospital. Weekly clinicopathological exercises. Case 25-2003. A newborn boy with petechiae and thrombocytopenia. N Engl J Med 2003; 349:691–700.
85. Miyahara M, Shimamoto Y, Yamada H, Shibata K, Matsuzaki M, Ono K. Cytomegalovirus-associated myelodysplasia and thrombocytopenia in an immunocompetent adult. Ann Hematol 1997; 74:99–101.
86. Osborn JE, Shahidi NT. Thrombocytopenia in murine cytomegalovirus infection. J Lab Clin Med 1973; 81:53–63.
87. Maciejewski JP, Bruening EE, Donahue RE, Mocarski ES, Young NS, St Jeor SC. Infection of hematopoietic progenitor cells by human cytomegalovirus. Blood 1992; 80:170–178.
88. Eisenberg MJ, Kaplan B. Cytomegalovirus-induced thrombocytopenia in an immunocompetent adult. West J Med 1993; 158:525–526.
89. Espinoza C, Kuhn C. Viral infection of megakaryocytes in varicella with purpura. Am J Clin Pathol 1974; 61:203–208.
90. Winiarski J. Platelet antigens in varicella associated thrombocytopenia. Arch Dis Child 1990; 65:137–139.
91. Feusner JH, Slichter SJ, Harker LA. Mechanisms of thrombocytopenia in varicella. Am J Hematol 1979; 7:255–264.
92. Young NS, Mortimer PP, Moore JG, Humphries RK. Characterization of a virus that causes transient aplastic crisis. J Clin Invest 1984; 73:224–230.
93. Anderson MJ, Higgins PG, Davis LR, et al. Experimental parvoviral infection in humans. J Infect Dis 1985; 152:257–265.
94. Timuragaoglu A, Surucu F, Nalcaci M, Dincol G, Pekcelen Y. Anemia and thrombocytopenia due to parvovirus B-19 infection in a pregnant woman. J Med 1997; 28:245–249.
95. Srivastava A, Bruno E, Briddell R, et al. Parvovirus B19-induced perturbation of human megakaryocytopoiesis in vitro. Blood 1990; 76:1997–2004.
96. Inoue S, Kinra NK, Mukkamala SR, Gordon R. Parvovirus B-19 infection: aplastic crisis, erythema infectiosum and idiopathic thrombocytopenic purpura. Pediatr Infect Dis J 1991; 10:251–253.
97. Lefrere JJ, Courouce AM, Kaplan C. Parvovirus and idiopathic thrombocytopenic purpura. Lancet 1989; 1:279.
98. Murray JC, Kelley PK, Hogrefe WR, McClain KL. Childhood idiopathic thrombocytopenic purpura: association with human parvovirus B19 infection. Am J Pediatr Hematol Oncol 1994; 16:314–319.
99. Heegaard ED, Rosthoj S, Petersen BL, Nielsen S, Karup Pedersen F, Hornsleth A. Role of parvovirus B19 infection in childhood idiopathic thrombocytopenic purpura. Acta Paediatr 1999; 88:614–617.

100. Duchin JS, Koster FT, Peters CJ, et al. Hantavirus pulmonary syndrome: a clinical description of 17 patients with a newly recognized disease. The Hantavirus Study Group. N Engl J Med 1994; 330:949–955.
101. Mackow ER, Gavrilovskaya IN. Cellular receptors and hantavirus pathogenesis. Curr Top Microbiol Immunol 2001; 256:91–115.
102. Corash L. Interactions of viruses and platelets and the inactivation of viruses in platelet concentrates prepared for transfusion. In: Gresele P, Page C, Fuster V, Vermylen J, eds. Platelets. Boston: Cambriidge Press, 2002.
103. Hudson JB, Weinstein L, Chang TW. Thrombocytopenia purpura in measles. J Pediatrics 1965; 48:48–52.
104. Bayer WL, Sherman FE, Michaels RH, Szeto IL, Lewis JH. Purpura in congenital and acquired rubella. N Engl J Med 1965; 273:1362–1366.
105. Hirsh EO, Gerdner FH. The transfusion of blood platelets with a note on the transfusion of granulocytes. J Lab Clin Med 1952; 39:556–560.
106. Morse EE, Zinckham WH, Jackson DP. Thrombocytopenic purpura following rubella infection in children and adults. Arch Intern Med 1966; 117:573–577.
107. Graham DY, Brown CH, III, Benrey J, Butel JS. Thrombocytopenia. A complication of mumps. JAMA 1974; 227:1162–1164.
108. Myllyla G, Vaheri A, Vesikari T, Penttinen K. Interaction between human blood platelets, viruses and antibodies. IV. Post-Rubella thrombocytopenic purpura and platelet aggregation by Rubella antigen-antibody interaction. Clin Exp Immunol 1969; 4:323–332.
109. Oski FA, Naiman JL. Effect of live measles vaccine on the platelet count. N Engl J Med 1966; 275:352–356.
110. Howson CP, Fineberg HV. Adverse events following pertussis and rubella vaccines. Summary of a report of the Institute of Medicine. JAMA 1992; 267:392–396.
111. Richards GA, Murphy S, Jobson R, et al. Unexpected Ebola virus in a tertiary setting: clinical and epidemiologic aspects. Crit Care Med 2000; 28:240–244.
112. La Russa VF, Innis BL. Mechanisms of dengue virus-induced bone marrow suppression. Baillieres Clin Haematol 1995; 8:249–270.
113. Wong RS, Wu A, To KF, et al. Haematological manifestations in patients with severe acute respiratory syndrome: retrospective analysis. BMJ 2003; 326:1358–1362.
114. Gerardin P, Rogier C, Ka AS, Jouvencel P, Brousse V, Imbert P. Prognostic value of thrombocytopenia in African children with falciparum malaria. Am J Trop Med Hyg 2002; 66:686–691.
115. Ladhani S, Lowe B, Cole AO, Kowuondo K, Newton CR. Changes in white blood cells and platelets in children with falciparum malaria: relationship to disease outcome. Br J Haematol 2002; 119:839–847.
116. Fajardo LF. Letter: Malarial parasites in mammalian platelets. Nature 1973; 243:298–299.
117. Fajardo LF. The role of platelets in infections. I. Observations in human and murine malaria. Arch Pathol Lab Med 1979; 103:131–134.
118. Skudowitz RB, Katz J, Lurie A, Levin J, Metz J. Mechanisms of thrombocytopenia in malignant tertian malaria. Br Med J 1973; 2:515–518.
119. Neva FA, Sheagren JN, Shulman NR, Canfield CJ. Malaria: host-defense mechanisms and complications. Ann Intern Med 1970; 73:295–306.

120. Hatcher JC, Greenberg PD, Antique J, Jimenez-Lucho VE. Severe babesiosis in Long Island: review of 34 cases and their complications. Clin Infect Dis 2001; 32:1117–1125.
121. Young EJ, Tarry A, Genta RM, Ayden N, Gotuzzo E. Thrombocytopenic purpura associated with brucellosis: report of 2 cases and literature review. Clin Infect Dis 2000; 31:904–909.
122. Stephan JL, Kone-Paut I, Galambrun C, Mouy R, Bader-Meunier B, Prieur AM. Reactive haemophagocytic syndrome in children with inflammatory disorders. A retrospective study of 24 patients. Rheumatology (Oxford) 2001; 40:1285–1292.
123. Francois B, Trimoreau F, Vignon P, Fixe P, Praloran V, Gastinne H. Thrombocytopenia in the sepsis syndrome: role of hemophagocytosis and macrophage colony-stimulating factor. Am J Med 1997; 103:114–120.
124. Baker GR, Levin J. Transient thrombocytopenia produced by administration of macrophage colony-stimulating factor: investigations of the mechanism. Blood 1998; 91:89–99.
125. Aguero-Rosenfeld ME. Laboratory aspects of tick-borne diseases: lyme, human granulocytic ehrlichiosis and babesiosis. Mt Sinai J Med 2003; 70:197–206.
126. Bakken JS, Aguero-Rosenfeld ME, Tilden RL, et al. Serial measurements of hematologic counts during the active phase of human granulocytic ehrlichiosis. Clin Infect Dis 2001; 32:862–870.
127. Dumler JS, Dawson JE, Walker DH. Human ehrlichiosis: hematopathology and immunohistologic detection of Ehrlichia chaffeensis. Hum Pathol 1993; 24:391–396.
128. Borjesson DL, Simon SI, Tablin F, Barthold SW. Thrombocytopenia in a mouse model of human granulocytic ehrlichiosis. J Infect Dis 2001; 184:1475–1479.
129. Turgut M, Sunbul M, Bayirli D, Bilge A, Leblebicioglu H, Haznedaroglu I. Thrombocytopenia complicating the clinical course of leptospiral infection. J Int Med Res 2002; 30:535–540.
130. Edwards CN, Nicholson GD, Hassell TA, Everard CO, Callender J. Thrombocytopenia in leptospirosis: the absence of evidence for disseminated intravascular coagulation. Am J Trop Med Hyg 1986; 35:352–354.
131. Alugupalli KR, Michelson AD, Barnard MR, et al. Platelet activation by a relapsing fever spirochaete results in enhanced bacterium-platelet interaction via integrin alphaIIbbeta3 activation. Mol Microbiol 2001; 39:330–340.
132. Kahn JB. A case of Weil's disease requiring steroid therapy for thrombocytopenia and bleeding. Am J Trop Med Hyg 1982; 31:1213–1215.
133. Perine PL, Parry EH, Vukotich D, Warrell DA, Bryceson AD. Bleeding in louse-borne relapsing fever. I. Clinical studies in 37 patients. Trans R Soc Trop Med Hyg 1971; 65:776–781.
134. Coburn J, Leong JM, Erban JK. Integrin alpha IIb beta 3 mediates binding of the Lyme disease agent Borrelia burgdorferi to human platelets. Proc Natl Acad Sci USA 1993; 90:7059–7063.
135. George JN, Raskob GE, Shah SR, et al. Drug-induced thrombocytopenia: a systematic review of published case reports. Ann Intern Med 1998; 129:886–890.
136. Silverstein MN, Petitt RM, Solberg LA, Jr., Fleming JS, Knight RC, Schacter LP. Anagrelide: a new drug for treating thrombocytosis. N Engl J Med 1988; 318:1292–1294.

137. Tomer A. Effects of anagrelide on in vivo megakaryocyte proliferation and maturation in essential thrombocy themia. Blood 2002; 99:1602–1609.
138. Shrestha R, McKinley C, Bilir BM, Everson GT. Possible idiopathic thrombocytopenic purpura associated with natural alpha interferon therapy for chronic hepatitis C infection. Am J Gastroenterol 1995; 90:1146–1147.
139. Lopez Morante AJ, Saez-Royuela F, Casanova Valero F, Yuguero del Moral L, Martin Lorente JL, Ojeda Gimenez C. Immune thrombocytopenia after alpha-interferon therapy in a patient with chronic hepatitis, C.. Am J Gastroenterol 1992; 87:809–810.
140. Monte D, Wietzerbin J, Pancre V, et al. Identification and characterization of a functional receptor for interferon-gamma on a megakaryocytic cell line. Blood 1991; 78:2062–2069.
141. Ganser A, Carlo-Stella C, Greher J, Volkers B, Hoelzer D. Effect of recombinant interferons alpha and gamma on human bone marrow-derived megakaryocytic progenitor cells. Blood 1987; 70:1173–1179.
142. Wang Q, Miyakawa Y, Fox N, Kaushansky K. Interferon-alpha directly represses megakaryopoiesis by inhibiting thrombopoietin-induced signaling through induction of SOCS-1. Blood 2000; 96:2093–2099.
143. Zuckerman AJ, Chazan AA. Agranulocytosis with thrombocytopenia following chlorthiazide therapy. Br Med J 1958; 2:13–38.
144. Dinin LR, Kim YS, Vander Veer JB. Clinical experience with chlorthiazide (Diuril) with particular emphasis on untoward responses. Am J Med Sci 1958; 236:533–545.
145. Chong BH, Chesterman C. Thrombocytopenia due to bone marrow disorders. In: Gresele P, Page C, Fuster V, Vermylen J, eds. Platelets in Thrombotic and non-Thrombotic Disorders. Cambridge, UK: Cambridge University Press, 2002.
146. Wallerstein RO, Condit PK, Kasper CK, Brown JW, Morrison FR. Statewide study of chloramphenicol therapy and fatal aplastic anemia. JAMA 1969; 208:2045–2050.
147. Custer RP. Aplastic anemia in soldiers treated with atabrine (quinacrine). Am J Med Sci 1946; 212:211–214.
148. Cowan DH, Hines JD. Thrombocytopenia of severe alcoholism. Ann Intern Med 1971; 74:37–43.
149. Lindenbaum J, Hargrove RL. Thrombocytopenia in alcoholics. Ann Intern Med 1968; 68:526–532.
150. Cowan DH. Thrombokinetic studies in alcohol-related thrombocytopenia. J Lab Clin Med 1973; 81:64–76.
151. Gewirtz AM, Hoffman R. Transitory hypomegakaryocytic thrombocytopenia: aetiological association with ethanol abuse and implications regarding regulation of human megakaryocytopoiesis. Br J Haematol 1986; 62:333–344.
152. Levine RF, Spivak JL, Meagher RC, Sieber F. Effect of ethanol on thrombopoiesis. Br J Haematol 1986; 62:345–354.
153. Yardley-Jones A, Anderson D, Parke DV. The toxicity of benzene and its metabolism and molecular pathology in human risk assessment. Br J Ind Med 1991; 48:437–444.
154. Rangan U, Snyder R. Scientific update on benzene. Ann N Y Acad Sci 1997; 837:105–113.
155. Fleming LE, Timmeny W. Aplastic anemia and pesticides. An etiologic association? J Occup Med 1993; 35:1106–1116.

156. Yin SN, Li GL, Tain FD, et al. Leukaemia in benzene workers: a retrospective cohort study. Br J Ind Med 1987; 44:124–128.
157. Kalf GF, Rushmore T, Snyder R. Benzene inhibits RNA synthesis in mitochondria from liver and bone marrow. Chem Biol Interact 1982; 42:353–370.
158. Rauch AE, Kowalsky SF, Lesar TS, Sauerbier GA, Burkart PT, Scharfman WB. Lindane (Kwell)-induced aplastic anemia. Arch Intern Med 1990; 150:2393–2395.
159. West RR, Stafford DA, White AD, Bowen DT, Padua RA. Cytogenetic abnormalities in the myelodysplastic syndromes and occupational or environmental exposure. Blood 2000; 95:2093–2097.
160. Rigolin GM, Cuneo A, Roberti MG, et al. Exposure to myelotoxic agents and myelodysplasia: case-control study and correlation with clinicobiological findings. Br J Haematol 1998; 103:189–197.
161. Gale RP. Immediate medical consequences of nuclear accidents. Lessons from Chernobyl. JAMA 1987; 258:625–628.
162. Gale RP. USSR: follow-up after Chernobyl. Lancet 1990; 335:401–402.
163. Richardson FL. Effect of Severe hemorrhage on the number of blood platelets in blood from the peripheral circulation of rabbits.. J Med Res 1904; 13:99.
164. Perlman MK, Schwab JG, Nachman JB, Rubin CM. Thrombocytopenia in children with severe iron deficiency. J Pediatr Hematol Oncol 2002; 24:380–384.
165. Berger M, Brass LF. Severe thrombocytopenia in iron deficiency anemia. Am J Hematol 1987; 24:425–428.
166. Soff GA, Levin J. Thrombocytopenia associated with repletion of iron in iron-deficiency anemia. Am J Med Sci 1988; 295:35–39.
167. Karpatkin S, Garg SK, Freedman ML. Role of iron as a regulator of thrombopoiesis. Am J Med 1974; 57:521–525.
168. Stabler SP, Allen RH, Savage DG, Lindenbaum J. Clinical spectrum and diagnosis of cobalamin deficiency. Blood 1990; 76:871–881.
169. Slichter SJ, Harker LA. Thrombocytopenia: mechanisms and management of defects in platelet production. Clin Haematol 1978; 7:523–539.
170. Kotilainen M. Platelet kinetics in normal subjects and in haematological disorders; with special reference to thrombocytopenia and to the role of the spleen. Scand J Haematol Suppl 1969; 5:5–97.
171. Ghosh K, Sarode R, Varma N, Varma S, Garewal G. Amegakaryocytic thrombocytopenia of nutritional vitamin B12 deficiency. Trop Geogr Med 1988; 40:158–160.
172. Poelmann AM, Aarnoudse JG. A pregnant woman with severe epistaxis—a rare manifestation of folic acid deficiency. Eur J Obstet Gynecol Reprod Biol 1986; 23:249–254.
173. Mant MJ, Connolly T, Gordon PA, King EG. Severe thrombocytopenia probably due to acute folic acid deficiency. Crit Care Med 1979; 7:297–300.
174. Garderet L, Maury E, Lagrange M, Najman A, Offenstadt G, Guidet B. Schizocytosis in pernicious anemia mimicking thrombotic thrombocytopenic purpura. Am J Med 2003; 114:423–425.

PART II: THROMBOCYTOPENIA DUE TO EXCESSIVE PLATELET DESTRUCTION

5

Platelet Clearance

Steven E. McKenzie and Michael P. Reilly

Cardeza Foundation for Hematologic Research, Thomas Jefferson University, Philadelphia, Pennsylvania, U.S.A.

NORMAL PHYSIOLOGY

Platelets play essential roles in hemostasis, immunity, and wound repair. The ability of platelets to perform these functions is related to the concentration of platelets in circulating blood. Normally there are 150,000 to 450,000 platelets per mm^3, or 1.5 to 4.4×10^{11}/L. At steady state, the number of platelets produced is equal to the number destroyed, i.e., that leave the circulation, and the platelet life span is approximately 9 days. Physiologically, platelets leave the circulation by two major mechanisms: (1) consumption at common sites of minor vascular injury, likely in the microcirculation, and (2) phagocytosis by macrophages, predominantly in the spleen and liver. The senescence signals for platelets to undergo phagocytosis by macrophages are incompletely characterized. There are a number of candidates (see below), and it is likely that several contribute. Pathologically, we refer to clearance in the broadest sense, namely, removal from the circulating pool in the bloodstream. Excess clearance, if removal is of sufficient magnitude to exceed the production of new platelets, results in thrombocytopenia. There are multiple mechanisms for pathologically increased clearance of platelets, as detailed below.

Measures of platelet clearance have included studies of radiolabeled platelets. ^{111}Indium labeling of platelets has been used for over two decades to ascertain the normal physiologic survival of platelets (1), and several key points have emerged from such studies. First, following injection, an average of 30% of autologous, labeled platelets is sequestered by the spleen. This proportion can vary widely, and needs to be explicitly accounted for in studies of altered clearance in pathologic conditions. Second, platelet survival is a function of the platelet count in that the measured survival decreases when the platelet count is in the thrombocytopenic range. These data have been interpreted to mean that there is a fixed component of platelet loss each day due to basal hemostatic function in the vasculature. As the platelet count decreases, an increasing proportion of the circulating mass is consumed by this basal need. Finally, nonlinear functions, including the so-called γ function, have been used to permit discrimination of the expected survival in thrombocytopenia secondary to marrow failure from the reduced survival in platelet destruction syndromes, such as immune thrombocytopenic purpura (ITP) (2–4).

More recently, other measures of platelet clearance include use of alternative labels, such as fluorescent dye CMFDA or biotin in animal models (5,6), and of surrogate biological markers of platelet clearance such as thrombopoietin or glycocalicin levels.

Platelet Senescence

Candidates for the platelet senescence signals include phosphatidylserine (PS) exposure on the outer leaflet of the plasma membrane, alterations in cell surface glycoproteins, alterations in cell surface proteoglycans, and gradual loss of platelet fragments or microparticles. PS is an anionic phospholipid that in resting platelets is kept on the inner (cytoplasmic side) leaflet of the plasma membrane by the combined actions of several energy-dependent protein complexes including flippase, translocase, and scramblase. Following platelet activation, there is a rise in intracellular Ca^{++} concentration associated with reduction in translocase activity and an increase in scramblase activity. PS on the platelet outer leaflet is important to platelet procoagulant activity, namely, the platform for the assembly of the Factor IXa/VIIIa tenase complex and the Factor Xa/Va prothombinase complex. The rare hemorrhagic disorder Scott syndrome is associated with defective exposure of PS and reduced to absent platelet procoagulant activity. Macrophages recognize either exposed PS directly, for example by the PS receptor PSR (7), or by way of bridging proteins which bind both PS and macrophage receptors. An example of a bridging protein in which there has been increasing interest is MFG-E8, a protein that binds to PS and to $\alpha_v\beta_3$ and $\alpha_v\beta_5$ integrins to facilitate phagocytosis (8,9).

By analogy to red blood cell senescence, another contributor to senescence could be formation of denatured or damaged platelet cell surface glycoproteins. These glycoproteins might undergo changes in glycosylation and/or exposure of neoepitopes recognized by naturally occurring antibodies.

Cold Storage Lesion

There has been exciting progress in delineating the mechanisms involved in the platelet cold storage lesion. Clearly, the inability to store platelets at 4 °C has had a profound impact on the safety of platelet transfusion therapy. It has now been demonstrated that hepatic macrophages use complement/scavenger receptor CR3 (also known as Mac-1 or $\alpha_M\beta_2$ integrin) to detect clustered GPIbα receptors on platelets that have been exposed to cold temperatures (10). Specific sugars (β-N-acetylglucosamine) on the clustered GPIbα molecules permit the recognition and engulfment of the cold-stored platelets. However, the platelets work well despite the clustering of the GPIbα receptors. Therefore, Hoffmeister, Hartwig, Stossel, and colleagues (11) identified a way to provide the murine platelet surface GPIbα glycoprotein with sugar groups (via enzymatic galactosylation) that are not recognized by the macrophages, and so circulate normally in recipient mice despite prior storage at 4 °C. Extension of these findings to human clinical trials is eagerly awaited. It is unclear at this time if the same mechanism, clustering of GPIbα receptors on platelets and recognition of β-N-acetylglucosamine, plays a role in physiologic senescence and clearance.

Inhibition of Phagocytosis

There has been an interesting twist in the concept of clearance and senescence with the discovery of several families of receptors that inhibit phagocytosis (12). Red blood cells and virtually all tissues examined express CD47 (also known as IAP, integrin-associated protein). CD47 engages a receptor on macrophages variously known as SIRPα or SHPS-1, and the interaction inhibits phagocytosis. It has been interpreted to mean that this is a signal to leave "self" alone. Mice deficient in CD47 have reduced survival of their red blood cells in the circulation of CD47-positive recipients. Furthermore, autoimmune hemolytic anemia is worsened in the absence of CD47 (13). With respect to platelets, mice expressing a truncated form of SHPS-1 have a moderate (25%) reduction in platelet count, which has been attributed to loss of the cytoplasmic motifs necessary to impart the phagocytosis-inhibiting signal (14). More developments in the CD47-SIRPα/SHPS-1 area with respect to platelets can be anticipated.

Microparticle Generation

When platelets circulate, there is gradual loss of platelet fragments or microparticles. Microparticle generation has assumed increasing importance to our understanding of normal hemostasis and pathologic thrombosis (15,16). Even healthy individuals have readily detected platelet-derived microparticles in their circulation. The concentration of platelet-derived particles increases in a number of inflammatory and prothrombotic conditions. How platelet microparticles are generated, how and where they are cleared, and what impact they have on platelet survival remain unanswered questions.

PATHOPHYSIOLOGY—IMMUNE THROMBOCYTOPENIA SYNDROMES

There are a number of immune thrombocytopenia syndromes, including ITP, drug-related immune thrombocytopenia, and alloimmune thrombocytopenia. ITP is an autoimmune condition that can manifest as isolated thrombocytopenia or be part of a systemic autoimmune disorder. While drug-related thrombocytopenia is common, there are a number of mechanisms for the resultant thrombocytopenia, including marrow suppression or increased clearance. In certain conditions, the offending drug forms a complex with a platelet surface glycoprotein, and the drug-glycoprotein complex is the antigenic target of autoantibodies that clear platelets in a way very similar to ITP. Offending drugs include quinine and quinidine, which form complexes with GPIb/V/IX, as well as the newer GPIIb/IIIa inhibitors, which in a small percentage of patients cause a drug-dependent conformational change that serves as a target for naturally occurring antibodies. Heparin-induced thrombocytopenia is a special condition that is discussed in the next section. Alloimmune thrombocytopenia falls into two major categories, neonatal alloimmune thrombocytopenia and alloimmunization following platelet transfusion. Neonatal alloimmune thrombocytopenia (NAIT) is relatively common, affecting 1 in 1000 to 1 in 2000 live births, sometimes with devastating consequences. In this syndrome, mothers generate antibodies to platelet epitopes that they lack, but which are present on fetal platelets by way of inheritance from the father. Though analogous to hemolytic disease of the newborn secondary to Rh immunization on red blood cells, NAIT differs in that up to 50% of cases are recognized in first pregnancies. Though not formally proven in experimental models, the weight of the evidence is that decreased platelet survival in NAIT is due to IgG anti-platelet antibodies that cross the placenta and use the same antibody effector mechanisms in the baby that are operational in ITP. Likewise, the survival of alloimmunized platelets is diminished due to IgG anti-platelet antibodies triggering the antibody effector mechanisms.

Phagocytic Fcγ Receptors

What these immune thrombocytopenia syndromes share is the presence of anti-platelet IgG antibody which binds to a platelet surface by way of the Fab domains. The free Fc domains of the IgG antibody are then positioned to be recognized by the Fcγ receptors of splenic macrophages as the platelets pass through the splenic cords in the sinusoids. The antibody-coated platelet is an example of a particulate immune complex, and the macrophages possess three classes of Fcγ receptors that participate in phagocytosis of these complexes (Fig. 1). There is little evidence to support a significant role for complement or complement receptors in human ITP or ITP mouse models (17,18).

Fcγ receptors that engage antibody-coated platelets and mediate phagocytosis are called activating receptors. On human splenic macrophages, these are FcγRI/γ (CD64), FcγRIIa (CD32a), and FcγRIIIa/γ (CD16a). FcγRI

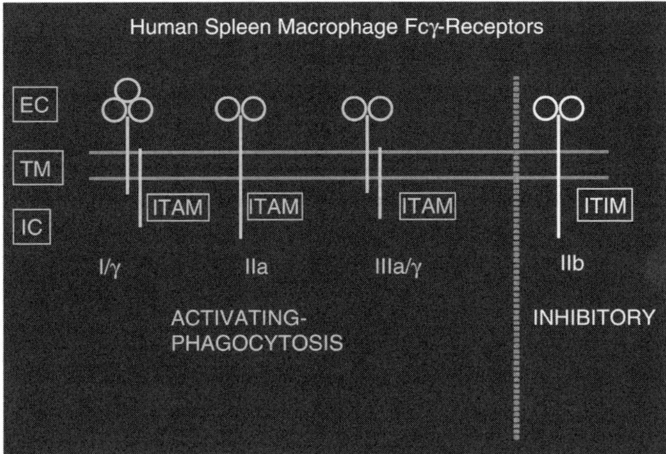

Figure 1 Fcγ receptors on human macrophages: the phagocytic Fcγ receptors (I/γ, IIa, and IIIa/γ) and the inhibitory Fcγ receptor (FcγRIIb) are depicted.

and FcγRIIIa are the ligand-binding subunits of a multimolecular receptor; the other component is the FcR γ-chain, a subunit associated with and used by multiple receptors to transmit activating signals. In contrast, FcγRIIa possesses both ligand-binding and activating signal transduction components within the same molecule. The basis of phagocytic activation by the FcR γ-chain and FcγRIIa is the intracytoplasmic ITAM (immunoreceptor tyrosine activation motif). Though there are several differences between the FcR γ-chain and the FcγRIIa ITAMs, both are subjected to tyrosine phosphorylation by members of the src family of non-receptor protein tyrosine kinases, and upon tyrosine phosphorylation both dock syk kinases to propagate activating intracellular signals. Some of the most prominent second messenger systems downstream of activating FcγR engagement include PI3K and PLCγ. There are data to support a role for each of these receptors in phagocytosis in vivo. Most of these data derive from genetically-manipulated mouse models, although some derive from clinical observations. In a small human clinical trial, an antibody directed against the FcγRIIIa molecule showed efficacy in improving the platelet counts in ITP (19).

In murine models, we have begun to dissect the relative roles of the various Fcγ receptors in ITP in vivo. We created FcγRIIa transgenic mice because mice and other non-primate mammals lack the gene, and thus the protein, for FcγRIIa. Mice do express FcγRI/γ and FcγRIII/γ on splenic macrophages. We established that the humanized repertoire (FcγRI/γ, FcγRIIa, and FcγRIII/γ) is more effective at clearance of antibody-coated platelets than that of wild-type mice, as assessed by the severity of the thrombocytopenia in animals treated with the same dose of exogenous antiplatelet antibody. We bred mice in which the FcR γ-chain was knocked out in the FcγRIIa transgenic line, and further established that FcγRIIa on its own is nearly as effective as having all three receptors in mediating ITP in vivo (18). Thus, our data support the contention that therapies directed at modulating the level of expression or function of the activating Fcγ spleen receptors ought to explicitly include FcγRIIa. Though much can be learned from murine models of Fcγ receptor function in wild-type mice, we believe that the pathophysiologic relevance to human disease is enhanced when the mice express the fully humanized repertoire of Fcγ receptors, including FcγRIIa.

Inhibitory Fcγ Receptors

An increasingly important area is that of inhibitory receptors, especially the inhibitory Fcγ receptor FcγRIIb. While other receptor-counter receptor systems such as CD47—SIRPα/SHPS-1 were discussed previously, inhibitory FcγRIIb is unique in that it is competing for binding of IgG immune complex ligand with the activating Fcγ receptors. Like FcγRIIa and FcγRIIIa/γ, FcγRIIb has minimal affinity for monomeric IgG, but moderate avidity for multimeric IgG. In fact, it is the co-crosslinking by ligand of activating FcγR simultaneously with inhibitory FcγR that results in the manifestation of the inhibition. There has been excellent progress in delineation of the mechanisms of inhibition. Activating FcγRs when clustered leads to phosphorylation of src family members. FcγRIIb can then be phosphorylated on its cytoplasmic tyrosine residues which form an ITIM, the immunoreceptor tyrosine inhibition motif. Specifically, the tyrosine-phosphorylated ITIM serves as docking site for the binding of protein tyrosine phosphatases (such as SHP-1, SHP2) and inositol phophatases (such as SHIP-1) which down-regulate the activity of a number of critical phosphorylated second messengers in the activation pathway. The net result, whether a particular cell is active in phagocytosis of antibody-coated platelets, is dependent on the balance of activating and inhibitory receptors. This balance of activating vs. inhibitory receptors is dynamic. Alterations in the balance may help to explain the clinical observation of exacerbations of chronic ITP accompanying infection, often viral, or by immunization with live attenuated viral vaccines. Certain pro-inflammatory cytokines may alter the balance to favor one in which activating receptors predominate over inhibitory receptors. In contrast, anti-inflammatory cytokines may create a balance in which inhibitory receptors predominate over activating receptors.

The FcRn System

It is logical that the degree of thrombocytopenia in ITP will also depend on the titer of the antiplatelet antibody. The HLA Class I-like FcRn receptors for IgG represent a saturable system on the endothelial cells of the vasculature. One normal function of the FcRn system is the ability to protect IgG molecules from catabolism, by way of endocytosis and recycling back to the extracellular milieu. Because of FcRn, IgG molecules have a long serum half-life, ranging from 21 to 28 days. The FcRn system can, however, be overwhelmed and lose its ability to protect IgG molecules from catabolism. This can be exploited to permit catabolism of disease-causing antibodies, such as antiplatelet antibodies (20,21).

The clearance mechanisms have implications for the mechanism of action of therapeutics in ITP. We now appreciate that corticosteroids have several mechanisms of action. These include down-regulation of activating FcγRs in addition to reduction in autoantibody production. Likewise, IVIG acts through multiple mechanisms, and recently two newer mechanisms have emerged as particularly important. First, IVIG upregulates monocyte-macrophage FcγRIIb, altering the balance of activating and inhibitory receptors to favor inhibition of phagocytosis of antibody-coated platelets. The effects of IVIG on up-regulation of phagocytic cell FcγRIIb appear to be indirect, and likely secondary to secretion of one or more anti-inflammatory cytokines by other IVIG-recognizing cell subpopulations. Second, IVIG overwhelms the saturable FcRn system, and thereby decreases the titer of the offending autoantibodies. Of interest, anti-D immune globulin works primarily by blockade of the activating Fcγ receptors. Since IVIG and anti-D thus have different mechanisms of action, they provide a rationale for their combined use in selected difficult patients.

Immune Complex–Mediated Thrombocytopenia

In some ITP patients, Fcγ receptors contribute to accelerated platelet clearance through an alternative mechanism. In systemic autoimmune disorders in which there is an increase in circulating immune complexes, there can also be increased platelet clearance due to spleen macrophage FcR interacting with the Fc domain of immune complexes (ICs) bound to platelets via platelet FcγRIIa, assuming the titer and valency of the IC is such that it does not activate the platelet. We have observed more severe thrombocytopenia in our mouse model of systemic autoimmunity, a human FcγRIIa transgenic on the NZW × BXSB F1 background, than in the wild-type NZW × BXSB F1 model. Interestingly, immune complex-mediated glomerulonephritis, another feature of the NZW × BXSB F1 model, is diminished by the concurrent presence of the FcγRIIa transgene. We have speculated that these data support a model in which platelets serve a physiologic role in handling and disposition of circulating immune complexes.

Another potentially confounding issue in the understanding of platelet clearance in ITP is the clearance of antibody-coated platelets by tissue macrophages outside the spleen, as well as the occurrence of accessory spleens. In addition, Fcγ receptor polymorphisms may influence disease severity in the setting of otherwise identical antibody targets and titers. Such polymorphisms include ligand-binding polymorphisms (22,23) and copy number polymorphisms (24,25). Another interesting area is the expression by platelets of what had originally been described as immune effectors, such as CD40 and CD40 ligand, as well as numerous potent chemokines.

Reduced Platelet Production in ITP

The thrombocytopenia in ITP is sometimes not due solely to increased platelet clearance. Since measurement of specific antiplatelet antibodies in ITP remains a complex procedure performed in research laboratories rather than in routine clinical laboratories, it is possible that some "refractory ITP" cases are in reality genetic thrombocytopenia syndromes (26), especially in the younger patient. In addition, there is appreciation of the fact that some refractory ITP cases are accompanied by reduced platelet production, whether due to autoantibody-mediated attack on megakaryocytes and megakaryocyte precursors or other mechanisms, such as nascent myelodysplastic syndrome. These patients will not manifest the reduced platelet lifespan seen in the most common form of ITP. The observation that there are ITP patients with poor platelet production has led to enthusiasm for use of TPO or TPO mimetics to treat them (27,28). Finally, studies in vitro have indicated that T-lymphocytes may specifically recognize platelets (29). Whether this mechanism has a basis in vivo for reduced platelet survival in ITP remains to be demonstrated.

HIV-related Thrombocytopenia

HIV-related thrombocytopenia warrants special consideration because it is clearly multifactorial. Immune-mediated platelet destruction is present in many affected patients, which responds to IVIG therapy in a similar manner as ITP. The association between HIV infection and ITP-like illness has led to the consensus that there be testing for HIV in new onset ITP in any individual at risk. Interesting new developments in a novel mechanism for anti-GPIIb/IIa-mediated platelet destruction have been determined by Nardi, Karpatkin, and colleagues. Generation of lytic reactive oxygen species following binding of the antibody to the platelet surface antigen has been seen (30). In addition, splenic sequestration can reduce platelet counts, as can reduced platelet production (31). HIV can infect megakaryocytes and their progenitors, and highly active antiretroviral therapy can also suppress megakaryopoiesis.

In summary, much of the pathologic burden in ITP and related immune thrombocytopenia syndromes is due to clearance of IgG-coated platelets by phagocytic splenic Fcγ receptors, and therapies to interrupt this pathology have proven successful. However, there remain subtle nuances that impact the course of individual patients, and new avenues exist for exploration of the role of inhibitory receptors and the benefit of pharmacologic stimulation of thrombopoiesis.

PATHOPHYSIOLOGY—THROMBOCYTOPENIA AND THROMBOSIS SYNDROMES

The key concept in HITT (heparin-induced thrombocytopenia with thrombosis) that distinguishes it from ITP is that intravascular platelet activation occurs in the presence of a physically intact endothelium (32–35); hence, the physiologic hemostatic route of platelet activation by exposure to the subendothelium is not operable. Intravascular platelet activation is prothrombotic and accelerates platelet clearance; the platelet count is diminished not because antibody-coated platelets move passively through the bloodstream where they are culled from the circulation by the spleen, but rather because the immune complexes generated in HITT (between heparin and platelet factor 4) activate platelets while they are still in the circulation. The circulating activated platelet then has several potential fates: (1) be incorporated into a thrombus that is localized at a site of inflamed endothelium, (2) be incorporated into a thrombus that is trapped at the next microcirculatory bed it encounters, or (3) travel to the spleen where the PS (and likely adhesion molecule) exposure triggers phagocytosis by macrophages.

We have created murine models of immune complex-triggered thrombocytopenia and thrombosis syndromes, including HITT. These models have produced several striking observations about the fate of platelets as a result of such pathology. First, immune complexes activate platelets via their Fcγ receptor, FcγRIIa, the only Fcγ receptor expressed by platelets. Activation requires a multimeric IgG immune complex, and few antiplatelet antibodies in non-thrombotic disorders such as ITP bind platelet targets with sufficient density to cause efficient crosslinking of FcγRIIa on neighboring platelets via the antibody Fc domains. However, consistent with the observations of Deckmyn and colleagues (36), Ahn and colleagues (37), and others, we recognized that a small subset of ITP patients indeed make antibodies to GPIIb/IIIa or to CD9 (high density antigens) of sufficient titer that their free Fc ends activate platelets via FcγRIIa. As stated earlier, we created FcγRIIa transgenic mice because mice and other non-primate mammals lack the gene, and thus the protein, for FcγRIIa. Anti-CD9 antibody in vitro activates platelets of FcγRIIa transgenic mice, but not wild-type mice, and in a manner dependent on FcγRIIa availability, as it was blocked by the anti-FcγRIIa blocking antibody IV.3. Anti-CD9 antibody in wild-type mice, with no platelet Fcγ receptor to cause platelet activation, but with FcγRI/γ and FcγRIII/γ on their spleen macrophages, caused simple ITP. In contrast, at the same dose of anti-CD9 antibody, FcγRIIa transgenic mice had severe thrombocytopenia and thrombus generation, especially in the lungs, resulting in respiratory distress and a shock phenotype. Thus, we modeled for the first time the effects of intravascular platelet activation in the setting of an anti-platelet antibody to a high density antigen. As expected, the severity of the phenotype depended on the titer of the antibody. Other investigators have also shown a dependence not just on antigen density, but also on the topography of the antibody bound to the antigen, in triggering Fcγ receptor responses (38). For these reasons (antigen density, antibody titer, antigen-antibody topography), it is very uncommon in ITP for there to be significant intravascular platelet activation, but in rare cases it can occur.

An intriguing additional observation concerning antiplatelet antibodies which activate platelets came when we took one of several measures to reduce splenic clearance. Though we initially hypothesized that the thrombocytopenia might be more mild, to our surprise not only was the thrombocytopenia more severe, but also the thrombosis was worse. The three different measures were quite distinct: genetic knockout of the splenic macrophage FcR γ-chain; anti-FcγRIII antibody blockade; and, splenectomy. Thus, we clearly established that antiplatelet antibody-mediated thrombocytopenia can be a consequence of intravascular platelet activation, not just splenic clearance. Furthermore, splenic clearance, while reducing the platelet count, is protective in that it reduces thrombus formation in the setting of activating antiplatelet antibodies. These mouse model findings have implications for thrombosis after splenectomy, as has been reported in some ITP patients, and perhaps also in HITT.

In contrast to the rare circumstance of ITP with activating antiplatelet antibodies, HITT is marked by the regular occurrence of an activating immune complex. We demonstrated that HITT in vivo depends on four necessary and sufficient components: heparin, PF4, anti-heparin/PF4 antibody, and platelet FcγRIIa (39).

We now appreciate that the HITT antigen in more than 90% of cases is a multimeric complex of heparin and PF4 (in other cases, heparin may interact with another cationic chemokine such as platelet basic protein (PBP) or IL-8, to form a neoantigen). Rauova, Sachais et al. have now clearly demonstrated the nature of the multimeric complex (40). The multimeric complex, size >600 kDa, shows optimal binding of anti-heparin/PF4 antibody, and the complex is most effective in activation of platelets in an FcγRIIa-dependent manner. The very large complexes fail to form at less-than-optimal molar ratios of heparin-to-PF4, whether too low or too high. This last finding, that of an optimal ratio for complex formation, is a nice parallel to the observation in the serotonin release assay (SRA) that an optimal heparin:PF4 ratio is required for serotonin release. Reilly et al. have extended this observation to demonstrate the critical role of the heparin:PF4 ratio in the murine HITT model in vivo, with respect to the thrombocytopenia and thrombosis phenotypes (39).

Medical conditions in which intravascular platelet activation occurs include HITT, APLS, TTP, and sepsis. Intravascular platelet activation can also accompany localized intravascular coagulation, for example, that due to a vascular malformation, disseminated intravascular coagulation, or flow through extracorporeal circuits.

How does intravascular platelet activation lead to platelet clearance? Following intravascular activation, platelets can be entrapped in thrombi. Because intravascular platelet activation is most often accompanied by inflammation, platelet-containing thrombi may become adherent to inflamed endothelial cells via newly expressed adhesive proteins. Alternatively, platelet-containing thrombi may embolize and be trapped in the microcirculation of downstream organs if generated on the arterial side, or in the pulmonary circulation if generated on the venous side of the circulation. We have demonstrated both organ microvascular thrombi and pulmonary thrombi in our murine model of HITT. As an alternative to entrapment in thrombi, activated platelets can circulate to organs such as the spleen and liver where macrophages of the reticuloendothelial system bind and phagocytose them. It remains undetermined whether the ligands and receptors which mediate binding and phagocytosis of activated platelets are the same as those that mediate clearance of senescent platelets. While it is likely that there is some overlap, it is also possible that platelet activation results in an additional distinct set of receptors and counter-receptors that ensure rapid removal from circulation.

SUMMARY AND FUTURE RESEARCH DIRECTIONS

In summary, clearance of platelets can be viewed as encompassing four major categories: senescence, cold storage lesion-induced, antibody-mediated, and activation-mediated. The extent to which the physiologic (senescence) and pathologic (cold-induced, antibody-mediated, activation-mediated) platelet clearance mechanisms overlap is unknown. If there is a finite set of platelet surface molecules and a corresponding set of macrophage and endothelial molecules used in clearance, the implications for therapy of the pathologic conditions are clear. Targeted modulation of platelet surface molecule expression or function, with or without modulation of the macrophage or endothelial cell surface molecule expression or function, should permit continued circulation of platelets. An attractive way to modulate clearance interactions is to pharmacologically down-regulate the phagocytic receptors while up-regulating inhibitory receptors.

There are, however, some precautionary notes. It may be better for the host to clear platelets that have become activated pathologically within the vasculature in the spleen, resulting in less end organ damage because of a reduction in thrombosis. The resulting thrombocytopenia is more adaptive for the host than the thrombosis. Likewise, if platelets bind immune complexes and in so doing remove them from the circulation, the host benefits from "sacrificing" platelets and avoiding immune complex disposition in end organs such as the kidney. We believe that careful consideration of the mechanisms of platelet clearance will be necessary in order for rational therapeutic decisions to be made about the benefits of modulating clearance.

Scientific frontiers that will enable greater understanding of the mechanisms of platelet clearance abound. They include further study of the PSR deficient mouse, study of the regulation of cholesterol/sphingolipid microdomains in PS exposure and microparticle release, studies of the role of platelets in systemic regulation of IC disposition, and, finally, studies of polymorphisms in the molecules mediating clearance for their relative contribution to human disease and its treatment.

ACKNOWLEDGMENTS

We would like to acknowledge the input of my coworkers and colleagues with whom we have pursued studies of ITP and HITT: Scott Taylor, Douglas Cines, Mortimer Poncz, Gow Arepally, Bruce Sachais, Anna Kowalska, Chunyan Zhang, and Lubica Raouva. The work herein has been supported by the Public Health Service, via NIH grants R01 HL61685 (McKenzie), R01 HL69471 (Reilly), R01 HL54749 (Poncz), and P01 HL40387 (McKenzie).

REFERENCES

1. Carter R, Smith K, Harker LA. Megakaryocytopoiesis and platelet kinetics. In: Anderson KC, Ness PM, eds. Scientific Basis of Transfusion Medicine, Implications for Clinical Practice. 2nd ed. Philadelphia, PA: W.B. Saunders Company, 2000:30–44.
2. Louwes H, Beekhuis H, Goedemans WT, Keijser SP, Schuurman JJ. ^{111}In-tropolonate labelled platelets; studies in normals and in patients with thrombocytopenia. Eur J Nucl Med 1987; 13:47–51.
3. Louwes H, Zeinali Lathori OA, Vellenga E, de Wolf JT. Platelet kinetic studies in patients with idiopathic thrombocytopenic purpura. Am J Med 1999; 106:430–434.
4. Tomer A, Hanson SR, Harker LA. Autologous platelet kinetics in patients with severe thrombocytopenia: discrimination between disorders of production and destruction. J Lab Clin Med 1991; 118:546–554.
5. Baker GR, Sullam PM, Levin J. A simple, fluorescent method to internally label platelets suitable for physiological measurements. Am J Hematol 1997; 56:17–25.
6. Rand ML, Wang H, Bang KW, Poon KS, Packham MA, Freedman J. Procoagulant surface exposure and apoptosis in rabbit platelets: association with shortened survival and steady-state senescence. J Thromb Haemost 2004; 2:651–659.
7. Hoffmann PR, deCathelineau AM, Ogden CA, et al. Phosphatidylserine (PS) induces PS receptor-mediated macropinocytosis and promotes clearance of apoptotic cells. J Cell Biol 2001; 155:649–659.
8. Hanayama R, Tanaka M, Miyasaka K, et al. Autoimmune disease and impaired uptake of apoptotic cells in MFG-E8-deficient mice. Science 2004; 304:1147–1150.
9. Zullig S. Tickling macrophages, a serious business. Science 2004; 304:1123–1124.
10. Hoffmeister KM, Felbinger TW, Falet H, et al. The clearance mechanism of chilled blood platelets. Cell 2003; 112:87–97.
11. Hoffmeister KM, Josefsson EC, Isaac NA, Clausen H, Hartwig JH, Stossel TP. Glycosylation restores survival of chilled blood platelets. Science 2003; 301:1531–1534.
12. Yamao T, Noguchi T, Takeuchi O, et al. Negative regulation of platelet clearance and of the macrophage phagocytic response by the transmembrane glycoprotein SHPS-1. J Biol Chem 2002; 277:39833–39839.

13. Oldenborg P-E, Gresham HD, Lindberg FP. CD47-Signal regulatory protein alpha (SIRPalpha) regulates Fcγ and complement receptor-mediated phagocytosis. J Exp Med 2001; 193:855–861.
14. Sato R, Ohnishi H, Kobayashi H, et al. Regulation of multiple functions of SHPS-1, a transmembrane glycoprotein, by its cytoplasmic region. Biochem Biophys Res Commun 2003; 309:584–590.
15. VanWijk MJ, VanBavel E, Sturk A, Nieuwland R. Microparticles in cardiovascular diseases. Cardiovasc Res 2003; 59:277–287.
16. Osterud B. The role of platelets in decrypting monocyte tissue factor. Dis Mon 2003; 49:7–13.
17. Ravetch JV. A full complement of receptors in immune complex diseases. J Clin Invest 2002; 110:1759–1761.
18. McKenzie SE, Taylor SM, Malladi P, et al. The role of the human Fc receptor Fcγ RIIA in the immune clearance of platelets: a transgenic mouse model. J Immunol 1999; 162:4311–4318.
19. Clarkson SB, Bussel JB, Kimberly RP, Valinsky JE, Nachman RL, Unkeless JC. Treatment of refractory immune thrombocytopenic purpura with an anti-Fcγ γ-receptor antibody. N Engl J Med 1986; 314:1236–1239.
20. Hansen RJ, Balthasar JP. Effects of intravenous immunoglobulin on platelet count and antiplatelet antibody disposition in a rat model of immune thrombocytopenia. Blood 2002; 100:2087–2093.
21. Hansen RJ, Balthasar JP. Intravenous immunoglobulin mediates an increase in anti-platelet antibody clearance via the FcRn receptor. Thromb Haemost 2002; 88:898–899.
22. Reilly AF, Surrey S, Rappaport EF, Schwartz E, McKenzie SE. Variation in human FCGR2C gene copy number. Immunogenetics 1994; 40:456.
23. Lehrnbecher T, Foster CB, Zhu S, et al. Variant genotypes of the low-affinity Fcγ receptors in two control populations and a review of low-affinity Fcγ receptor polymorphisms in control and disease populations. Blood 2001; 98:1634–1635.
24. Sebat J, Lakshmi B, Troge J, et al. Large-scale copy number polymorphism in the human genome. Science 2004; 305:525–528.
25. Reilly AF, Norris CF, Surrey S, et al. Genetic diversity in human Fc receptor II for immunoglobulin G: Fcγ receptor IIA ligand-binding polymorphism. Clin Diagn Lab Immunol 1994; 1:640–644.
26. Drachman JG. Inherited thrombocytopenia: when a low platelet count does not mean ITP. Blood 2004; 103:390–398.
27. Nomura S, Dan K, Hotta T, Fujimura K, Ikeda Y. Effects of pegylated recombinant human megakaryocyte growth and development factor in patients with idiopathic thrombocytopenic purpura. Blood 2002; 100:728–730.
28. Inagaki K, Oda T, Naka Y, Shinkai H, Komatsu N, Iwamura H. Induction of megakaryocytopoiesis and thrombocytopoiesis by JTZ-132, a novel small molecule with thrombopoietin mimetic activities. Blood 2004; 104:58–64.
29. Olsson B, Andersson PO, Jernas M, et al. T-cell-mediated cytotoxicity toward platelets in chronic idiopathic thrombocytopenic purpura. Nat Med 2003; 9:1123–1124.
30. Nardi M, Feinmark SJ, Hu L, Li Z, Karpatkin S. Complement-independent Ab-induced peroxide lysis of platelets requires 12-lipoxygenase and a platelet NADPH oxidase pathway. J Clin Invest 2004; 113:973–980.

31. Cole JL, Marzec U, Gunthel CJ, et al. Ineffective platelet production in thrombocytopenic human immunodeficiency virus-infected patients. Blood 1998; 91:3239–3246.
32. Arepally G, Cines DB. Pathogenesis of heparin-induced thrombocytopenia and thrombosis. Autoimmun Rev 2002; 1:125–132.
33. Reilly MP, Taylor SM, Hartman NK, et al. Heparin-induced thrombocytopenia/thrombosis in a transgenic mouse model requires human platelet factor 4 and platelet activation through FcγRIIA. Blood 2001; 98:2442–2447.
34. Warkentin TE, Greinacher A. Heparin-induced Thrombocytopenia. 2nd ed. New York, NY: Marcel Dekker, Inc, 2001.
35. Visentin GP. Heparin-induced thrombocytopenia: molecular pathogenesis. Thromb Haemost 1999; 82:448–456.
36. Deckmyn H, Vanhoorelbeke K, Peerlinck K. Inhibitory and activating human antiplatelet antibodies. Baillieres Clin Haematol 1998; 11:343–359.
37. Ahn YS, Horstman LL, Jy W, Jimenez JJ, Bowen B. Vascular dementia in patients with immune thrombocytopenic purpura. Thromb Res 2002; 107:337–344.
38. Kumpel BM, van de Winkel JG, Westerdaal NA, Hadley AG, Dugoujon JM, Blancher A. Antigen topography is critical for interaction of IgG2 anti-red-cell antibodies with Fcγ receptors. Br J Haematol 1996; 94:175–183.
39. Reilly MP, Chien CD, Poncz M, Cines DB, Kowalska MA, McKenzie SE. Dependence of heparin induced thrombocytopenia on the heparin:platelet factor 4 ratio *in vivo*. Blood 2002; 100:15a.
40. Rauova L, Poncz M, McKenzie SE, Reilly MP, Cines DB, Sachias B. Ultralarge complexes of heparin and PF4 are central to the pathogenesis of heparin-induced thrombocytopenia. Blood 2004; 105:131–138.

6

Idiopathic Thrombocytopenic Purpura

Douglas B. Cines
Department of Pathology and Laboratory Medicine, University of Pennsylvania School of Medicine, Philadelphia, Pennsylvania, U.S.A.

Victor Blanchette
Division of Haematology and Oncology, Department of Paediatrics, Hospital for Sick Children, Toronto, Ontario, Canada

INTRODUCTION

Idiopathic thrombocytopenic purpura (ITP) is an autoimmune disorder caused by platelet-reactive antibodies that lead to the development of thrombocytopenia and eventuate in mucosal bleeding (1). The exact incidence is uncertain. It is estimated that approximately 100 new cases are diagnosed per 1,000,000 persons each year (2–5), divided roughly equally between adults and children. Although adult-onset ITP and ITP manifesting in early childhood are both caused by platelet autoantibodies, their natural histories and possibly their etiologies differ. In adults, ITP occurs more commonly in females and the disorder tends to run a chronic course, whereas in children both sexes are equally affected and spontaneous remissions are common. There are also important differences in the differential diagnosis and management. Therefore, we will consider ITP diagnosed in these two age groups separately. Another important distinction is between ITP that occurs as an isolated condition (primary ITP) and ITP that occurs in the context of several well-described predisposing conditions (secondary ITP). This chapter will focus on primary ITP, but the salient features of common forms of secondary ITP will be noted where appropriate. Several recent reviews have appeared (5a,5b).

PATHOGENESIS

Involvement of a transmissible plasma factor in ITP had long been suspected based on the observation that affected women often gave birth to children with transient thrombocytopenia. The immunological basis of the disease was affirmed when it was found that ITP plasma and its IgG fraction caused transient thrombocytopenia when infused into healthy recipients. Platelets coated with IgG autoantibodies are recognized by Fcγ receptors on tissue macrophages in the spleen and elsewhere and are prematurely cleared from the circulation. Platelet production is increased in many patients, but not others (6–8) in whom megakaryocyte development (9) and platelet production (10) are impaired, or megakaryocytes may undergo apoptosis (11) or intramedullary destruction of nascent platelets may occur (12). T-cell mediated cytotoxicity towards platelets has recently been reported (13). Thrombopoietin levels are normal, reflecting the normal to increased megakaryocyte mass (14).

Circulating B cells synthesizing antiplatelet antibodies (15) and circulating antibodies that bind to the glycoprotein IIb/IIIa, Ib/IX, or Ia/IIa complex, glycoprotein IV, V, and in some cases to other components of the platelet surface, are found in most patients (16) and it is common for antibodies to several components to be detected (17). There is some evidence that platelet-autoantibodies originate from a limited number of B cell clones based on light chain and V_H gene usage (18,19), likely by antigen-driven affinity selection and somatic mutation (20). Why certain individuals demonstrate this propensity is unknown. Familial ITP is rare and a consistent relationship between MHC-I and MHC-II polymorphisms and the incidence of ITP has not been demonstrated. T-cells tolerized to platelet glycoproteins have been identified in healthy individuals (21), whereas ITP-T cells stimulate antibody synthesis when exposed to fragments of glycoprotein IIb/IIIa (22). Increased platelet-associated CD154 has been noted (23) and a cytokine profile compatible with activation of Th0/Th1 cells (24), characterized by elevated IL-2 and IFNγ, reduced to absent 1L-10, and a reduced Th3 response (25), have been reported both in adults and children (26,27). B7-costimulation (28) and cytokine-driven activation of antigen-presenting cells, e.g., in the spleen (29) and elsewhere, likely contribute to antibody production. However, the fundamental mechanism underlying the loss of tolerance and the subsequent emergence of platelet-specific T- and B-cell clones remains enigmatic (25).

ITP IN ADULTS

Presentation

ITP occurs most commonly in women during the second and third decades of life (30,31), but it can develop in either sex and at any age and the disorder is being increasingly recognized in older individuals of both sexes (2,5). Patients typically present with petechiae, purpura, or ecchymoses developing over the course of several days. Platelet counts are generally between 1 and 20×10^9/L. When platelet counts are below 10,000/μL, widespread cutaneous bleeding, epistaxis, gingival bleeding, hematuria, menorrhagia, or melena occur more commonly. Spontaneous intracranial hemorrhage or bleeding at other internal sites is rare (see below). Individuals with platelet counts between 30×10^9/L and 50×10^9/L may give a history of easy bruising, while platelet counts above 50×10^9/L are likely to be discovered incidentally. Most patients are otherwise in their usual state of health, although some complain of easy fatigability. A few show evidence of a systemic disorder associated with immune thrombocytopenia (see below).

Diagnosis

The diagnosis of primary ITP remains one of exclusion. A careful history to exclude inadvertent or surreptitious exposure to drugs that have been implicated in causing thrombocytopenia is important, as is a thorough family history, inquiry for systemic disorders associated with ITP (see below), or a recent history of transfusions (to exclude post-transfusion purpura). The physical examination shows only evidence of bleeding. The blood counts are normal except for the platelet count unless significant bleeding has occurred. Thrombocytopenia determined by an automated analyzer must be confirmed by reviewing the peripheral blood smear to exclude pseudothrombocytopenia, i.e., in vitro platelet clumping caused by antibody upon chelation of calcium (32), and other hematological conditions. The platelets are often large; however, platelets approaching the size of red cells and the finding of unusually small platelets should prompt attention to the possibility of an inherited thrombocytopenia, especially in children and young adults (33). The marrow reveals normal to increased numbers of megakaryocytes with no dysplastic features when an aspirate or biopsy is performed, but these procedures are not required to establish the diagnosis. Even when the presentation is typical, bone marrow aspiration and biopsy are indicated in older individuals (34). No additional diagnostic studies are required to make a diagnosis of ITP in the typical case (4,34), but the response to therapy provides important diagnostic clues.

Serological evaluation for HIV and/or hepatitis C infection is indicated in at-risk populations (35–37). Testing for infection with *H. pylori* remains controversial because the outcome of treatment has been highly variable (see below). ITP may also occur in the context of SLE, anti-phospholipid syndrome, B-cell neoplasms (most commonly chronic lymphocytic and large granular lymphocytic leukemias), immune thyroid disorders, pernicious anemia, and common variable hypogammaglobulinemia, and after allogeneic or autologous bone marrow or stem cell transplantation, among others. The presence of these disorders, other than subclinical thyroid disease, is usually evident. Extensive serological or other testing in the absence of suggestive signs and symptoms is of limited utility, although it has recently been reported that concurrent

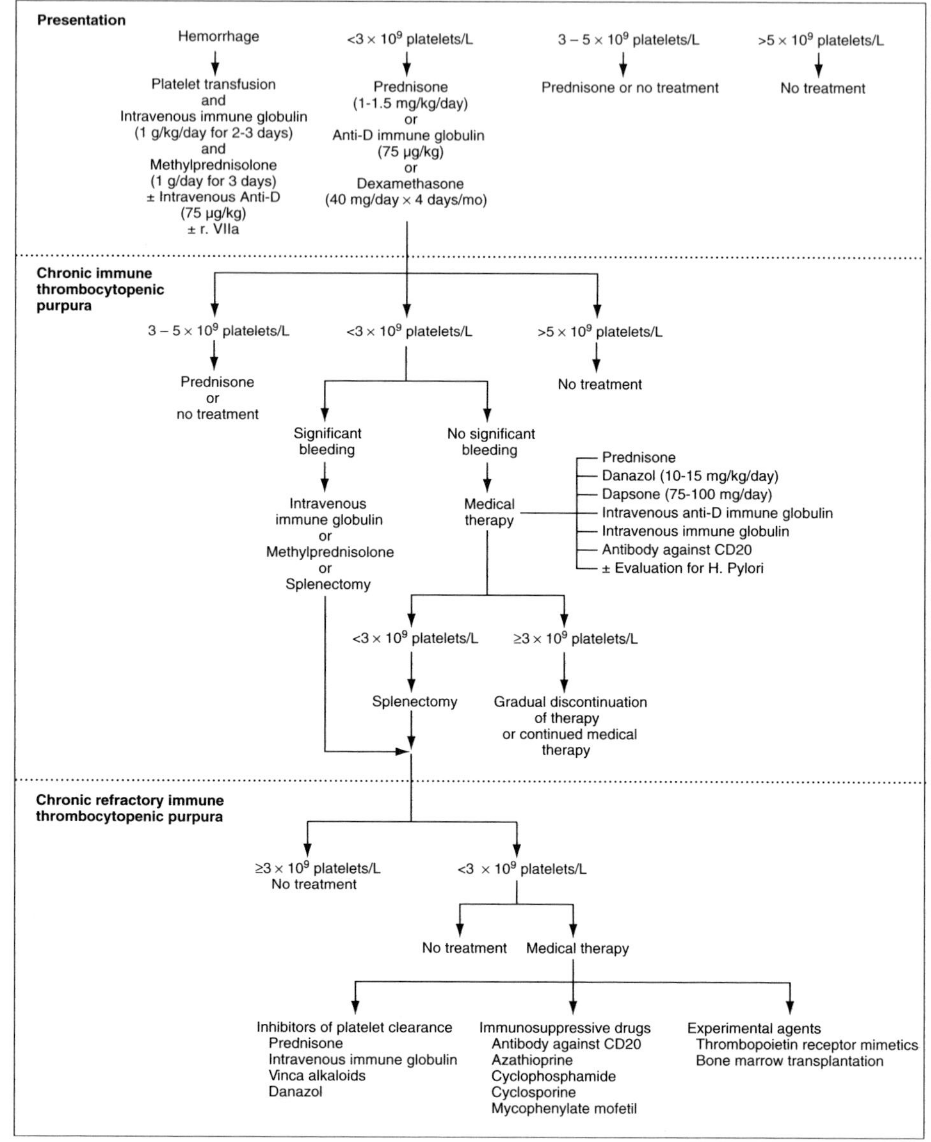

Figure 1 (*caption on facing page*)

antiphospholipid antibodies identify a subpopulation at risk for thrombosis when the platelet count exceeds 100×10^9/L in response to therapy (38). Approximately 1% of patients with ITP have co-existing immune hemolytic anemia (Evans syndrome) and a smaller percentage have immune neutropenia.

Measurement of Platelet Antibodies

The clinical utility of laboratory testing to measure platelet antibodies remains an area where opinions differ. Techniques have been developed that permit antibodies to several of the most abundant surface glycoproteins to be measured (39). The finding of platelet-bound autoantibodies has an estimated sensitivity of 49–66%, a specificity of 78–92%, and a positive predictive value of 80–83% (40,41) when comparing patients with ITP to healthy individuals. Inter-laboratory agreement is 55–67% (42) and a negative test cannot yet be used to rule out the diagnosis of ITP (40,43). Detection of antiplatelet antibody in plasma is less useful. The utility of the test may be lower when the differential diagnosis includes chronic liver disease, myelodysplasia, and systemic lupus erythematosus (SLE). Test results do not presage chronicity versus spontaneous recovery in children (44). No studies have been reported in which test results were used to alter the diagnosis or to determine therapy.

Initial Management

Management is predicated on the severity of the thrombocytopenia and associated bleeding. The goal of treatment is to attain a hemostatic platelet count (>20–30×10^9/L in most patients) while minimizing toxicity, although some authorities accept even lower thresholds (45). Most patients are treated initially with prednisone (1–1.5 mg/kg/day). Anti-D (0.5–0.75 μg/kg/iv) can be used in Rh(+) individuals intolerant of steroids (46,47) (Fig. 1). Anti-D causes a mild hemolytic anemia which is generally well-tolerated, although

Figure 1 (*figure on facing page*) Treatment algorithm for managing adult ITP. Schemas in Figs. 1 and 2 are based in part on published literature, expert opinion, ASH guidelines, and authors' experience. *Presentation*: Some advocate the use of 2×10^9/L as a guideline for therapy. There is no consensus as to duration of steroid therapy. The use of anti-D as initial therapy is appropriate only for Rh(+) individuals. The choice of intravenous immune globulin (IVIG) or anti-D as initial therapy depends on the severity of thrombocytopenia and the extent of mucocutaneous bleeding. *Chronic ITP*: The decision to treat depends on comorbid risk factors for bleeding and risk of trauma. Higher platelet counts may be appropriate for surgery or after trauma. IVIG or methylprednisolone may help increase the platelet count immediately prior to splenectomy. Medications can be used individually, but either danazol or dapsone can be combined with the lowest dose of prednisone required to attain a hemostatic platelet count. IVIG and anti-D are generally reserved for severe thrombocytopenia or unresponsive to oral agents. The decision to proceed to splenectomy in patients responding to medical therapy depends upon the intensity of therapy required, tolerance to side effects, risk of surgery, and patient preference. *Chronic refractory ITP*: The decision to treat refractory patients involves assessing the risk of hemorrhage versus the side effects of each form of therapy (see text). Drugs are often used in combination. Patients receiving protracted courses of corticosteroids should be monitored for osteopenia and cataracts.

acute and severe intravascular hemolysis, disseminated intravascular coagulation and renal failure have been reported on rare occasions (48,48a). Intravenous immunoglobulin (IVIG; 1 g/kg/day for 2 days) (49) should be used with IV methylprednisolone (30 mg/kg up to 1 g) when platelet counts remain below 5×10^9/L despite several days of corticosteroids or when bleeding is more widespread. One recent study reporting a high rate of durable remissions in patients given high dose dexamathasone (40 mg qd for 4 days/mo) requires confirmation (9). Therapy is generally not required at platelet counts above 30×10^9/L in the absence of bleeding or predisposing comorbid conditions (34).

Consideration should be given to hospitalizing adults who present for the first time with platelet counts $<10\text{–}20\times10^9$/L and those with widespread purpura or serious mucosal bleeding until the condition has been stabilized. Emergent therapy should be given to patients with profound mucocutaneous or internal bleeding and general measures to reduce the risk of bleeding should be instituted, including avoidance of drugs that impair platelet function, control of blood pressure, measures to minimize the risk of trauma, and local treatments where indicated, e.g., amicar for epistaxis, progesterone for vaginal bleeding. Treatment is initiated immediately with IVIG (1 g/kg/day for 1–3 consecutive days) and/or intravenous methylprednisolone (1–2 g/day for 1–3 consecutive days) until the platelet count exceeds 50 x 10^9/L (34,51,52). It is unknown whether addition of anti-D will improve outcome. Platelet transfusions are to be given as needed for life- or organ-threatening bleeding (53–55). Recombinant factor VIIa has been used in addition in true emergencies (56). Strong consideration should be given to performing a bone marrow aspiration and biopsy in this setting to exclude other hematological disorders.

There is no consensus as to the optimal duration of treatment. We generally continue treatment with corticosteroids for a minimum of three to four weeks or until a response is seen by which time toxicity is usually apparent. Response rates of 50–90% have been reported based on intensity and duration of therapy (34,57–59). Durable responses of 10–30% are reported with prednisone (34,57,59,60) and perhaps higher with dexamethasone (50) or anti-D (61). Therefore, most patients will relapse as the dose of prednisone is lowered over the next one to four months or when anti-D is discontinued (62) and will therefore require alternative forms of intervention. Failure to respond to prednisone, anti-D, and IVIG should prompt reevaluation of the diagnosis and consideration of a bone marrow evaluation if not previously performed.

Splenectomy

Splenectomy remains the mainstay of subsequent therapy in adults. The timing of splenectomy depends on disease severity, side effects of therapy, extent of physical activity, and patient preference. Most hematologists recommend splenectomy within three to six months if more than 10–20 mg of prednisone/day is required to maintain a hemostatic platelet count, although others recommend a more protracted period of watchful waiting. IVIG, anti-D, or pulse doses of corticosteroids are used to boost the platelet count immediately prior to surgery, although splenectomy has been performed safely at exceedingly low platelet counts. Use of prophylactic platelet transfusions is discouraged in most situations. Approximately 75–85% of patients attain an initial hemostatic response after splenectomy (34,57,63,64,64a), 25–40% of whom will relapse within 5–10 years (57,65). Responses cannot be predicted through routinely available measures (64a,66), though in our experience and in some studies, patients totally refractory to prior treatment fare less well, as do the elderly (63), patients with secondary forms of ITP (especially SLE and anti-phospholipid syndrome), patients with Evans syndrome (67), and perhaps those with a purely hepatic sequestration process (68). The outcomes of laparascopic and conventional transabdominal approaches are comparable (69) and the former hastens recovery. Splenic irradiation is reserved for the elderly and others in whom splenectomy is indicated but hazardous (70).

The major risk of splenectomy is overwhelming bacterial sepsis, which occurs in less than 1% of otherwise healthy adults with uncomplicated ITP managed appropriately (71). Immunization with polyvalent pneumoccocal, *Hemophilus influenzae type b*, and quadrivalent meningococcal polysaccharide vaccines, depending on age and immunization history, should be given at least two weeks prior to splenectomy (72,73). Life-long use of phenoyxmethylpenicillin (250–500 mg BID) or erythromycin (500 mg BID) has been recommended in a recent guideline from the United Kingdom (4), but is not routine in the United States. Some argue for the availability of antibiotics at home and the use of a MedAlert bracelet. At the least, any febrile illness demands careful evaluation and IV antibiotics should be strongly considered at the onset of a systemic illness with fever $\geq$101°F.

Chronic ITP

Approximately 30–40% of adults require additional therapy after splenectomy (57), while others eventually attain a hemostatic platelet count (5,74) (Fig. 1). Published guidelines recommend that platelet counts be maintained between 30 and 50×10^9/L, if possible without significant therapy-related toxicity, as a practical surrogate marker of the risk of severe bleeding (34). Platelet counts in this range are generally adequate for simple dental extractions and minor surgery; a platelet count above 80×10^9/L is generally recommended for most major surgery (4), but higher counts are preferable for bypass surgery.

The guiding principles in treating chronic ITP are that many patients who relapse after splenectomy will eventually attain a hemostatic platelet count although this may take many years to occur (75), while on the other hand, for the minority who require treatment to maintain a hemostatic platelet count, many die of hemorrhage (75) and the incidence of intracerebral hemorrhage approaches

2–3% per year in those totally refractory to all interventions (65,76,77). This risk is influenced by the patient's age, bleeding history, comorbid conditions and response to therapy (77–80). These factors must be balanced against the risk of potential complications associated with each treatment modality. Elderly patients are more likely to bleed and to be exposed to medications that impair platelet function, but also are more likely to suffer debilitating side effects from therapy. Moreover, published response rates, especially those involving newer forms of therapy, are likely to be optimistic, as they are sometimes based on small numbers of selected patients with short follow-up. Indeed, the benefit of treating asymptomatic patients has not been formally proven (81). Therefore, treatment must be individualized, and intangibles such as intensity of physical activity, other medical conditions, and life expectations must be taken into consideration. Therapies are often used in combination to achieve synergy and to limit toxicity.

The initial treatment of symptomatic relapse typically follows the same approach as was used on presentation, with primary reliance being placed on corticosteroids and IVIG, as anti-D has little efficacy after splenectomy. Approaches that showed limited success initially may be more effective post-splenectomy. Repetitive injections of IVIG may be life saving, but refractoriness may develop (82,83). Infusions are repeated as needed every 7–21 days. IVIG impairs the clearance of IgG-coated platelets (84,85), perhaps indirectly through the inhibitory receptor FcRγIIb (86–88). There is no evidence that commercial preparations differ in efficacy. Patients may complain of headache and a few develop aseptic meningitis (89). Other major side effects include thrombosis (90), pulmonary or renal failure (91), and anaphylactoid reactions in IgA-deficient patients with IgE anti-IgA antibodies in whom IgA-depleted preparations should be used (92,93). Antiviral antibodies (94) can be passively acquired, but there are no documented cases of HIV or hepatitis A, B, or C transmission with currently available preparations. Positive antiglobulin tests may develop in the same way. Overt hemolytic anemia from infused isoagglutinins occurs rarely (95), but isoagglutinins may form in response to transfer of blood group A substance (96).

Few patients attain a durable response to accessory splenectomy (97) and few can be maintained on low doses of corticosteroids alone. Therefore, drugs that have a slower onset of action are often introduced concomitantly as a steroid-sparing measure many of which, like corticosteroids, impede platelet clearance. Danazol (10–15 mg/kg/day) is beneficial in 20–40% of patients if given for three to six months (98), but few steroid-refractory patients respond. Side effects include hepatotoxicity, rash, and masculinization. Dapsone (75 mg/day) has been used successfully in 40–50% of relapsed patients (99) but, again, severely affected patients are less responsive. Vinca alkaloids are now used infrequently because the response rate is low (3–30%) and generally transient, and therapy is often complicated by neuropathy (100). Occasional responses occur with ex vivo perfusion of plasma over a staphylococcal protein A column (101), but severe side effects have been reported.

Rituximab, a chimeric antibody to the B cell co-stimulatory model CD20 (375 mg/m^2 IV weekly $\times$ 4), induces complete remissions that have been durable in approximately 25% of patients; partial, often transient, responses occur in another 25%. Responses may occur after the initial dose or may not occur until the entire course has been completed (102–104). Successful treatment of patients with CLL and secondary ITP has also been reported (105). The prevalence and duration of unmaintained remission is unknown. The drug is generally well tolerated. Prolonged B-cell depletion may increase the risk of opportunistic infection, but such complications have been rare in patients with primary ITP to date. Agranulocytosis, serum sickness, and interstitial pneumonitis have been reported in patients treated with rituximab for other conditions.

Other forms of immunosuppression are generally reserved for patients with platelet counts $<20 \times 10^9$/L who are intolerant or unresponsive to the above-mentioned measures. Responses are seen in 20–40% of patients treated for two to six months with azathioprine (57,106,107) (1–4 mg/kg po daily) or cyclophosphamide (57,108) (1–2 mg/kg po daily) with the dose adjusted to cause mild neutropenia. Cyclophosphamide has been given as an intravenous bolus as a single agent (1.0–1.5 g/m^2 every 4 wk for 1–5 doses) or in combination with prednisone, a vinca alkaloid, and/or other drugs (57,109). Liver function tests should be monitored in patients treated with azathioprine, which is generally well tolerated. The potential risk of malignancy should be discussed, but is not known to have occurred in ITP. Cyclophosphamide can cause marrow suppression, hemorrhagic cystitis, bladder fibrosis, alopecia, infertility, teratogenicity, and myeloid leukemia and is generally not the preferred agent in young individuals. Anecdotal responses have been reported in patients treated with cyclosporine alone or in combination with cyclophosphamide (110,111), with mycophenolate mofetil (112,113), etanercept (114), or anti-CD154 monoclonal antibody (115). Azathioprine or other immunosuppressive agents may be combined with danazol and prednisone in severely affected individuals. Thrombopoietin (116) and thrombopoietic receptor agonists (117,118) have been used successfully in some patients and larger trials are underway. In one series, high dose immunosuppression followed by autologous stem cell transplantation resulted in durable complete and partial remission in 6 and 2 of 12 treated patients, respectively (119). Recombinant IL-11 was ineffective and toxic in one study (120).

The role of infection with *H. pylori* remains a matter of considerable debate based on as yet unexplained wide variation in the rate of response to documented successful eradication of infection in patients with severe thrombocytopenia (121–127,127a). Anti-retroviral therapy is indicated in HIV-infected individuals (35). Many, but not all, patients with ITP and chronic hepatitis C infection respond to the typical therapeutic approach used to treat primary ITP (36,128,129) and the utility of adjunctive anti-viral therapy has not been proven.

ITP and Pregnancy

ITP is estimated to occur in 0.1–1/1000 pregnancies and to account for approximately 3% of women found to be thrombocytopenic at delivery (130). Pregnancy is generally not discouraged, but maternal and fetal complications do occur and additional monitoring and therapy may be needed (see refs. 131,132 for comprehensive reviews). The major differential diagnosis of thrombocytopenia during pregnancy includes pregnancy-induced hypertension and related conditions such as HELLP, microangiopathic hemolytic processes, hereditary thrombocytopenias, and gestational thrombocytopenia (also referred to as incidental or benign thrombocytopenia of pregnancy) (133).

Gestational thrombocytopenia accounts for approximately 75% of cases of thrombocytopenia at term in healthy women after an uneventful pregnancy (134). Thrombocytopenia is generally mild (platelet counts greater than 70×10^9/L in 95% of cases) and there is no impact on the health of the mother or fetus. Platelet counts generally return to normal within two months post-partum. ITP should be suspected if severe isolated thrombocytopenia is detected early in pregnancy, but the distinction may be problematic in the absence of a prenatal platelet count as both are diagnoses of exclusion.

Platelet counts typically fall during even uneventful pregnancy and should be monitored at least monthly through the first two trimesters, biweekly in the third, and weekly as term approaches. Corticosteroids can exacerbate gestational diabetes, bone loss, and hypertension. Splenectomy should be avoided, if at all possible, and deferred if necessary to the second trimester to avoid abortion. Danazol, cyclophosphamide, vinca alkaloids, and other potentially teratogenic therapy (with the possible exception of azathioprine) are also to be avoided. Experience with anti-D is limited but appears safe and effective (135). Therefore, IVIG tends to be used more commonly than in non-parous patients. Ideally, maternal platelet counts should be maintained above 30×10^9/L throughout pregnancy and above 50×10^9/L near term to minimize platelet transfusions (4,34,136).

Approximately 4% of neonates are born with profound thrombocytopenia (platelets $<20 \times 10^9$/L), but few have platelet counts below 5×10^9/L in the absence of concurrent alloantibodies (137). There may be a marked discrepancy between the neonatal and maternal platelet count. No antenatal measures reliably predict neonatal status and maternal response to intervention does not guarantee a favorable neonatal outcome. Only prior neonatal outcome provides a useful predictor of the neonatal platelet count in the subsequent pregnancy (138). The risk of intracranial hemorrhage is estimated to be less than 1%, which is likely less than that of percutaneous umbilical vein sampling in severely affected neonates (4,130). There is no evidence that this risk can be reduced by cesarean section (139) or maternal therapy, and current practice is not to alter the mode of delivery (4,130). Opinions vary concerning the minimal platelet count ($50–100 \times 10^9$/L) required for epidural anesthesia (4,140). ITP is not a contraindication to breast-feeding.

The platelet count should be measured in every neonate at birth and repeated during the first few days; the nadir often occurs two to five days post-delivery. An ultrasound of the head should be obtained to exclude intracranial hemorrhage in thrombocytopenic infants. IVIG and/or high-dose corticosteroids should be considered for neonates with platelet counts less than 30×10^9/L and certainly if there is evidence of bleeding. Platelet transfusions should be considered in the face of life-threatening hemorrhage or for severe thrombocytopenia if other risk factors for bleeding are present. Thrombocytopenia generally resolves within days to weeks.

ITP IN CHILDREN

Acute ITP

Childhood ITP is typically an acute, self-limited illness (141,142). Most affected children are young (peak age 5 yr) and in previous good health (143). In approximately two-thirds of cases, ITP occurs several days to a few weeks after an infectious illness, most often an upper respiratory tract infection (Table 1); a minority of cases are preceded by other viral illness, e.g., varicella, or immunization with a live virus vaccine (144). Physical examination is remarkable for the cutaneous manifestations of severe thrombocytopenia with bruising and petechiae present in almost all cases. Epistaxis is a presenting feature in approximately one-third of affected children; hematuria occurs less frequently. Significant lymphadenopathy or gross hepatosplenomegaly are atypical; however, the finding of small, mobile lymph nodes in the neck is not uncommon and a spleen tip may be palpable in 5 to 10% of cases (141,142). The key laboratory features of childhood

Table 1 Presenting Features in Children with Acute ITP

				Hemorrhagic manifestations		
Investigator	Number of cases	Male: female ratio	Preceding infectious illness	Purpura/ petechiae	Epistaxis	Hematuria
Lusher, J (141) (1956–1964)[a]	152	69:83	122/146	–	46/152	8/152
Choi, S (142) (1950–1964)	239	117:122	119/239	235/239	76/239	20/239
Blanchette, V[b]	80	37:43	58/80	75/80	20/80	3/80
	471	223:248	299/465 (64%)	310/319 (97%)	142/471 (30%)	31/471 (7%)

[a] Period of observation.

[b] Data for 80 consecutive newly diagnosed childhood ITP seen at the Children's Hospital of Eastern Ontario, Ottawa, Canada during the period 1974–1982 Unpublished observations.

acute ITP are the same as in adults with the exception of eosinophilia, which is a relatively common finding (141). In at least two-thirds of cases, platelet counts at presentation are $<20\times10^9$/L (Fig. 3) (142). The differential diagnosis includes primarily acute leukemia and aplastic anemia. Clues to these diagnoses include symptoms such as bone pain, presence of clinically significant hepatosplenomegaly and adenopathy, and the finding of anemia, neutropenia, atypical white blood cells, or macrocytosis for which there is not an obvious explanation (e.g., anemia secondary to epistaxis). A bone marrow aspirate should be performed in all such cases. A careful family history and a diligent search for exposure to medication are indicated.

Natural History of Childhood Acute ITP

The outcome of children with typical acute ITP is excellent. Approximately 75% of children will attain a complete remission (CR; a platelet count of $>150\times10^9$/L) within six months of initial diagnosis and without the need for platelet-enhancing therapy. This excellent outcome appears to be independent of management strategy. As an example, in a prospective study of 2190 children with newly diagnosed ITP, remission rates of 68%, 73%, and 66% were reported in children who received no treatment, IVIG, or corticosteroids, respectively (143). These data are similar to the 76% complete remission rate reported in a review of 12 case series involving 1597 children with acute ITP (34).

Management of Childhood ITP

Management of children with acute ITP is dominated by the long-standing and ongoing controversy "to treat or not to treat." The case for treatment relates to the very small but finite risk of intracranial hemorrhage (ICH), which is probably on the order of 1 per 500 cases (145). Approximately 40% of reported cases of ICH occurred within two weeks of diagnosis and affected children almost always had platelet counts of $<20\times10^9$/L (34,145,146). Head trauma, exposure to antiplatelet drugs such as aspirin (146), cerebral arteriovenous malformations, and coexisting vasculitis may place children with severe thrombocytopenia at greater risk for ICH. The case for non-treatment rests on the fact that acute ITP in children is a benign self-limited condition in the vast majority of cases, and there are no studies that clearly document a decrease in the incidence of ICH associated with treatment (80,147).

Since this debate cannot be resolved by a prospective clinical trial (the number of subjects required being prohibitively large), and because of the significant morbidity and mortality associated with ICH and the availability of highly effective platelet-enhancing therapies (discussed below), it is our recommendation that families of young children "at-risk" for ICH (those with platelet counts $<20\times10^9$/L) be offered the option of treatment using the minimum therapy necessary to rapidly increase the platelet count to a safe hemostatic level. It is important that recommendations regarding management take into consideration clinical symptoms in addition to cutaneous signs and not the platelet count alone. Recent recommendations from a Working Party of the British Committee for Standards in Hematology (General Hematology Task Force) considered it appropriate to manage a child with acute ITP and mild clinical disease expectantly, with supportive advice and a 24 hr contact point in all cases (4). Based on these guidelines, intervention would be reserved for overtly hemorrhagic children with platelet counts below 20×10^9/L, or those with organ or life-threatening bleeding irrespective of platelet count (4,148). This select non-interventionist approach is supported by other studies (149).

If treatment is given, the most rapid platelet responses are achieved with IVIG (150), although impressive responses occur with oral prednisone given in a dose of 4 mg/kg/day $\times$ 4 days (151) or, for Rhesus-positive subjects, anti-D in a dose of 75 μg/kg (47). Initial platelet responses to conventional dose oral corticosteroids (prednisone 1–2 mg/kg/day) appear to be slower, although these two corticosteroid regimens have not been compared in a prospective, randomized trial. A single dose of 0.8 g/kg IVIG is as effective as the traditional dose of 1.0 g/kg given daily for 2 consecutive days (152). Most would caution against use of anti-D if the starting hemoglobin level was < 100 g/dL. One factor influencing the choice of plasma-based therapies (IVIG, anti-D) over oral corticosteroids for initial treatment is the generally and often strongly held opinion among pediatric hematologists that a bone marrow aspirate should be obtained before starting corticosteroid therapy in order to avoid inappropriate treatment of a child with acute leukemia (153,154). However, the frequency of misdiagnosis is extremely low for children with a history, physical examination, and initial complete blood count typical for acute ITP (155,156).

As the debate "to treat or not to treat" remains unresolved (150), it is important that the risks, benefits, and alternative of observation alone be discussed with the parents/guardians and child, if of an appropriate age. The decision to hospitalize a child, with newly diagnosed ITP should take into consideration the history, findings on physical examination, initial platelet count, decision to treat, and whether a bone marrow aspirate will be performed. For those children not admitted, a point of contact to the health care facility should be provided and parents/children should be warned to avoid use of aspirin or other platelet inhibitory medications, as well as high-risk contact activities. Most children with acute ITP respond rapidly to minimal platelet-enhancing therapy or do well with observation alone (Fig. 2).

For those who fail such an approach, and especially those with clinically significant bleeding and platelet counts $< 20 \times 10^9$/L, a more aggressive management approach is warranted. Options include IVIG 1 g/kg/day for up to 2 consecutive days with or without high-dose corticosteroids often given in the form of intravenous methylprednisolone 30 mg/kg (to a maximum of 1 g) on three consecutive days (158). It should be cautioned, however, that platelet responses in

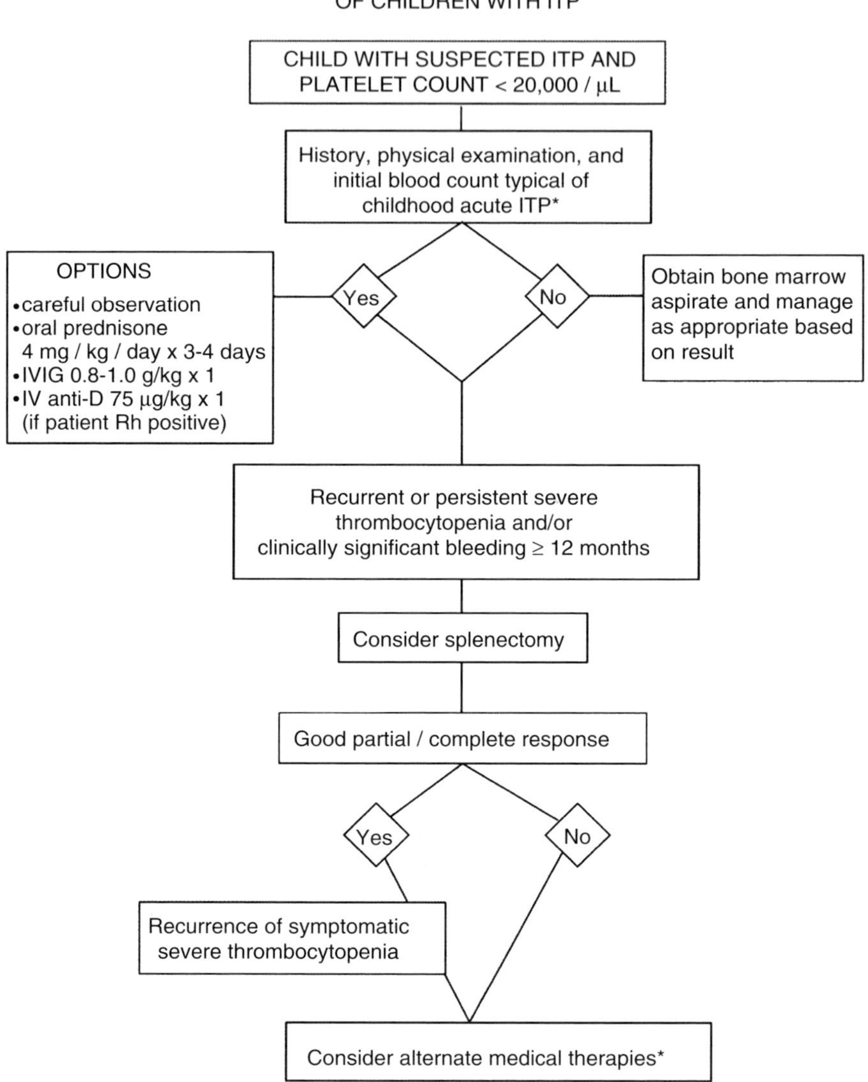

Figure 2 Treatment algorithm for managing childhood ITP.

this small subgroup are often suboptimal and may be delayed (159). In the case of life- or organ-threatening bleeding, a commonly used approach involves the immediate administration of a larger (2–3 fold) than usual infusion of donor platelets plus the intravenous administration of IV methylprednisolone 30 mg/kg (maximum dose 1 g/kg) over 20–30 min and IVIG (1 g/kg) daily as needed, generally for at least one to two days (55,158). There is anecdotal experience with recombinant factor VIIa (56). Emergency splenectomy may need to be considered if not previously performed.

Chronic ITP

Approximately 25% of an unselected cohort of children with acute ITP will have platelet counts of $<150\times10^9$/L six months after initial diagnosis and are considered to have chronic ITP (157). Predictors for chronicity include an insidious presentation and age greater than 10 years (160–162). The goal of therapy in these patients should be to maintain a hemostatically "safe" platelet count based on the circumstances present for the individual child while avoiding the potential toxicities and cost of overtreatment, in particular the well known adverse affects of protracted corticosteroid therapy. Our practice is to use either short courses of relatively high doses of oral prednisone (4 mg/kg/day for 4 days, maximum daily dose 180 mg), IVIG (0.8–1.0 g/kg once), or IV anti-D (75 μg/kg once) for children who are Rh positive with treatment given intermittently based on clinical need. Treatment is, in the main, out-patient-based and parents and children (if of an appropriate age) are counseled about benefits and alternatives to treatment as well as the risks, including the remote risk of transfusion-transmitted infection from virus-inactivated, plasma-based therapies such as IVIG and anti-D. The advantage of anti-D over IVIG in this setting relates to ease of administration (anti-D can be infused over 5–10 min as compared to several hours for IVIG), lower cost, and a comparable efficacy (46,163). Approximately 20–30% of children respond to pulsed high-dose oral dexamethasone (164,165). However, the regimen is commonly associated with prominent mood changes including irritability and sleep disturbances.

Approximately one-third of children with chronic ITP develop a spontaneous CR (34,157), most within six to 24 months of diagnosis and which are often preceded by a period of relatively stable mild to moderate thrombocytopenia not requiring platelet enhancing therapy. On the other hand, approximately 5% of children continue to have platelet counts of $<20\times10^9$/L six months from diagnosis and require ongoing treatment (Figs. 3 and 4) (142,166). The frequency of spontaneous, sustained CRs in this small subgroup of severely affected cases is unknown, but is, in our opinion, considerably less than 30–40% and splenectomy may need to be considered.

Splenectomy

Medical management is preferred over splenectomy for children who have had ITP for less than 12 months. In 1992, the British Paediatric Haematology

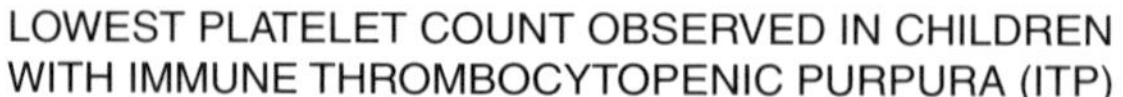

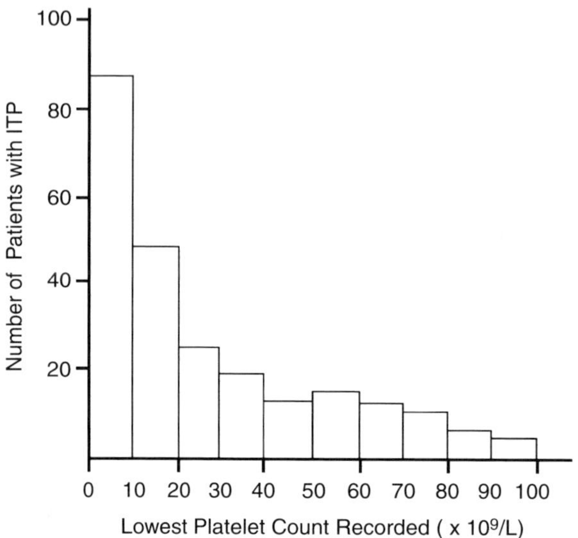

Figure 3 Lowest platelet count in 239 children with idiopathic thrombocytopenic purpura presenting to the Hospital for Sick Children (Toronto) during the period 1950–1964. *Source*: From Ref. 142.

Group, recommended that "splenectomy should not be considered before at least six months and preferably 12 months from the time of diagnosis, unless there are very major problems" (154). An update of these guidelines published in 2003 stated that splenectomy is rarely indicated in children with ITP and commented that: "severe lifestyle restrictions, crippling menorrhagia and life-threatening hemorrhage may give good reason for the procedure..." (4). Practice guidelines developed for the American Society of Hematology and published in 1996 are similarly conservative (34); the expert panel reached consensus on only selected indications for elective splenectomy in children with ITP, such as persistence of disease 12 months after diagnosis with bleeding symptoms and a platelet count of $<10\times10^9$/L (ages 3–12 yr) or $10–30\times10^9$/L (ages 8 to 12 yr). Other experts recommend splenectomy for children older than 5 years with symptomatic ITP of greater than 6 months duration whose quality of life is adversely affected by hemorrhagic manifestations, constant fear of bleeding, or complications of medical therapies (167). These guidelines reflect the significant rates of spontaneous remission that have been reported in children with chronic ITP, and the small but life-long risk of overwhelming sepsis post-splenectomy, a risk that is especially worrisome in children under six years of age.

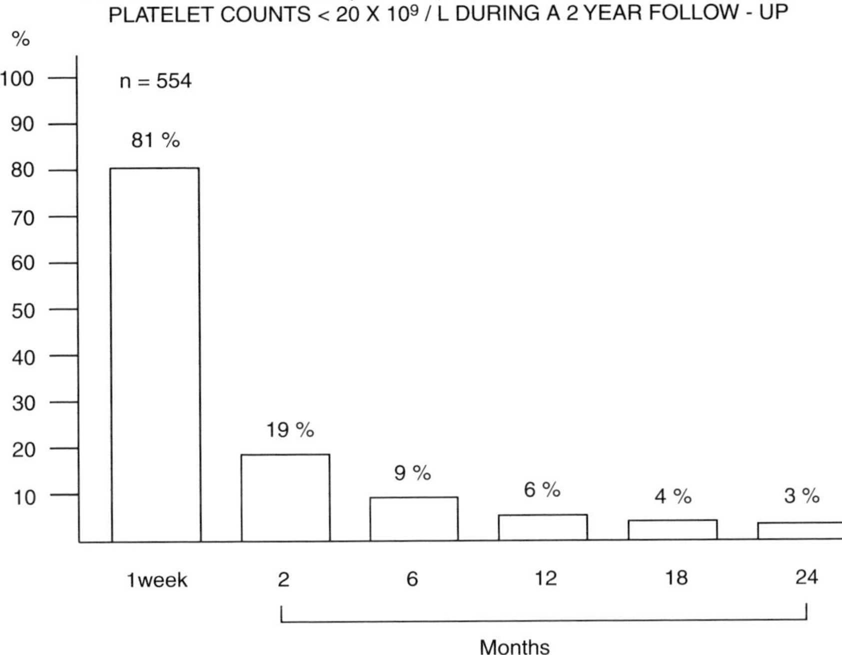

Figure 4 Percent of children (n = 554) with platelet counts below 20×10^9/L at 1 wk. and 2, 6, 12, 18 and 24 mo. following the diagnosis of acute ITP. *Source*: From Ref. 184.

Laparoscopic splenectomy is preferred in centers with an experienced surgeon (168,169). Advantages of laparoscopic over open splenectomy include reduced operative trauma, less post-operative pain, superior cosmetic outcome, earlier discharge from hospital (most within 48 hr), and the ability to resume normal activity within 7–10 days of the procedure (169). In skilled hands, the need to convert to an open approach is very small. Pre-operative treatment with corticosteroids, IVIG, or anti-D is appropriate to reduce the risk of intraoperative and/or post-operative bleeding if the platelet count is $<30\times 10^9$/L (34).

The outcome after splenectomy in children with primary ITP is good. Of 271 children reported in 16 case series, 72% achieved a CR (34). In our experience with 41 children, the incidence of initial and durable (>6 mo.) CR was 85% and 81%, respectively (160). Similar results have been reported by others (Table 2) (167,170). The role of partial splenectomy in selected cases merits further study (171). The results of imaging studies are insufficiently specific (68), and the reports of prior response to medical therapies too conflicting (172,173), to recommend that this information be used to determine whether or not a splenectomy should be performed.

Table 2 Complete Remission (CR) Rates Following Splenectomy in Children

	Number of cases	% CR
ASH review	271	72
Blanchette, V (1992) (160)	21	81
Ben-Yehuda D (1994) (170)	27	67
Mantadakis E (2000) (167)	38	76
	357	72.5 (259/357)

Protection Against Overwhelming Post-Splenectomy Infection

At least two weeks before elective splenectomy, patients should be immunized with Haemophilus influenzae type b and pneumococcal vaccines depending on their age and immunization history (72,73); meningococcal vaccine is also recommended. Because the protection provided by vaccines is incomplete, daily prophylaxis of penicillin (or an equivalent antibiotic if the child is allergic to penicillin) is recommended for patients up to five years of age for at least one year after splenectomy (174). Physicians in the United Kingdom recommend continuing antibiotic prophylaxis into adulthood (154). All febrile episodes should be carefully assessed, and the urgent use of parenteral antibiotics should be considered because overwhelming post-splenectomy infection can occur despite vaccination and antibiotic prophylaxis (175). An explanatory letter, a supply of antibiotics, and a Medic Alert bracelet may be helpful to patients when they are traveling.

Management of Post-Splenectomy Failures

Management of children with chronic ITP who fail to respond, or who relapse after splenectomy, and who manifest symptomatic, severe thrombocytopenia remains a challenge. Therapeutic options include corticosteroids and IVIG plus an extensive list of diverse therapies used singly or in combination. The sustained remission rate with monotherapy (azathioprine, 6-mercaptopurine, cyclophosphamide, vinca alkaloids, cyclosporine, danazol, colchicine, dapsone, ascorbic acid) is disappointing and controlled trials have not been performed (176). The response rate to anti-CD20 (rituximab) is encouraging and merits further study (177). Combination therapy may offer the potential of improved outcomes (178). In one study, 10 children (ages 10 to 18 yr) were treated with a combination of vincristine (1.5 mg/M^2/wk, maximum 2 mg/dose), IV methylprednisolone (100 mg/M^2/wk) and oral cyclosporine (5–7 mg/kg twice daily adjusted to a target cyclosporine trough level of 100–200 mg/mL) (179). Vincristine and methylprednisolone were given weekly until the platelet count was $>50 \times 10^9$/L (minimum 2 doses, maximum 4 doses). Cyclosporine was continued until the platelet count was normal for 3 to 6 mo in most patients. Four patients had Evans syndrome and 3 had been splenectomized. Continuous CRs were obtained in 7 patients and a partial response in 1; the median time to response was 7 days (range 7–67 days).

Childhood Chronic Secondary ITP

Management decisions in children with chronic secondary ITP present additional challenges. As a working rule, long-term treatment should be focused on the underlying conditions (e.g., antiretroviral therapy in cases of HIV associated ITP). Platelet enhancing therapies, singly or in combination, should be used in like manner to the treatment of chronic, primary ITP with the caveat that protracted use of corticosteroids should be avoided in children with immune deficiency disorders. The response rates may be lower than in children with multiple autoimmune cytopenias e.g., Evans' syndrome, than in primary ITP. An important, albeit very rare, cause of ITP in children is autoimmune lymphoproliferative syndrome (ALPS). The disorder is characterized by chronic, non-malignant proliferation of lymphoid tissues (lymphadenopathy, splenomegaly), autoimmune cytopenias, and an increased incidence of lymphomas (180,181). Key laboratory findings include hypergammaglobulinemia; increased circulating CD3 positive, CD4/CD8 negative T lymphocytes; elevated serum interleukin 10; and defective Fas-mediated programmed cells. Mutations in the Fas gene have been reported in the majority of affected subjects (182). Rarely, mutations in the Fas ligand or caspase 10 genes may cause APLS (181,182). The immunosuppressive agent mycophenalate mofetile (MMF) and the antimalarial drug pyrimethamine/sulfadoxine (112,181,182) or combination therapy with anti-CD20 and vincristine (183) has been used successfully to treat this rare, but often difficult to manage, condition.

REFERENCES

1. Cines DB, Blanchette V. Immune thrombocytopenic purpura. N Engl J Med 2002; 364:995–1008.
2. Frederiksen H, Schmidt K. The incidence of idiopathic thrombocytopenic purpura in adults increases with age. Blood 1999; 94:909–913.
3. George JN, el Harake MA, Aster RH. Thrombocytopenia due to enhanced platelet destruction by immunologic mechanisms. In: Beutler E, Lichtmann MA, Coller BA, Kipps TJ, eds. Williams Hematology. New York: McGraw-Hill, 1995:1315–1355.
4. Povan D, Newland A, Bolton-Maggs P, et al. Guidelines for the investigation and management of idiopathic thrombocytopenic purpura in adults, children and in pregnancy. Br J Haematol 2003; 120:574–596.
5. Neylon AJ, Saunders PWG, Howard MR, Proctor SJ, Taylor PRA, on behalf of the Nortner Regional Haematology Group. Clinically significant newly presenting autoimmune thrombocytopenic purpura in adults: a prospective study of a population-based cohort of 245 patients. Br J Haematol 2003; 122:966–974.

5a. Cines DB, R McMillian. Management of adult idiopathic thrombocytopenic purpura. Annu Rev Med 2005; 56:425–442.

5b. Cines DB, Bussel JB. How I treat Idiopathic thrombocytopenic purpura (ITP). Blood 2005; 106:2244–2251.

6. Stoll D, Cines DB, Aster RH, Murphy S. Platelet kinetics in patients with idiopathic thromobcytopenic purpura and moderate thrombocytopenia. Blood 1985; 65:584–588.
7. Heyns AP, Badenhorst PN, Lotter MG, Pieters H, Wessels P, Kotze HF. Platelet turnover and kinetics in immune thrombocytopenic purpura: results with autologous 111-In-labeled and homologous 51-Cr-labeled platelets differ. Blood 1986; 67:86–92.
8. Ballem PJ, Segal GM, Stratton JR, Gernsheimer T, Adamson JW, Slichter SJ. Mechanisms of thrombocytopenia in chronic autoimmune thrombocytopenic purpura: evidence of both impaired platelet production and increased platelet clearance. J Clin Investig 1987; 80:33–40.
9. McMillan R, Wang L, Tomer A, Nichol J, Pistillo J. Suppression of in vitro megakaryocyte production by antiplatelet autoantibodies from adult patients with chronic ITP. Blood 2004; 103:1364–1369.
10. Chang M, Nakagawa PA, Williams SA, et al. Immune thrombocytopenic purpura (ITP) plasma and purified ITP monoclonal autoantibodies inhibit megakaryopoieses in vitro. Blood 2003; 102:887–895.
11. Houwerzijl EJ, Blom NR, van der Want JJL, et al. Ultrastructural study shows morphological features of apoptosis and para-apoptosis in megakaryocytes from patients with idiopathic thrombocytopenic purpura. Blood 2003; 103:500–506.
12. Gernsheimer T, Stratton J, Ballem PJ, Slichter SJ. Mechanisms of response to treatment in autoimmune thrombocytopenic purpura. N Engl J Med 1989; 320:974–980.
13. Olsson B, Andersson P-O, Jernas M, Jacobsson S, Carlsson LMS, Wadenvik H. T-cell mediated cytotoxicity toward platelets in chronic idiopathic thrombocytopenic purpura. Nat Med 2003; 9:1123–1124.
14. Emmons RVB, Reid DM, Cohen RL, et al. Human thrombopoietin levels are high when thrombocytopenia is due to megakaryocyte deficiency and low when due to increased platelet destruction. Blood 1996; 87:4068–4071.
15. Kuwana M, Pokazaki Y, Kaburaki J, Ikeda Y. Detection of circulating B cells secreting platelet-specific autoantibody is useful in the diagnosis of autoimmune thrombocytopenia. Am J Med 2003; 114:322–325.
16. McMillan R. Autoantibodies and autoantigens in chronic immune thrombocytopenic purpura. Semin Hematol 2000; 2000:239–248.
17. He R, Reid DM, Jones CE, Shulman NR. Spectrum of Ig classes, specificities, and titers of serum glycoproteins in chronic idiopathic thrombocytopenic purpura. Blood 1994; 83:1924–1932.
18. McMillan R, Lopez-Dee J, Bowditch R. Clonal restriction of platelet-associated anti-gpIIb/IIIa autoantibodies in patients with chronic ITP. Thromb Haemost 2001; 85:821–823.
19. Bussel J, Wissert M, Oates B, Scaramucci J, Nadeau K, Adelman B. Humanized monoclonal anti-CD40 ligand antibody (hu5c8) rescue therapy of 15 adults with severe chronic refractory ITP. Blood 1999; 96:646a.
20. Roarke J, Bussel JB, Cines DB, Siegel DL. Genetic analysis of autoantibodies idiopathic thrombocytopenic purpura reveals evidence of clonal expansion and somatic mutation. Blood 2000; 100:1388–1398.

21. Filion MC, Proulx C, Bradley AJ, et al. Presence in peripheral blood of healthy individuals to a membrane antigen present on bone marrow-derived cells. Blood 1996; 88:2144–2150.
22. Kuwana M, Kaburaki J, Ikeda Y. Autoreactive T cells to platelet GPIIb-IIIa in immune thrombocytopenic purpura. Role in production of anti-platelet autoantibody. J Clin Investig 1998; 102:1393–1402.
23. Solanilla A, Pasquet JM, Viallard JF, et al. Platelet-associated CD154 in immune thrombocytopenic purpura. Blood 2005; 105:215–218.
24. Panitsas FP, Theodoropoulou M, Kouraklis A, et al. Adult chronic idiopathic thrombocytopenic purpura (ITP) is the manifestation of a type-1 polarized immune response. Blood 2004; 103:2645–2647.
25. Andersson P-O, Olsson A, Wadenvik H. Reduced transforming growth factor-b1 production by mononuclear cells from patients with active chronic idiopathic thrombocytopenic purpura. Br J Haematol 2002; 116:862–867.
26. Semple JW, Milev Y, Cosgrave D, et al. Differences in serum cytokine levels in acute and chronic autoimmune thrombocytopenic purpura: relationship to platelet phenotype and antiplatelet T-cell reactivity. Blood 1996; 87:4245–4254.
27. Mouzaki A, Theodoropoulou M, Gianakopoulos I, Vlaha V, Kyrtsonis M, Maniatis A. Expression patterns of Th1 and Th2 cytokine genes in childhood idiopathic thrombocytopenic purpura (ITP) at presentation and their modulation by intravenous immunoglobulin G (IVIg) treatment: their role in prognosis. Blood 2002; 100:1774–1779.
28. Peng J, Liu C, Liu D, et al. Effects of B7-blocking agent and/or CsA on induction of platelet-specific T-cell anergy in chronic autoimmune thrombocytopenia purpura. Blood 2003; 101:2721–2726.
29. Kuwana M, Okazaki Y, Kabukari J, Kawakami Y, Ikeda Y. Spleen is the primary site for activation of platelet-reactive T and B cells in patients with immune thrombocytopenic purpura. J Immunol 2002; 168:3675–3682.
30. Doan CA, Bouroncle BA, Wiseman BK. Idiopathic and secondary thrombocytopenic purpura: clinical study and evaluation of 381 cases over a period of 28 years. Ann Intern Med 1960; 53:861–876.
31. Mueller-Eckhardt C. Idiopathic thrombocytopenic purpura. Clinincal and immunologic considerations. Semin Thromb Hemost 1977; 3:125–162.
32. Bizzao N. EDTA-dependent pseudothrombocytopenia: A clinical and epidemiological study of 112 cases, with 10 year follow-up. Am J Hematol 1995; 50:103–109.
33. Drachman JG. Inherited thrombocytopenia: when a low platelet count does not mean ITP. Blood 2004; 103:390–398.
34. George JN, Woolf SH, Raskob GE, et al. Idiopathic thrombocytopenic purpura: A practice guideline developed by explicit methods for the American Society of Hematology. Blood 1996; 88:3–46.
35. Hoxie JA. Heamtologic manifestations of HIV infection. In: Hoffman R, Benz EJ, Jr., Shattil SJ et al, eds. Hematology: Basic Principals and Practice. Philadelphia: Churchill Livingstone, 2000:2430–2458.
36. Zhang L, Li H, Zhao H, Ji L, Yang R. Hepatitits C virus-related adult chronic idiopathic thrombocytopenic purpura: experience from a single Chinese center. Eur J Haematol 2004; 70:196–197.

37. Streiff MB, Mehta S, Thomas DL. Peripheral blood count abnormalities among patients with hepatitis C in the United States. Hepatology 2002; 35:947–952.
38. Diz-Kucukkaya R, Hacihanefioglu A, Yeneri M, et al. Antiphospholipid antibodies and antiphospholipid syndrome in patients presenting with immune thrombocyopenic purpura: a prospective cohort study. Blood 2001; 98:1760–1764.
39. Chong BH, Keng TB. Advances in the diagnosis of idiopathic thrombocytopenic purpura. Semin Hematol 2000; 37:249–260.
40. Brighton TA, Evans S, Castaldi PA, Chesterman CN, Chong BH. Prospective evaluation of usefulness of an antigen-specific assay (MAIPA) in idiopathic thrombocytopenic purpura and other immune thrombocytopenia. Blood 1996; 88:194–201.
41. Warner MN, Moore JC, Warkentin TE, Santos AV, Kelton JG. A prospective study of protein-specific assays used to investigate idiopathic thrombocytopenic purpura. Br J Haematol 1999; 104:442–447.
42. Berchtold P, Muller D, Beardsley D, et al. International study to compare antigen-specific methods used for the measurement of antiplatelet autoantibodies. Br J Haematol 1997; 96:477–481.
43. Raife TJ, Olseon JD, Lentz SR. Platelet antibody testing in idiopathic thrombocytopenic purpura. Blood 1996; 88:1112–1113.
44. Taub JW, Warrier I, Holtkamp C, Beardsley DS, Lusher JM. Characterization of autoantibodies against the platelet glycoproteins IIb/IIIa in childhood idiopathic thrombocytopenic purpura. Am J Hematol 1995; 48:104–107.
45. Imbach P, Kuhne T. Sequelae of treatment of ITP with anti-D (Rho) immunoglobulin. Lancet 2000; 356:447–448.
46. Scaradavou A, Woo B, Woloski BMR, et al. Intravenous anti-D treatment of immune thrombocytopenic purpura: experience in 272 patients. Blood 1997; 89:2689–2700.
47. Newman GC, Novoa MV, Fodero EM, Lesser ML, Woloski BMR, Bussel JB. A dose of 75 μg/kg/d of IV anti-D increases the platelet count more rapidly and for a longer period of time that does 50 μg/kg/d in adults with immune thrombocytopenic purpura (ITP). Br J Haematol 2001; 112:1076–1078.
48. Gaines AR. Acute onset of hemoglobinemia and/or hemoglobinuria and sequelae following Rho(D) immune globulin intravenous administration in immune thrombocytopenic purpura patients. Blood 2000; 95:2523–2529.
48a. Gaines AR. Disseminated intravascular coagulation associated with acute hemoglobinemia or hemoglobinuria following Rho(D) Immune globulin intravenous administration for Immune thrombocytopenic pupura. Blood 2005; 106:1532–15377.
49. Bussel JB, Fitzgerald-Pedersen J, Feldman C. Alternation of two doses of intravenous gammaglobulin in the maintenance treatment of patients with immune thrombocytopenic purpura. Am J Hematol 1990; 33:184–188.
50. Cheng Y, Wong RSM, Soo YOY, et al. Initial treatment of immune thrombocyopenic purpura with high-dose dexamethasone. N Engl J Med 2003; 349:831–836.
51. Akoglu T, Paydas S, Bayik M, Lawrence R, Firatli T. Megadose methylprednisolone pulse therapy in adult idiopathic thrombocytopenic purpura. Lancet 1991; 337:56.
52. von dem Borne AEGK, Vos JJE, Pegels JG, Thomas LLM, van der Lelie H. High dose intravenous methylprednisolone or high dose intravenous gammaglobulin for autoimmune thrombocytopenia. Br Med J 1988; 296:249–260.

53. Lacey JV, Penner JA. Management of idiopathic thrombocytopenic purpura in the adult. Semin Thromb Hemost 1977; 3:160–174.
54. Carr AM, Kruskal M, Kaye J, Robinson S. Efficacy of platelet transfusions in immune thrombocytopenia. Am J Med 1986; 80:1051–1054.
55. Baumann MA, Menitove JE, Aster RH, Anderson T. Urgent treatment of idiopathic thrombocytopenic purpura with single-dose gammaglobulin infusion followed by platelet transfusion. Ann Intern Med 1986; 104:808–809.
56. Culic S. Recombinant Factor VIIa for refractory haemorrhage in autoimmune idiopathic thrombocytopenic purpura. Br J Haematol 2003; 120:909–910.
57. McMillan R. Therapy for adults with refractory chronic immune thrombocytopenic purpura. Ann Intern Med 1997; 126:307–314.
58. den Ottolander GJ, Gratama JW, de Koning J, Brand A. Long-term follow-up study of 168 patients with immune thrombocytopenic purpura. Scand J Haematol 1984; 32:101–110.
59. DiFino SM, Lachant NA, Kirshner JJ, Gottlieb AJ. Adult idiopathic thrombocytopenic purpura: clinical findings and response to therapy. Am J Med 1980; 69:430–442.
60. den Ottolander GJ, Gratama JW, de Koning J, Brand A. Long-term follow-up study of 168 patients with immune thrombocytopenia: implications for therapy. Scand J Haematol 1984; 32:101–110.
61. Cooper N, Woloski BMR, Fodero EM, Novoa M, Leber M, Bussel JB. Does treatment with intermittent infusions of IV anti-D allow a proportion of adults with recently diagnosed immune thrombocytopenic purpura (ITP) to avoid splenectomy? Blood 2002; 99:1922–1927.
62. George JN, Raskob GE, Vesely SK, et al. Initial management of immune thrombocytopenic purpura in adults: a randomized controlled trial comparing intermittent anti-D with routine care. Am J Hematol 2003; 74:161–169.
63. Fabris F, Tassan T, Ramon R, et al. Age as the major predictor of long-term response to splenectomy in immune thrombocytopenic purpura. Br J Haematol 2001; 112:637–640.
64. Radaelli F, Faccini P, Goldaniga M, et al. Factors predicting response to splenectomy in adult patients with idiopathic thrombocytopenic purpura. Haematologia 2002; 85:1040–1044.
64a. Kojouri K, Vesely SK, Terrell DR, George JN. Splenectomy for adult patients with Idlopathic thrombocytopenic purpura: a systematic review to assess long-term platelet count responses, prediction of response, and surgical complications. Blood 2004; 104:2623–2634.
65. Stasi R, Stipa E, Masi M, et al. Long-term observation of 208 adults with chronic idiopathic thrombocytopenic purpura. Am J Med 1995; 98:436–442.
66. Kojouri K, Vesely SK, Terrell DR, George JN. Splenectomy for adult patients with idiopathic thrombocytopenic purpura: a systematic review to assess long-term platelet count responses, prediction of response, and surgical complications. Blood 2004; 104:2623–2634.
67. Bussel J, Cines DB. Idiopathic thrombocytopenic purpura, neonatal alloimmune thrombocytopenia, and post-transfusion purpura. In: Hoffman R, Benz EJ, Jr., Shattil SJ et al., eds. Hematology: Basic Principals and Practice. Philadelphia: Churchill Livingstone, 2004:2269–2286.

68. Najean Y, Rain J-D, Billotey C. The site of destruction of autoloogous ^{111}In-labelled platelets and the efficiency of splenectomy in children and adults with idiopathic thrombocytopenic purpura: a study of 568 patients with 268 splenectomies. Br J Haematol 1997; 97:547–550.
69. Marcaccio MJ. Laparoscopic splenectomy in chronic idiopathic thrombocytopenic purpura. Semin Hematol 2000; 37:267–274.
70. Calverley DC, Jones GW, Kelton JG. Splenic radiation for corticosteroid-resistant immune thrombocytopenia. Ann Intern Med 1992; 116:977–981.
71. Lortan JE. Management of asplenic patients. Br J Haematol 1993; 84:566–569.
72. American Academy of Pediatrics. Committee on Infectious Diseases. Recommendations of the advisory committee on immunization practices (ACIP): use of vaccines and immune globulins in persons with altered immunocompetence. MMWR 1993; 42:1–11.
73. American Academy of Pediatrics. Committee on Infectious Diseases. Recommendations for the prevention of pneumococcal infections, including the use of pneumococcal conjugate vaccine (Prevnar), pneumococcal polysaccharide vaccine, and antibiotic prophylaxis. Pediatrics 2000; 106:362–366.
74. Bourgeois E, Caulier MT, Delarozee C, Brouillard M, Bauters F, Fenaux P. Long-term follow-up of chronic autoimmune thrombocytopenic purpura refractory to splenectomy: a prospective analysis. Br J Haematol 2003; 120:1079–1088.
75. McMillan R, Durette C. Long-term outcomes in adults with chronic ITP after splenectomy failure. Blood 2004; 104:956–960.
76. Berchtold P, McMillan R. Therapy of chronic idiopathic thrombocytopenic purpura in adults. Blood 1989; 74:2309–2317.
77. Cohen YC, Djulbegovic B, Shamai-Lubovitz O, Mozes B. The bleeding risk and natural history of idiopathic thrombocytopenic purpura in patients with persistent low platelet counts. Arch Int Med 2000; 160:1630–1638.
78. Cortelazzo S, Finazzi G, Buelli M, Molteni A, Viero P, Barbui T. High risk of severe bleeding in aged patients with chronic idiopathic thrombocytopenic purpura. Blood 1991; 77:31–33.
79. Gutherie TH, Brannan DP, Prisant LM. Idiopathic thrombocytopenic purpura in the older patient. Am J Med Sci 1988; 296:17–21.
80. Lee MS, Kim WC. Intracranial hemorrhage associated with idiopathic thrombocytopenic purpura: Report of seven patients and a meta-analysis. Neurology 1998; 50:1160–1163.
81. Portiejle JEA, Westendorp RGJ, Kluin-Nelemans HC, Brand A. Morbidity and mortality in adults with idiopathic thrombocytopenic purpura. Blood 2001; 97:2549–2554.
82. Bussel JB, Pham LC. Intravenous treatment with gammaglobulin in adults with immune thrombocytopenic purpura: review of the literature. Vox Sanguinis 1987; 51:264–269.
83. Bussel J. Intravenous immunoglobulin therapy for treatment of idiopathic thrombocytopenic purpura. Prog Thromb Hemost 1986; 8:103–125.
84. Bussel JB, Kimberly RP, Inman RD, et al. Intravenous gammaglobulin treatment of chronic idiopathic thrombocytopenic purpura. Blood 1983; 62:480–486.

85. Fehr J, Hoffman V, Kappeler U. Transient reversal of thrombocytopenia in idiopathic thrombocytopenic purpura by high dose intravenous immunoglobulin. N Engl J Med 1982; 306:1242–1258.
86. Samuelsson A, Towers TL, Ravetch JV. Anti-inflammatory activity of IVIG mediated through the inhibitory Fc receptor. Science 2001; 291:484–486.
87. Crow AR, Song S, Freedman J, et al. IVIg-mediated amelioration of murine ITP via FcγRIIB is indepdent of SHIP1, SHP-1, and Btk activity. Blood 2003; 102:558–560.
88. Siragam V, Brinc D, Crow AR, Song S, Freedman J, Lazarus AH. Can antibodies with specificity for soluble antigens mimic the therapeutic effects of intravenous IgG in the treatment of autoimmune disease? J Clin Investig 2005; 115:155–160.
89. Vera-Ramirez M, Charlet M, Parry GJ. Recurrent aseptic meningitis complicating intravenous immunoglobulin therapy for chronic inflammatory demyelinating polyradiculoneuropathy. Neurology 1992; 42:1636–1637.
90. Woodruff RK, Grigg AP, Firkin FC, Smith IL. Fatal thrombotic events during treatment of autoimmune thrombocytopenia with intravenous immunoglobulin in elderly patients. Lancet 1986; 2:217–218.
91. Rault R, Piraino B, Johnston JR, Oral A. Pulmonary and renal toxicity of intravenous immunoglobulin. Clin Nephrol 1991; 36:83–86.
92. Burks AW, Sampson HA, Buckley RH. Anaphylactic reactions after gamma globulin administration in patients with hypogammaglobulinemia. Detection of IgE antibodies to IgA. N Engl J Med 1986; 314:560–564.
93. Cunningham-Rundles C, Zhou C, McKarious S, Courter S. Long term use of IgA-depleted intravenous immunoglobulin in immunodeficiency subjects with anti-IgA antibodies. J Clin Immunol 1992; 13:271–278.
94. Garcia L, Huh YO, Fisher HE, Lichtiger B. Positive immunohematologic and serologic test results due to high-dose intravenous immune globulin administration. Transfusion 1987; 27:503.
95. Copelan EA, Strohm PL, Kennedy MS, Tutschka PJ. Hemolysis following intravenous immune globulin therapy. Transfusion 1986; 26:410–412.
96. Potter M, Stockley R, Storry J, SLade R. ABO alloimunization after intravenous immunoglobulin infusion. Lancet 1988; 1:932–933.
97. Rudowski WJ. Accessory spleens: clinical significance with particular reference to the recurrence of idiopathic thrombocytopenic purpura. World J Surg 1985; 9:422–430.
98. Ahn YS, Rocha R, Mylvaganam R, Garcia R, Duncan R, Harrington WJ. Long-term danazol therapy in autoimmune thrombocytopenia: Unmaintained remission and age-dependent response in women. Ann Intern Med 1989; 111:723–729.
99. Godeau B, Durand J-M, Roudot-Thoraval F, et al. Dapsone for chronic autoimmune thrombocytopenic purpura: a report of 66 cases. Br J Haematol 1997; 97:336–339.
100. Facon T, Caulier MT, Wattel E, Jouet JP, Auters F, Fenaux P. A randomized trial comparing vinblastine in slow infusion and by bolus i.v. injection in idiopathic thrombocytopenic purpura: a report on 42 patients. Br J Haematol 1994; 86:678–680.
101. Snyder HW, Jr., Cochran SK, Balint JP, Jr., et al. Experience with Protein A-Immunoadsorption in treatment-resistant adult immune thrombocytopenic purpura. Blood 1992; 79:2237–2245.

102. Stasi R, Pagano A, Stipa E, Amadori S. Rituximab chimeric anti-CD20 monoclonal antibody treatment for adults with chronic idiopathic thrombocytopenic purpura. Blood 2001; 98:952–957.
103. Dunkley SM, Manoharan A, Kwan YL. Variable patterns of response to rituximab treatment in adults with chronic idiopathic thrombocytopenic purpura. Blood 2002; 99:3872–3873.
104. Giagounidis AAN, Anhuf J, Schneider P, et al. Treatment of relapsed idiopathic thrombocytopenic purpura with the anti-CD20 monoclonal antibody rituximab: a pilot study. Eur J Haematol 2002; 69:95–100.
105. Hedge U, Wilson W, White T, Cheson B. Rituximab treatment of refractory fludarabine-associated immune thrombocytopenia in chronic lymphocytic leukemia. Blood 2002; 100:2260–2262.
106. Quiquandon I, Fenaux P, Caulier MT, Pagniez D, Huart JJ, Bauters F. Re-evaluation of the role of azathioprine in the treatment of adult chronic idiopathic thrombocytopenic purpura: a report on 53 cases. Br J Haematol 1990; 74:223–228.
107. Pizzuto J, Ambriz R. Therapeutic experience on 934 adults with idiopathic thrombocytopenic purpura: Multicentric trial of the cooperative Latin American Group on Hemostasis and Thrombosis. Blood 1984; 64:1179–1183.
108. Verlin M, Laros RK, Jr., Penner JA. Treatment of refractory thrombocytopenic purpura with cyclophosphamide. Am J Hematol 1976; 1:97–104.
109. Figueroa M, Gehlsen J, Hammond D, et al. Combination chemotherapy in refractory immune thrombocytopenic purpura. N Engl J Med 1993; 328:1226–1229.
110. Webert KE, Kelton F, Coull D, Hayward CPM, Warkentin TE, Kelton JG. Treatment of chronic refractory idiopathic thrombocytopenic purpura with cyclophosphamide and cyclosporine. Blood 2000; 96:253a.
111. Kappers-Klunne MC, van't Veer MB. Cyclosporin A for the treatment of patients with chronic idiopathic thrombocytopenia purpura refractory to corticosteroids or splenectomy. Br J Haematol 2001; 114:121–125.
112. Howard J, Hoffbrand AV, Prentice HG, Mehta A. Mycophenolate mofetil for the treatment of refractory auto-immune haemolytic anemia and auto-immune thrombocytopenia purpura. Br J Haematol 2002; 117:712–715.
113. Hou P, Pang J, Shi Y, et al. Mycophenylate mofetil (MMF) for the treatment of steroid-resistant idiopathic thrombocytopenic purpura. Eur J Haematol 2003; 70:353–357.
114. McMinn JJ, Cohen S, Moore J, et al. Complete recovery from immune thrombocytopenic purpura in three patients treated with etanercept. Am J Hematol 2003; 73:135–140.
115. Kuwana M, Nomura S, Fujimura K, et al. Effect of a single injection of humanized anti-CD154 monoclonal antibody on the platelet-specific autoimmune response in patients with immune thrombocytopenic purpura. Blood 2004; 103:1229–1236.
116. Nomura S, Kazuo D, Tomomitsu H, Fujimura K, Ikeda Y. Effects of pegylated recombinant human megakaryocyte growth and development factor in patients with idiopathic thrombocytopenic purpura. Blood 2002; 100:728–730.

117. Kuter D, Bussel JB, Aledort LM, et al. A phase 2 placebo controlled study evaluating the platelet response and safety of weekly dosing with a novel thrombopoietic potein (AMG531) in thrombocytopenic adult patients (pts) with immune thrombocytopenic purpura (ITP). Blood 2004; 114:148a.
118. Newland A, Caulier MT, Schipperus MR, et al. An open-label, unit dose-finding study evaluating the safety and platelet response of a novel thrombopoietic protein (AMG531) in thrombocytopenic adult patients (pts) with immune thrombocytopenic purpura (ITP). Blood 2004; 104:567a.
119. Huhn RD, Fogarty PF, Nakamura R, et al. High-dose cyclophosphamide with autologous lymphocyte-depleted peripheral blood (PBSC) support for treatment of refractory chronic autoimmune thrombocytopenia. Blood 2002; 101:71–77.
120. Bussel JB, Mukherjee R, Stone AJ. A pilot study of rhuIL-11 treatment of refractory ITP. Am J Hematol 2001; 66:172–177.
121. Emilia G, Longo G, Luppi M, et al. *Heliobacter pylori* eradication can induce platelet recovery in idiopathic thrombocytopenic purpura. Blood 2001; 97:812–814.
122. Jarque I, Andreu R, Llopis I, et al. Absence of platelet response after eradication of *Helicobacter pylori* infection in patients with chronic idiopathic thrombocytopenic purpura. Br J Haematol 2001; 115:1002–1003.
123. Kohda K, Kuga T, Kogawa K, et al. Effect of Helicobacter pylori eradication on platelet recovery in Japanese patients with chronic idiopathic thrombocytopenic purpura and secondary autoimmune thrombocytopenic purpura. Br J Haematol 2002; 118:584–588.
124. Michel M, Khellaf M, Desforges L, et al. Autoimmune thrombocytopenic purpura and *Helicobactor* pylori infection. Arch Intern Med 2002; 162:1033–1036.
125. Rajantie J, Klemola T. *Heliobactor pylori* and idiopathic thrombocytopenic purpura in children. Blood 2003; 101:1660.
126. Hino M, Yamani T, Park K, et al. Platelet recovery after eradication of *Helicobacter pylori* in patients with idiopathic thrombocytopenic purpura. Ann Hematol 2003; 82:30–32.
127. Michel M, Cooper N, Jean C, Frissora C, Bussel JB. Does *Helicobacter pylori* initiate or perpetuate immune thrombocytopenic purpura. Blood 2003; 103:890–896.
128. Pockros PJ, Duchini A, McMillan R, Nyberg LM, McHutchison J, Viernes E. Immune thrombocytopenic purpura in patients with chronic hepatitis C infection. Am J Gastroenterol 2002; 97:2040–2045.
129. Sakuyara M, Murakami H, Uchiumi H, et al. Steroid-refractory chronic idiopathic thrombocytopenic purpura associated with hepatitis C virus infection. Eur J Haematol 2002; 68:48–53.
130. Gill KK, Kelton JG. Management of idiopathic thrombocytopenic purpura in pregnancy. Semin Hematol 2000; 37:275–289.
131. Fujimura K, Harada Y, Fujimoto T, et al. Nationwide study of idiopathic thrombocytopenic purpura in pregnant women and the clinical influence on neonates. Int J Hematol 2001; 75:426–433.
132. Webert KE, Mittal R, Sigouin C, Heddle NM, Kelton JG. A retrospective, 11-year analysis of obstetrical patients with idiopathic thrombocytopenic purpura. Blood 2003; 102:4306–4311.

133. McCrae KR, Samuels P, Schreiber AD. Pregnancy-associated thrombocytopenia: Pathogenesis and management. Blood 1992; 80:2697–2714.
134. Burrows RF, Kelton JG. Fetal thrombocytopenia and its relation to maternal thrombocytopenia. N Engl J Med 1993; 329:1463–1466.
135. Michel M, Novoa MV, Bussel JB. Intravenous anti-D as a treatment for immune thrombocytopenic purpura (ITP) during pregnancy. Br J Haematol 2003; 123:142–146.
136. Letsky EA, Greaves M. Guidelines on the investigation and management of thrombocytopenia in pregnancy and neonatal alloimmune thrombocytopenia. Br J Haematol 1996; 95:21–26.
137. Burrows RF, Kelton JG. Pregnancy in patients with idiopathic thrombocytopenic purpura: Assessing the risks for the infant at delivery. Obstet Gynecol Survey 1993; 46:781–788.
138. Christiaens GCML, Niewenhuis HK, Bussel JB. Comparison of platelet counts in first and second newborns of mothers with immune thrombocytopenic purpura. Obstet Gynecol 1997; 97:893–898.
139. Payne SD, Resnik R, Moore TR, Hedriana HL, Kelly TF. Maternal characteristics and risk of severe neonatal thrombocytopenia and intracranial hemorrhage in pregnancies complicated by autoimmune thrombocytopenia. Am J Obstet Gynecol 1997; 177:149–155.
140. Beilin Y, Zahn J, Comerford M. Safe epidural analgesia in thirty parturients with platelet counts between 69,000 and 98,000 mm^{-3}. Anesthesia and Analgesia 1997; 85:385–388.
141. Lusher JM, Zueltzer WW. Idiopathic thrombocytopenic purpura in childhood. J Pediatr 1966; 68:971–978.
142. Choi SI, McClure PD. Idiopathic thrombocytopenic purpura in childhood. Can Med Assoc J 1967; 97:562–568.
143. Kuhne T, Imbach P, Bolton-Maggs PHB, et al. Newly diagnosed idiopathic thromboctyopenic purpura in childhood: an observational study. Lancet 2001; 358:2122–2125.
144. Miller E, Waight P, Farrington P, Andrews N, Stowe J, Taylor B. Idiopathic thrombocytopenic purpura and MMR vaccine. Arch Dis Childhood 2001; 84:224.
145. Lilleyman JS. Intracranial haemorrhage in idiopathic thrombocytopenic purpura. Arch Dis Childhood 1994; 71:251–253.
146. Woerner SJ, Abildgaard CF, French BN. Intracranial hemorrhage in children with idiopathic thrombocytopenic purpura. Pediatrics 1981; 67:453–460.
147. Bolton-Maggs PHB, Dickerhoff R, Vora AJ. The nontreatment of childhood ITP (or "The art of medicine consists of amusing the patient until nature cures the disease"). Semin Thromb Hemost 2001; 27:269–275.
148. Lilleyman JS. Management of childhood idiopathic thrombocytopenic purpura. Br J Haematol 1999; 105:871–875.
149. Dickeroff R, von Ruecker A. The clinical course of immune thrombocytopenic pupura in children who did not receive intravenous immune globulins or sustained prednisone treatment. J Pediatr 2000; 137:629–632.
150. Blanchette VS, Carcao M. Childhood acute immune thrombocytopenic purpura: 20 years later. Semin Thromb Hemost 2003; 29:605–617.

151. Carcao MD, Zipursky A, Butchart S, Leaker M, Blanchette VS. Short-course oral prednisone therapy in children presenting with acute immune thrombocytopenic purpura (ITP). Acta Paediatr Suppl 1998; 484:71–74.
152. Blanchette V, Imbach P, Andrew M, et al. Randomized trial of intravenous immunoglobulin G, intravenous anti-D and oral prednisone in childhood acute immune thrombocytopenic purpura. Lancet 1994; 344:703–706.
153. Dubansky AS, Oski FA. Controversies in the management of acute idiopathic thrombocytopenic purpura: a survey of specialists. Pediatrics 1986; 77:49–52.
154. Eden OB, Lilleyman JS. Guidelines for management of idiopathic thrombocytopenic purpura. Arch Dis Children 1992; 67:1056–1058.
155. Halperin DS, Doyle JJ. Is bone marrow examination justified in idiopathic thrombocytopenic purpura? Am J Dis Childhood 1988; 142:508–511.
156. Calpin C, Dick P, Foon A, Feldman W. Is bone marrow aspiration needed in acute childhood idiopathic thrombocytopenic purpura to rule out leukemia? Arch Pediatr Adolescent Med 1998; 152:345–347.
157. Blanchette VS, Price V. Childhood chronic immune thrombocytopenic purpura: unresolved issues. J Pediatr Hematol Oncol 2003; 25:S28–S33.
158. van Hoff J, Ritchey AK. Pulse methylprednisolone therapy for acute childhood idiopathic thrombocytopenic purpura. J Pediatr 1988; 113:563–566.
159. Medeiros D, Buchanan GR. Major hemorrhage in children with idiopathic thrombocytopenic purpura: immediate response to therapy and long-term outcome. J Pediatr 1998; 133:334–339.
160. Blanchette VS, Kirby MA, Turner C. Role of intravenous immunoglobulin G in autoimmune hematologic disorders. Semin Hematol 1992; 29:72–82.
161. Simons SM, Main CA, Yaish HM, Rutzky J. Idiopathic thrombocytopenic purpura in children. J Pediatr 1975; 87:216–225.
162. Robb LG, Tiederman K. Idiopathic thrombocytopenic purpura: predictors of chronic disease. Arch Dis Childhood 1990; 65:502–506.
163. Andrew M, Blanchette VS, Adams M, Ali K, Bernard D, Chan KW. A multicenter study of the treatment of childhood chronic idiopathic thrombocytopenic purpura with anti-D. J Pediatr 1992; 120:522–527.
164. Kuhne T, Freedman J, Semple JW, Doyle J, Butchart S, Blanchette VS. Platelet and immune responses to oral cyclic dexamethasone therapy in childhood chronic immune thrombocytopenic purpura. J Pediatr 1997; 19:526–529.
165. Hedlund-Treutiger I, Henter JI, Elinder G. Randomized study of IVIg and high-dose dexamethasone therapy for children with chronic idiopathic thrombocytopenic purpura. J Pediatr Hematol/Oncol 2003; 25:139–144.
166. Lusher JM, Rathi I. Idiopathic thrombocytopenic purpura in children. Semin Thromb Hemost 1977; 3:175–199.
167. Mantadakis E, Buchanan GR. Elective splenectomy in children with idiopathic thrombocytopenic purpura. J Pediatr Hematol/Oncol 2000; 22:148–153.
168. Park A, Heniford BT, Hebra A, Fitzgerald P. Pediatric laparoscopic splenectomy. Surg Endosc 2000; 14:527–531.
169. Szold A, Schwartz J, Abu-Abeid S, Bulvik S, Eldor A. Laparoscopic splenectomies for idiopathic thrombocytopenic purpura: experience of sixty cases. Am J Hematol 2000; 63:7–10.

170. Ben-Yehuda D, Gillis S, Eldor A. Group TIIS. Clinical therapeutic experience in 712 Israeli patients with idiopathic thrombocytopenic purpura. Acta Haematol 1994; 91:1–6.
171. Monpoux F, Kurzenne JY, Sirvent N, Cottalorda J, Boutte P. Partial splenectomy in a child with human immunodeficiency virus-related immune thrombocytopenia. J Pediatr Hematol/Oncol 1999; 21:441–443.
172. Holt D, Brown J, Terrill K, et al. Response to intravenous immunoglobulin predicts splenectomy response in children with immune thrombocytopenic purpura: a study of 578 patients with 268 splenectomies. Pediatrics 2003; 111:87–90.
173. Bussel JB, Kaufmann CP, Ware RE, Woloski BMR. Do the acute platelet responses of gammaglobulin predict response to subsequent splenectomy? Am J Hematol 2001; 67:27–33.
174. Infectious diseases and immunization committee CPS. Prevention and therapy of bacterial infections for children with asplenia or hyposplenia. Paediatrics Child Health 1999; 4:416–421.
175. Klinge J, Hammersen G, Scharf J, Lutticken R, Reinert RR. Overwhelming post-splenectomy infection with vaccine-type streptococcus pneumoniae in a 12 year old girl despite vaccination and antibiotic prophylaxis. Infection 1997; 25:368–371.
176. Blanchette V, Garvey B. Management of chronic immune thrombocytopenic purpura in children and adults. Semin Hematol 1999; 35:35–51.
177. Wang J, Wiley JM, Luddy R, Greenberg J, Feuerstein MA, Bussel JB. Chronic Immune thrombocytopenic purpura in children: assessment of rituximab treatment. J Pediatr 2005; 146:217–221.
178. Scaradavou A, Bussel J. Evans syndrome. Results of a pilot study utilizing a multiagent treatment protocol. J Pediatr Hematol Oncol 1995; 17:290–295.
179. Williams JA, Boxer MD. Combination therapy for refractory idiopathic thrombocytopenic purpura (ITP) in adolescents. J Pediatr Hematol/Oncol 2003; 25:232–235.
180. Straus SE, Sneller M, Lenardo MJ, Puck JM, Strober W. The autoimmune lymphoproliferative syndrome. Ann Intern Med 1999; 130:591–601.
181. Ten Bosch J. Autoimmune lyphoproliferative syndrome: Etiology, diagnosis and management. Pediatr Drugs 2003; 5:185–193.
182. Straus SE, Jaffe ES, Puck JM, Dale JK, Elkon KB. The development of lymphomas in families with autoimmune lymphoproliferative syndrome with germline FAS mutations and defective lymphocyte apoptosis. Blood 2001; 98:194–200.
183. Heelan BT, Tormey V, Amlot P, Payne E, Mehta A, Webster DB. Effect of anti-CD20 (rituximab) on resistant thrombocytopenia in autoimmune lymphoproliferative syndrome. Br J Haematol 2002; 118:1078–1081.
184. Imbach P, Akatsuka J, Blanchette VS, et al. Immune thrombocytopenic purpura as a model for pathogenesis and treatment of autoimmunity. Eur J Pediatr 1995; 154:S60–S64.

7

Drug-Induced Thrombocytopenia

Richard H. Aster
Department of Medicine and Pathology, Medical College of Wisconsin, and Blood Research Institute, BloodCenter of Wisconsin, Milwaukee, Wisconsin, U.S.A.

James N. George
Hematology-Oncology Section, Department of Medicine, College of Medicine, University of Oklahoma Health Sciences Center, Oklahoma City, Oklahoma, U.S.A.

INTRODUCTION

Acute onset of thrombocytopenia and bleeding symptoms in patients taking quinine was first described 140 years ago (1). Similar findings were made subsequently in patients exposed to many other drugs (2–4). Clinical and laboratory investigations conducted during the past century to explain the relationship between drug exposure and thrombocytopenia have identified various mechanisms, both immune and non-immune, by which drugs cause platelet destruction. In this chapter, we review current understanding of the ways in which drugs cause thrombocytopenia, identify medications that have been shown with reasonable certainty to cause this complication, and consider diagnostic criteria and clinical aspects of drug-induced thrombocytopenia. Special emphasis will be placed on immune-mediated thrombocytopenia because this condition is a common clinical problem, presenting challenges for diagnosis and also for characterization of responsible mechanisms. We will not consider heparin-induced thrombocytopenia, a unique condition characterized principally by thrombotic complications; this is described separately in Chapter 8. Additional information about drug-induced thrombocytopenia can be found in several recent reviews (2,3,5,6).

PATHOPHYSIOLOGY OF DRUG-INDUCED THROMBOCYTOPENIA

Drug-Induced Suppression of Platelet Production

General Suppression of Hematopoiesis

(1) *Chemotherapeutic and immunosuppressive medications.* Many chemotherapeutic and immunosuppressive drugs suppress hematopoiesis. Although these agents affect all hematopoietic elements, their effect on platelet levels often governs the acceptable therapeutic dose. A model to identify patients at particularly high risk to develop severe thrombocytopenia when given chemotherapeutic or immunosuppressive agents has been described (7). IL-11 has been approved for amelioration of thrombocytopenia in patients with bone marrow failure (8).

(2) *Idiosyncratic aplastic anemia.* Hundreds of seemingly unrelated compounds are thought to be capable of causing idiosyncratic aplastic anemia (9). This complication does not appear to be related in any obvious way to dose or duration of exposure. Drugs implicated most often include anticonvulsants, gold salts, sulfonamides, and non-steroidal anti-inflammatory drugs (NSAIDS) (10). Although both immune and non-immune mechanisms have been implicated, the pathogenesis of idiosyncratic drug-induced aplastic anemia is poorly understood (11).

Specific Suppression of Megakaryocytopoiesis

A few drugs appear to inhibit megakaryocyte development in relatively specific ways, although underlying mechanisms are poorly understood.

(1) *Anagrelide.* The quinazolin compound, anagrelide, can cause isolated thrombocytopenia without anemia or neutropenia (12,13). From in vivo and in vitro studies, it appears that anagrelide perturbs megakaryocyte development, but the underlying molecular mechanisms have not been fully defined. Anagrelide is an accepted treatment for thrombocythemia in myeloproliferative syndromes (14,15). It is important to titrate the dose administered because profound thrombocytopenia following anagrelide treatment has been described (16).

(2) *Valproic acid.* Up to 30% of adults given valproate for treatment of epilepsy develop some degree of thrombocytopenia (17) on a dose-related basis (18). In some patients, thrombocytopenia resolves despite continued treatment with the drug (19). Experimental studies suggest valproate may inhibit megakaryocyte development and platelet production, (20–22) but a few cases of acute, profound thrombocytopenia have been reported, consistent with the possibility that drug-

induced antibodies may cause platelet destruction in some patients (23,24).

(3) *Alcohol.* Excessive ingestion of alcohol for long periods of time can lead to thrombocytopenia of various degrees of severity (25). Although vitamin deficiencies and/or alcoholic cirrhosis may be contributory, ethanol appears to have a relatively specific effect on megakaryocyte development in some individuals. Thrombocytopenia in patients with chronic alcoholism is rarely severe enough to cause bleeding, but profound thrombocytopenia with hemorrhage has been described (26). After withdrawal of alcohol, platelets usually return to normal in weeks or months.

(4) *Interferons.* Interferon therapy is known to inhibit hematopoiesis, and moderate thrombocytopenia is common in patients treated with this class of drugs (27–31). Although thrombocytopenia is usually mild, a profound drop in the platelet count has been described in patients given alpha interferon for treatment of hepatitis C (32,33). Experimental studies have shown that interferons alfa and gamma inhibit megakaryocyte proliferation in vitro and stem cell differentiation in vivo (30,34). The biochemical basis for this effect is not fully understood, but could be related to interference with signaling pathways critical to hematopoiesis (35). Paradoxically, many patients with hepatitis C-associated thrombocytopenia experience a rise in platelet levels after alfa interferon treatment (36,37).

Non-Immune, Drug-induced Platelet Destruction

Protamine Sulfate

About 30–40% of patients given protamine to neutralize heparin after cardiac surgery experience thrombocytopenia, usually mild, and this effect can be reproduced in an animal model (38). Protamine-associated thrombocytopenia may be the result of a direct action of heparin-protamine complexes on circulating platelets (39). Recent reports indicate that protamine perturbs the interaction between platelet membrane glycoprotein Ib (GP Ib) and von Willebrand factor (40,41), but whether this affects platelet survival is uncertain.

Leukokines and Hematopoietic Growth Factors

Acute thrombocytopenia has been described in patients given GM-CSF (42,43), M-CSF (44), tumor necrosis factor alpha with interferon gamma (45), and interleukin 2 (46,47) for treatment of hematopoietic disorders and cancer. Rapid onset of thrombocytopenia in such cases suggests that these agents sometimes act directly on platelets to trigger their destruction, but the responsible mechanism(s) have not been defined.

Porcine Factor VIII

Most patients given porcine Factor VIII for treatment of bleeding in the presence of Factor VIII inhibitors experience at least mild thrombocytopenia (48). Accompanying symptoms of hypersensitivity such as fever, urticaria, and chills sometimes occur, and evidence for platelet activation has been described (49). Possibly, immune complexes formed by the interaction of Factor VIII inhibitors and the infused xenoprotein interact with platelet Fc receptors to induce platelet destruction.

Desmopressin (DDAVP®)

In patients with Type 2B von Willebrand disease (vWD), treatment with desmopressin to raise vWF levels can lead to mild and, occasionally, severe thrombocytopenia (50,51). Desmopressin sometimes induces a mild and, rarely, a severe (52) drop in platelet levels in patients with normal vWF when given to ameliorate the bleeding tendency in patients with renal failure. Patients with "platelet-type" von Willebrand disease, in which a mutant vWF platelet receptor has abnormally high affinity for vWF (53,54), also may become thrombocytopenic after treatment with cryoprecipitate or DDAVP (55).

Snake Venom

Envenomation resulting from the bites of various poisonous snakes can produce severe thrombocytopenia (56,57). Although disseminated intravascular coagulation is common in such patients, a direct action of venom constituents on platelets appears to contribute importantly to platelet destruction (56,57).

Immune-Mediated Drug-Induced Platelet Destruction

Background

Dozens, possibly hundreds, of drugs have been implicated in the pathogenesis of antibody-mediated thrombocytopenia (2,3,58,59). Classes of drugs implicated most often include cinchona alkaloids (quinine and quinidine), antibiotics (sulfonamides, penicillin derivatives, and others), nonsteroidal inflammatory drugs (NSAIDs), and sedatives and anticonvulsants (carbamazepine, phenytoin). Among all of these drugs, quinine may now be the most common cause of drug-induced thrombocytopenia (3,60). In patients sensitive to certain drugs such as quinine and sulfamethoxazole, drug-dependent, platelet-reactive antibodies have been identified unequivocally by many investigators and are generally considered to be the causative agents. With other drugs, the role of antibodies in causing platelet destruction is less well documented. Mechanisms by which drugs are thought to cause immune-mediated thrombocytopenia are summarized in Table 1. In this section, we will review what is known about drug-induced, platelet-reactive antibodies and the mechanisms by which they are thought to cause platelet

Table 1 Mechanisms of Drug-Induced Thrombocytopenia

Antibody type	Mechanism	Example
Hapten-dependent antibodies	Drug binds covalently to a platelet membrane glycoprotein and functions as a hapten to induce an antibody response	Penicillin
Quinine-type antibodies	Drug binds non-covalently to a platelet surface glycoprotein to cause a compound epitope or to induce a conformational change that is antigenic Antibodies only bind to platelets in the presence of soluble drug	Quinine, sulfonamides
Antibodies induced by ligand-mimetic inhibitors of GP IIb/IIIa	Drug binds to GP IIb/IIIa to induce a conformational change that induces an antibody response	Tirofiban, eptifibatide
Abciximab-dependent antibodies	Antibodies recognize the drug itself when it is bound to platelets	Abciximab
Autoantibodies	Drug induces true autoantibodies that bind to platelet membrane glycoproteins without need for added drug	Gold salts

destruction. In later sections, we will cover criteria for the diagnosis of drug-induced thrombocytopenia and the clinical aspects of this group of disorders.

Hapten-Dependent Antibodies

In a classic series of studies done more than 50 years ago, Ackroyd showed that patients who experienced profound thrombocytopenia when treated with the sedative sedormid (allylisopropyl-acetylurea) had antibodies which, when incubated with platelets in vitro, caused platelet agglutination, complement-dependent lysis, and inhibition of clot retraction if the drug was present (61,62). Application of sedormid to the skin of such individuals produced local purpura in some patients, and challenge with the drug following recovery caused acute, severe thrombocytopenia. It was known at the time that, although low molecular weight compounds such as drugs are not ordinarily immunogenic, they can stimulate drug-specific antibodies when covalently linked to autologous proteins prior to immunization. Ackroyd postulated that drugs capable of inducing immune thrombocytopenia might become covalently linked to membrane proteins of circulating platelets and act as haptens to trigger antibody formation. According to this view, an ingested drug would "coat" autologous platelets, rendering them susceptible to destruction in a patient with a drug-specific antibody. As will be described, it is now thought that this mechanism rarely, if ever, accounts for drug-induced immune thrombocytopenia. Possible exceptions are patients treated with large doses of penicillinoid antibiotics, which are capable of linking covalently to autologous proteins by virtue of their labile beta lactam ring (63,64). Persons given large doses of penicillin for an extended time (65,66) and those with prior evidence of penicillin sensitivity (67) may be more likely to experience this complication. It should not be assumed that all patients who experience thrombocytopenia after treatment with penicillin, penicillin derivatives, or second-and third-generation cephalosporins have hapten-dependent antibodies because drug-dependent antibodies of the quinine-type (see below) have been identified in such individuals.

Quinine-Type Antibodies

Background: Quinine-type drug-induced immune thrombocytopenia is caused by an unusual class of antibodies that reacts with specific targets on the platelet membrane only in the presence of soluble drugs (4,68). Many drugs are capable of triggering such antibodies but, for unknown reasons, quinine, quinidine, and sulfonamide antibiotics are more likely to do so than others. Drug metabolites (see Section on Metabolite-Dependent Antibodies of the quinine-type) may be as likely to induce this type of antibody as primary drugs (69,70), but the range of metabolites capable of causing sensitization has not been defined. When quinine-type antibodies were first identified, it was assumed that they were hapten-specific, and therefore recognized the sensitizing drug covalently linked to one or more platelet membrane proteins. However, studies done more than 40 years ago by Shulman showed that: (i) binding of these antibodies to their targets is not inhibited by soluble drug at the highest achievable concentration, as would be expected of a hapten-dependent antibody; (ii) the antibodies do not recognize drug-treated platelets when soluble drug is not present; and (iii) the reaction between the drug and platelet is weak and reversible, and therefore unlikely to be capable of stimulating drug-specific antibodies (71,72). For some time, it was thought that quinine-type antibodies reacted with the drug for which they were specific to form immune complexes that somehow reacted with platelets to cause their destruction (73). However, it was later found that binding of the antibodies to their targets occurs by way of the Fab, rather than the Fc, domain (74,75). Many publications still refer to "immune complex" or "innocent bystander" mechanisms as being responsible for quinine-type immune thrombocytopenia. In the absence of any evidence to support this concept and in light of observations showing that antibody binding occurs by way of the Fab domain, use of these terms should be discontinued.

Although the immune complex mechanism has been discounted as an explanation for drug-dependent antibody binding, how soluble drugs at pharmacologic concentration promote tight binding of quinine-type antibodies to a specific target on a membrane glycoprotein is not yet understood. Two principal mechanisms have been proposed (Fig. 1). One calls for the sensitizing drug to react non-covalently with one or more platelet membrane glycoproteins

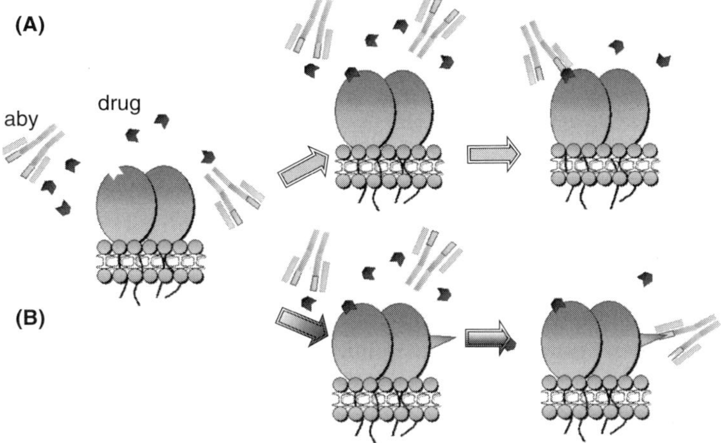

Figure 1 Two schemes by which soluble drug may promote tight binding of a drug-dependent antibody (aby) to a membrane glycoprotein (GP) complex. (**A**) Drug binds directly to a preferred site on GP, creating an epitope consisting of drug + adjacent peptide residues for which aby is specific. (**B**) Drug binds to a preferred site on GP and induces a conformational change elsewhere in the molecule, creating a "neotope" for which aby is specific.

to create a target epitope comprised of both drug and adjacent peptide residues that is recognized directly by the antibody (Fig. 1**A**). Many drugs that cause quinine-type thrombocytopenia are amphipathic, that is, they contain both hydrophilic and hydrophobic structural elements and are normally transported in plasma bound to hydrophobic sites on albumin (76,77). It would not be surprising, therefore, if such drugs react with hydrophobic domains on platelet glycoproteins. One study has shown that binding of quinine-dependent antibodies to platelets causes quinine to be trapped on the target glycoprotein, consistent with the possibility that the drug is in direct contact with the antibody (78). An alternative possibility is that when the drug interacts with a target protein, it induces a structural modification elsewhere in the molecule, creating an epitope for which the antibody is specific (Fig. 1**B**). An additional possible mechanism is that the drug reacts with the antigen-combining site of the antibody and reconfigures it in such a way that it acquires specificity for a site on the target; however, this concept is not supported by any experimental evidence.

Targets recognized by quinine-type antibodies: In the expectation that information about epitopes recognized by quinine-type antibodies might facilitate understanding of the mechanism(s) of drug-dependent antibody binding, studies have been done to characterize antibody binding sites at the molecular level. Antibodies induced by quinine, or its diastereoisomer quinidine, generally recognize epitopes on the platelet glycoprotein (GP) Ib/IX/V and/or IIb/IIIa complexes (79–82). It is not uncommon for two or more distinct drug-dependent antibodies, each recognizing a different target, to be present in the same patient (79,80). Some antibodies recognize isolated components of the glycoprotein complexes, such as the peptide GP IIIa, while others require the intact glycoprotein complexes for binding (80). Antibodies induced by sulfamethoxazole preferentially recognize the GP IIb/IIIa complex (83), whereas those induced by the antibiotic rifampicin may be relatively specific for GP Ib/IX/IV (84,85). Antibodies from patients with thrombocytopenia induced by the anti-thyroid drug carbimazole were specific for platelet endothelial cell adhesion molecule-1 (PECAM-1, CD31) (86). In the same study, evidence for weak reactivity against PECAM-1 by antibodies from patients with quinidine-induced thrombocytopenia was described (86).

In several studies, more precise localization of antibody binding sites has been achieved. The binding site for carbimazole-dependent antibodies was localized to the second of six extracellular domains of PECAM-1 (86). A family of quinine-dependent antibodies was found to be specific for a 17-amino acid sequence in the newly recognized hybrid and PSI homology domains GP IIIa (81). Three specific amino acid residues in this sequence appeared to be critical for antibody binding. In a third study, a group of quinine-dependent antibodies was found to be specific for amino acid residues 64–135 in the proximal half of the GP IX component of the GP Ib/IX/V complex (82); two particular amino acids appeared to be essential for this interaction. A single quinine-dependent antibody recognized a peptide sequence in the glycocalicin domain of GP Ibα (79). Although there appears to be no common link between the binding sites identified in these studies, further investigations to establish the molecular character of epitopes recognized by drug-dependent antibodies may help to resolve the question of how drugs promote binding of these antibodies to their targets and cause platelet destruction.

Induction of quinine-type antibodies: Although covalent association between drug and protein appears not to be a requirement for drug-dependent binding of quinine-type antibodies to their targets, it is possible that the drug or a drug metabolite covalently linked to some autologous protein creates the immunogen that triggers antibody formation. In drug metabolism, it is common for reactive intermediates to be formed that can spontaneously establish covalent linkages to intracellular proteins (87–89). Many drug metabolites become conjugated to glucuronide, in which form their urinary secretion is facilitated (90). Drug-glucuronide esters can spontaneously rearrange to form reactive intermediates capable of linking covalently to amino groups on proteins (91,92) and drug-protein adducts created by this reaction are immunogenic in animals (93). Autologous proteins linked to drug metabolites have been implicated in the pathogenesis of several drug-induced immune disorders in man (87,94,95).

How the immune response to a drug metabolite covalently coupled to an autologous protein or peptide might lead to production of antibodies of the type seen in patients with quinine-type thrombocytopenia is unknown. It is of interest that many of the drugs that cause thrombocytopenia have been implicated as triggers for immune disorders affecting other organs (96–98). Although platelets are by far the most common target among blood cells, it is not rare for multiple drug-dependent antibodies, some reactive with platelets and others with neutrophils and/or erythrocytes, to be present simultaneously in the same patient. Why multiple classes of blood cells should be targeted by drug-induced antibodies in some individuals is unresolved. It is known that enzymes of the cytochrome P450 (CYP) system, the major catalysts for drug biotransformation, are highly polymorphic and that certain genetic variants can predispose to adverse drug reactions (99,100). Polymorphisms of enzymes responsible for glucuronidation (90) are also of interest in light of the fact that glucuronide-conjugates of drugs can induce immune cytopenia (70,101). In view of the likely role of reactive drug metabolites in triggering drug sensitivity reactions (88,94), it seems possible that polymorphisms in enzyme systems responsible for drug metabolism could predispose individuals to produce drug-dependent antibodies of the quinine-type, but there is as yet no experimental support for this possibility.

Antibodies Induced by Ligand-Mimetic GP IIb/IIIa Inhibitors

Acute, often severe, thrombocytopenia is a recognized complication of treatment with a new class of anti-thrombotic agents, the ligand-mimetic GPIIb/IIIa inhibitors (102,103). These agents are designed to mimic the ligand arginine-glycine-aspartic acid (RGD) that is recognized by GP IIb/IIIa and are thus capable of inhibiting fibrinogen binding and platelet aggregation. Intravenous ligand-mimetic drugs are usually given only for a day or two to prevent restenosis after coronary angioplasty. Oral drugs, designed to be given for longer periods of time, are in development. Recent studies indicate that thrombocytopenia in patients sensitive to these agents is caused by antibodies specific for ligand-occupied GP IIb/IIIa (103–105). In patients given oral agents, thrombocytopenia is most likely to occur after one or two weeks of exposure (104,105), but can develop after several months (105). Acute thrombocytopenia can also occur within a few hours of first exposure to oral or intravenous agents (103–105) and appears to be caused by preexisting, naturally-occurring antibodies. This is in distinct contrast to antibodies in patients with quinine-type thrombocytopenia that require prior drug exposure to induce sensitization.

Not surprisingly, antibodies in patients sensitive to GP IIb/IIIa ligand-mimetic drugs are specific for the GP IIb/IIIa complex to which these drugs bind (103–105). Ligand-mimetic compounds are known to induce conformational changes (ligand-induced binding sites or LIBS) in GP IIb/IIIa that are recognized by certain monoclonal antibodies (106,107). It seems possible that antibodies causing thrombocytopenia in patients sensitive to ligand-mimetic drugs are human analogues of LIBS-specific murine monoclonals, but this has not yet been confirmed experimentally. Why such antibodies should be naturally occurring is an intriguing question that deserves further study. It may be possible to prevent thrombocytopenia in patients given ligand-mimetic drugs by prescreening serum for drug-dependent antibodies (108), but whether routine screening is practical is uncertain.

Abciximab-Dependent Antibodies

Abciximab is the Fab fragment of a chimeric (human/mouse) monoclonal antibody that inhibits fibrinogen binding to the platelet GP IIb/IIIa complex by virtue of recognizing an epitope close to the fibrinogen binding site (109) and has been shown to be effective in preventing secondary complications in patients undergoing percutaneous transluminal coronary angioplasty (110). About 4% of patients given abciximab a second time (111) and 1% of those treated for the first time (112,113) experience acute thrombocytopenia. Patients with abciximab-induced thrombocytopenia may be asymptomatic, but severe bleeding complications and fatalities have been reported (114–116). Although non-immune mechanisms have been postulated (117), a recent report suggests that abciximab-dependent antibodies are an important cause of abciximab-induced thrombocytopenia (114). Experimental evidence suggests that the antibodies in patients who develop thrombocytopenia after a second exposure to abciximab recognize murine sequences incorporated into the abciximab molecule to confer specificity for GP IIb/IIIa (114). Thus, abciximab-induced thrombocytopenia appears to be caused by antibodies that recognize the drug itself (Fig. 2). The possibility that some antibodies are specific for conformational changes induced in GP IIb/IIIa by

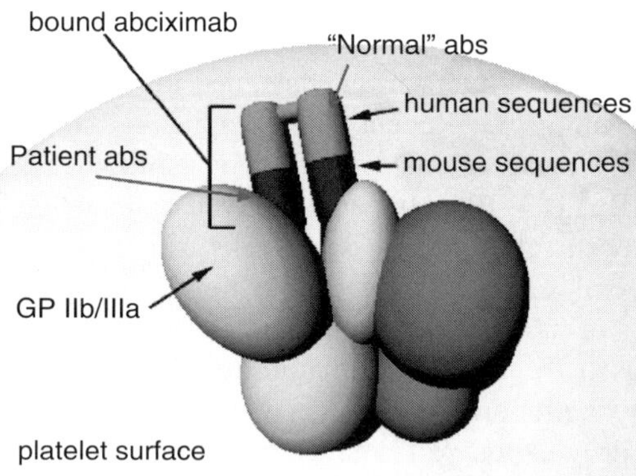

Figure 2 Reactions of antibodies with abciximab-coated platelets. Antibodies from patients who developed acute thrombocytopenia following abciximab administration appear to be specific for murine peptide sequences (black) incorporated into the abciximab molecule. "Normal" antibodies found commonly in plasma of persons who have never been exposed to abciximab recognize the C-terminus of abciximab at the site where the Fab fragment is cleaved from the chimeric IgG molecule by papain.

abciximab has not been unequivocally ruled out, however. Whether acute thrombocytopenia in patients given abciximab for the first time is caused by preexisting (naturally-occurring?) antibodies is not yet fully established.

Platelet-Specific Autoantibodies

Several drugs are known to cause autoimmune hemolytic anemia (118,119), but whether drugs sometimes induce platelet-specific autoantibodies capable of causing thrombocytopenia is less certain. About 1% of patients given gold salts for treatment of rheumatoid arthritis develop laboratory and clinical findings consistent with autoimmune thrombocytopenia (ITP) (120,121) and there are anecdotal reports of ITP following treatment with other drugs such as levodopa and procaine amide (122). Patients with quinine-type drug-induced thrombocytopenia sometimes produce transient autoantibodies that bind to platelets in the absence of the drug (123). A patient who presented with sulfamethoxazole-induced thrombocytopenia had drug-dependent antibodies initially, but later had chronic thrombocytopenia apparently caused by true autoantibodies, possibly induced by the drug (122) (Fig. 3). Although various mechanisms have been suggested (122), how medications might induce platelet-reactive autoantibodies is unknown. Nonetheless, it seems reasonable to consider the possibility that

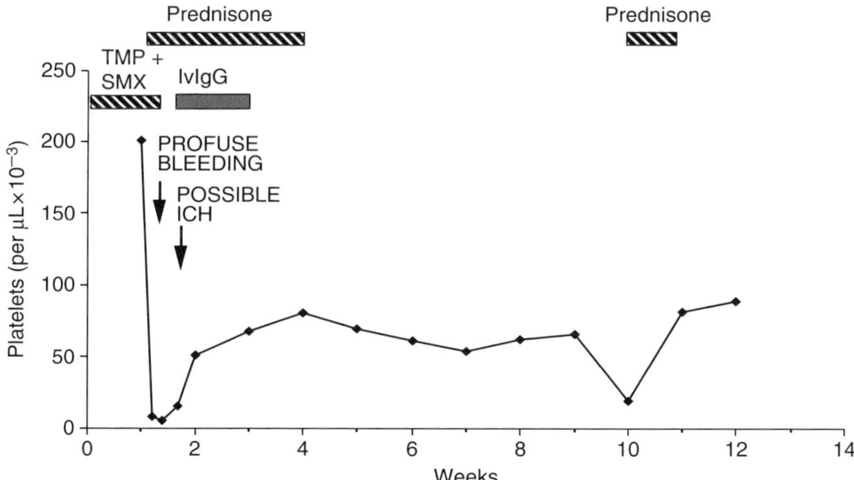

Figure 3 Clinical course of a patient in whom sulfamethoxazole (SMX)-induced immune thrombocytopenia apparently evolved into chronic immune (autoimmune) thrombocytopenia (ITP). After one week of treatment for a urinary tract infection, the patient presented with severe thrombocytopenia and was found to have an IgG, SMX-dependent antibody specific for the platelet GP IIb/IIIa complex. Improvement followed treatment with prednisone and IV IgG, but thrombocytopenia recurred after prednisone was discontinued. At this time, she was found to have an IgG antibody that reacted with GP IIb/IIIa on autologous platelets in the absence of SMX. *Source*: From Ref. 122.

sensitization to exogenous agents might be the underlying cause of autoimmune thrombocytopenia in some individuals.

LABORATORY DIAGNOSIS OF DRUG-INDUCED THROMBOCYTOPENIA

Background

It is not uncommon for patients suspected of having drug-induced thrombocytopenia to be taking numerous medications that may be critical to their medical management. Accordingly, sensitive and specific assays to identify the responsible medication could be extremely useful. Unfortunately, a specific laboratory diagnosis is possible only in a minority of patients. Reasons for this include: (1) some drugs that cause thrombocytopenia are relatively insoluble in water and are therefore difficult to work with in in vitro assays; (2) a metabolite formed in vivo, rather than the primary drug, can be the sensitizing agent (69,70,124–126); (3) the possibility that available methods are not sufficiently sensitive to detect the responsible antibodies; and (4) in any particular case, thrombocytopenia may have been unrelated to drug exposure. Whether detection of an antibody that recognizes platelets in the presence of a suspect drug proves that the antibody caused the thrombocytopenia can also be argued because of a lack of studies showing that such antibodies: (1) are rare in the general population and (2) are not commonly produced by patients taking the same drug who do not develop thrombocytopenia. Limited information of this type is available for the drugs sulfamethoxazole (83), the GP IIb/IIa inhibitors tirofiban and eptifibitide (103), the nonsteroidal anti-inflammatory drug naproxen (70), and acetaminophen (70), but comparable studies are needed to document the role of antibodies induced by other drugs as causes of platelet destruction. However, if suitable controls are negative, demonstration of an antibody that binds to platelets in the presence of a suspect drug at pharmacologic concentrations provides support for the possibility that the medication caused the thrombocytopenia. Therefore, useful information can be obtained by laboratories skilled in performance of the appropriate assays. We will here briefly review assays that appear to be useful for the diagnosis of drug-induced immune thrombocytopenia by the mechanisms shown in Table 1. Readers can refer to cited publications for technical details.

Hapten-Dependent Antibodies

As already noted, hapten-dependent antibodies rarely, if ever, cause immune thrombocytopenia. In one study of a patient with apparent penicillin-induced thrombocytopenia, washed, normal platelets were pretreated with penicillin at high concentration, washed again, and then used as targets for detection of the antibody using radiolabeled antiglobulin (127). However, an antibody from a patient with acute thrombocytopenia induced by the second generation cephalosporin, cefotetan, failed to react with cefotetan-treated platelets but did so when soluble cefotetan was present, suggesting that this antibody was of the quinine-type (128). Similar findings were made in a patient who experienced acute thrombocytopenia while taking the second generation cephalosporin drug, loracarbef (129). Numerous examples of immune hemolytic anemia induced by penicillin and penicillin derivatives have been described (63,130,131). Some of the antibodies present in such patients recognize drug-treated red cells (130,131), but those induced by second and third generation cephalosporin antibiotics more often require the drug to be present in solution throughout the assay and may, therefore, be of the quinine type. A protocol optimal for coating red cells with penicillin and penicillin derivatives has been described (131). Whether the same conditions are suitable for coating platelets is uncertain. Occasionally, antibodies induced by drugs other than those of the penicillin family can be detected using drug-coated red cells (132,133).

Quinine-Type Antibodies

As already noted, quinine-type antibodies react with their targets only when drug is present in soluble form. Accordingly, it is important that drug be present at all stages of any assay used to detect them. A reasonable concentration of drug, one that will assure a high molar ratio of drug to antibody, is 1.0 mM. Satisfactory concentrations of drugs that are poorly soluble in water can sometimes be achieved by dissolving the drug in 1% albumin or in DMSO (83). Quinine-type antibodies can sometimes be detected using complement fixation (71), complement-dependent platelet lysis (134), enzyme-linked immunospecific assay (ELISA) using immobilized platelet glycoproteins as targets (135,136), reverse passive hemagglutination in which indicator red cells coated with anti-Ig are allowed to interact with antibody-coated platelets (137), monoclonal antibody immobilization of platelet antigens (MAIPA) (86,138), and flow cytometry (83,135). In some studies, flow cytometry was found to be convenient and at least as sensitive as other methods (83,103,135). If a patient has non-drug-dependent antibodies, such as antibodies specific for HLA alloantigens, these will reduce the sensitivity of the assay unless removed by pre-absorbing patient serum in the absence of the drug with the same platelets that are to be used for detection of drug-dependent antibodies. Rarely, a serum sample drawn soon after the onset of thrombocytopenia will contain enough residual drug to give a positive reaction without adding more drug. In such cases, a drug-dependent antibody can sometimes be identified by dialyzing the serum sample prior to testing. Examples of quinine-type antibodies detected by several methods are shown in Figs. 4 and 5.

Metabolite-Dependent Antibodies of the Quinine-Type

As already noted, drug-metabolites produced in vivo can sometimes produce the stimulus for quinine-type antibodies. In studies done more than 30 years ago, Eisner and colleagues described a patient who experienced profound thrombocytopenia after taking acetaminophen and had an antibody that reacted with normal target

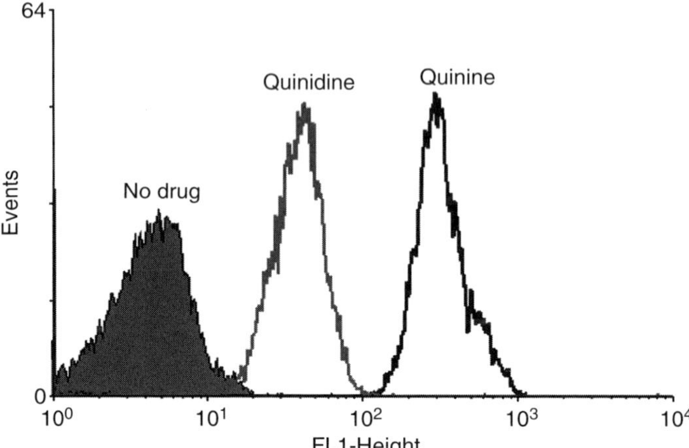

Figure 4 Flow cytometric detection of a strong, quinine-dependent, platelet-reactive IgG antibody in a patient who developed acute thrombocytopenia after taking quinine for treatment of nocturnal leg cramps. No reaction occurred in the absence of drug (gray). The antibody reacted weakly in the presence of quinidine, the diastereoisomer of quinine.

platelets when a major metabolite, acetaminophen sulfate, was present, but not with acetaminophen itself (124). A similar patient who appeared to be sensitive to an unidentified metabolite of para-aminosalicylic acid (PAS) was subsequently described (125). Later studies documented platelet-reactive antibodies dependent on metabolites of the drugs sulfamethoxazole (126) and naproxen (70).

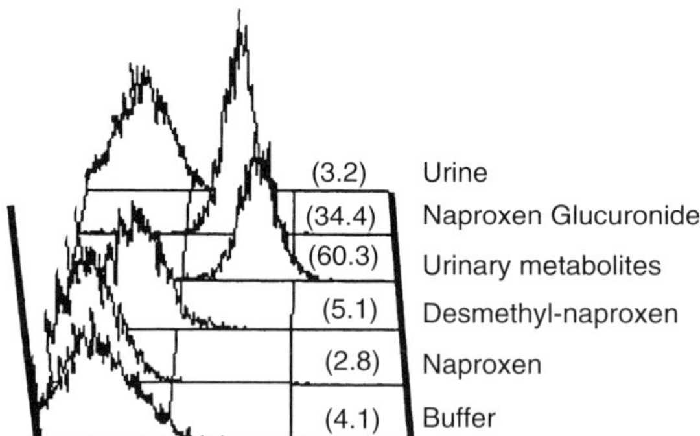

Figure 5 Reactions against normal platelets of serum from a patient who experienced acute thrombocytopenia while taking the non-steroidal anti-inflammatory drug, naproxen. No reaction occurred in the presence of naproxen or one of its metabolites, desmethyl naproxen. However, strong positive reactions (IgG) were obtained when metabolites isolated and concentrated from urine of a normal person taking naproxen or naproxen glucuronide were used as the source of "drug" in the reaction mixture. *Source*: From Ref. 70.

Metabolite-dependent, platelet-reactive antibodies can sometimes be demonstrated by using urine from a patient or a normal subject taking the suspect drug as the source of "drug" in antibody assays (69,139). Specific identification of the sensitizing agent can be achieved by testing with known metabolites of the suspect drug or by extracting metabolites from the urine of someone taking the drug and identifying the active substance by chemical analysis (70,124,125). Metabolite-dependent antibodies specific for red cells have been convincingly demonstrated in a number of patients with drug-induced immune hemolytic anemia (101,140,141). Since drug-induced immune thrombocytopenia is far more common than drug-induced immune hemolysis, it is important that the range of drug metabolites capable of causing immune thrombocytopenia be characterized more fully.

Antibodies Induced by Ligand Mimetic GP IIb/IIIa Inhibitors

This class of drug-dependent antibodies can be detected using platelets treated with the suspect ligand mimetic drug as targets for antibody, followed by identification of the bound immunoglobulin by flow cytometry (103–105). Since calcium is required for optimal binding of these antibodies to ligand-occupied GP IIb/IIIa, platelets isolated from blood anticoagulated with citrate (not EDTA) should be used for testing and calcium chelators should be excluded from the reaction mixtures (103). As with quinine-dependent antibodies, it is important that soluble drug be present throughout the test procedure. This type of antibody can also be detected using isolated GP IIb/IIIa as a target and ELISA for detection of bound immunoglobulin (103,108). On occasion, antibodies are undetectable in patients with a history strongly suggestive of thrombocytopenia induced by ligand mimetic drugs. A study in Rhesus monkeys suggests that clinically significant antibodies may be present at a concentration too low to be detected in conventional assays but can be identified by serially absorbing serum aliquots with ligand-coated platelets to concentrate antibodies on the target (142). Since this class of antibodies was identified very recently, it is likely that more sensitive and specific methods for their detection will be described in the future.

Abciximab-Dependent Antibodies

Patients with abciximab-induced thrombocytopenia usually have antibodies that react with abciximab-coated platelets and can be detected by flow cytometry (114). However, apparently similar antibodies are present in many normal individuals. Although these "normal," naturally-occurring, antibodies are usually weaker than those found in patients, there is overlap between the two groups (114). Experimental evidence indicates that antibodies from patients with abciximab-induced thrombocytopenia differ from antibodies commonly present in normal persons in two ways: (1) "normal" antibodies can be inhibited with Fab fragments isolated from pooled normal plasma, whereas patient antibodies cannot, and (2) the patient antibodies react preferentially with platelets coated with 7E3, the monoclonal antibody from which variable sequences that confer specificity on abciximab were derived (114). Differing behavior of the "normal," naturally-occurring) antibodies and antibodies found in patients with thrombocytopenia can perhaps be explained by the fact that the former are specific for the papain cleavage site at the N-terminus of the of the abciximab molecule (143) while the latter recognize murine-derived amino acid sequences incorporated into the abciximab molecule (114). Why one type of antibody causes thrombocytopenia while the other apparently does not is uncertain.

Drug-Induced, Platelet-Specific Autoantibodies

Drug-induced autoantibodies specific for platelets generally behave like those in patients with immune (idiopathic) thrombocytopenic purpura (ITP). Details of assays for platelet autoantibody detection can be found in several recent publications (144–147). Unfortunately, these methods have limited sensitivity and specificity.

CLINICAL DIAGNOSIS OF DRUG-INDUCED THROMBOCYTOPENIA

The causal relationship of a drug in a patient with suspected drug-induced thrombocytopenia can also be documented by clinical evidence (Table 2). Clinical evidence may be obtained from reports of individual patients or from randomized, controlled clinical trials. A method for establishing levels of certainty in individual patient reports is described in Table 2 (3). For some drugs, definite evidence of a causal relationship to thrombocytopenia has not been determined from reports of individual patients, but is clearly documented in randomized, controlled clinical trials in which thrombocytopenia is documented as an adverse event (148). These clinical data are important since sensitive and specific tests for identification of drug-dependent antibodies are not routinely available in clinical laboratories. Furthermore, the inability to identify a drug-dependent antibody does not exclude the drug as the etiology for the thrombocytopenia, as described above.

Evidence from Case Reports of Individual Patients

Table 2 describes four criteria used to evaluate case reports of patients with suspected drug-induced thrombocytopenia (3). A definite causal relation of the drug to the thrombocytopenia (Level I evidence) is established when all four criteria are met, including reexposure to the candidate drug that results in recurrent thrombocytopenia. When criteria 1–3 are met, but the patient is not reexposed to the suspected drug, the level of evidence is described as probable, Level II. When only criterion 1 is fulfilled, the level of evidence is described as possible, Level III. When the case report does not even provide a convincing

Table 2 Criteria to Document a Causal Relationship in Patients with Suspected Drug-Induced Thrombocytopenia

Criteria	Description
Case report criteria	
1	Therapy with the candidate drug preceded thrombocytopenia and Recovery from thrombocytopenia was complete and sustained after therapy with the drug was discontinued
2	The candidate drug was the only drug used before the onset of thrombocytopenia or Other drugs were continued or reintroduced after discontinuation of therapy with the candidate drug with a sustained normal platelet count
3	Other causes for thrombocytopenia were excluded
4	Re-exposure to the candidate drug resulted in recurrent thrombocytopenia
Level of evidence	
I	Definite: Criteria 1,2,3, and 4 met
II	Probable: Criteria 1,2, and 3 met
III	Possible: Criterion 1 met
IV	Unlikely: Criterion 1 not met
Randomized clinical trial criteria	
Significantly different frequency of thrombocytopenia as an adverse event	
Laboratory criteria	
Demonstration of drug-dependent antibodies	

Case report criteria are *Source*: Adapted from Ref. 3

description that fulfills criterion 1, the level of evidence is described as unlikely, Level IV.

Case reports may be difficult to interpret because of incomplete information. For the assessment of case reports (Table 2), criterion 2 is often the most difficult to accurately assess (3,148,149). Whether the patient has taken other drugs is often not mentioned, even though drug-induced thrombocytopenia typically occurs in older patients (3), and older patients typically take many different drugs (150). If other drugs were taken, whether they were continued or reintroduced, with no effect on the platelet count, is often not described.

Therefore when assessing case reports, the reader is often required to choose between accepting the author's implicit suggestion that the candidate drug was the only potential cause for thrombocytopenia or excluding the report for insufficient data. The assessment of other potential causes for thrombocytopenia (criterion 3, Table 2) is also often unclear. In some patients, systemic illnesses are described that could be associated with thrombocytopenia, potentially obscuring the role of the drug as the etiology for the thrombocytopenia. Fulfillment of criterion 4, reexposure to the candidate drug, is often unintentional though in some case reports intentional reexposure with careful observation is reported. This definitive diagnostic test may be dangerous, but in some situations it may be important. For example, when it is suspected that thrombocytopenia may be caused by acetaminophen, a very common ingredient of many over-the-counter compounds, conclusive documentation is important to insure that the patient subsequently avoids all remedies that include acetaminophen.

Evidence from Randomized Controlled Clinical Trials

Two drugs used extensively to inhibit platelet function in patients with acute coronary syndromes, abciximab and eptifibatide, have been conclusively documented to cause thrombocytopenia in clinical trials (148). These data are important because individual case reports describing thrombocytopenia with these agents are difficult to interpret since the patients were taking multiple additional drugs and, in addition, were often critically ill.

DRUGS THAT CAUSE THROMBOCYTOPENIA

Evidence from Case Reports of Individual Patients

All articles describing patients with drug-induced thrombocytopenia through July 2002 were retrieved and analyzed (3,148,149) using previously described systematic literature review methodology (151). The literature search strategy included a comprehensive search of the Medline database, plus a complete search of the bibliography of each retrieved article to identify additional reports, especially reports published before 1966 and therefore not included in the Medline database. In this search, articles reporting thrombocytopenia associated with heparin and heparin analogs were not retrieved. Two reviewers independently reviewed each retrieved article. This dual independent review was critical because data in the case reports was often not explicitly described, requiring interpretation based on the reviewer's judgment. When the initial two reviewers disagreed in their interpretation, adjudication was performed by a third reviewer.

The literature searches identified 846 articles that described 1232 individual patients and 250 individual drugs (3,148,149); 438 (36%) of the patient case reports were excluded from further review based on six a priori criteria: (1) insufficient clinical data with which to evaluate the relation between drug administration and thrombocytopenia; (2) nadir platelet count not less than 100,000/μL, to exclude patients with equivocal thrombocytopenia; (3) use of a cytotoxic agent or vaccine that predictably causes marrow suppression; (4) case reports in which the patient was exposed to a non-therapeutic agent or used an agent in the non-therapeutic manner (for example, environmental toxins, illicit drugs, drug overdose, and drugs not currently in use); (5) drug-induced disease that included thrombocytopenia but predominantly involved other abnormalities, such as aplastic anemia or the thrombotic thrombocytopenic purpura-hemolytic uremic syndrome; and (6) patient age of 16 years or younger.

The age criterion was established because idiopathic thrombocytopenic purpura in children is typically an acute, spontaneously resolving illness that may not be distinguishable from drug-induced thrombocytopenia. Although reports of cytotoxic agents were excluded from review, recent case reports have documented that cytotoxic, chemotherapeutic agents may cause sudden and severe thrombocytopenia (152,153) due to drug-dependent antibodies (154).

After exclusion of the 438 patient case reports, 794 individual patients who had thrombocytopenia reported to be caused by 187 different drugs were evaluated (3,148,149). Sixty (32%) drugs were considered to be definite causes of thrombocytopenia (Table 3) since they were described in reports fulfilling all four criteria and therefore had Level I evidence (Table 2). Table 3 also lists 25 additional drugs for which the causal relationship to thrombocytopenia was described in two or more case reports with Level II (probable) evidence. Although this evidence is not as strong as evidence supported by reexposure to the drug with recurrence of thrombocytopenia, a second case report with probable evidence provides confirmation. Table 3 also lists the number of individual patient case reports with Level I or Level II evidence.

Two agents, quinidine and quinine, are reported more often than any other drug. Since quinidine has been replaced in common usage by more effective and less toxic cardiac anti-arrhythmic agents, it may be anticipated that the frequency of quinidine-induced thrombocytopenia will diminish. However, the frequency of quinine-induced thrombocytopenia will remain common because quinine has continued to be the traditional remedy for the very common occurrence of nocturnal leg cramps (155,156) for more than 60 years (157). In a recent cohort study of patients with suspected ITP documented drug-induced thrombocytopenia as a common alternative diagnosis, quinine was the most common cause of drug-induced thrombocytopenia (60). Although over-the-counter sale of quinine sulfate tablets was banned by the U.S. Food and Drug Administration in 1994 (158) because of reports of severe adverse effects and insufficient evidence for efficacy, use of quinine may not have significantly diminished. Several remedies containing quinine, or the parent natural compound, cinchona, are readily available in markets and nutrition stores where they are advertised for treatment of leg cramps (159). These alternative remedies are widely discussed in internet "chat rooms" devoted to problems with leg cramps. Even the very small amount of quinine present in

Table 3 Drugs Causing Thrombocytopenia, Supported by Patient Case Reports with Level I (Definite) Evidence or Level II (Probable) Clinical Evidence

	Patient case reports		Severity of bleeding	
Drug (Generic name)	Level I Evidence	Level II Evidence	Major	Minor
Quinidine	20	29	5	17
Quinine	10	12	5	11
Rifampin	6	5	1	6
Para-Aminosalicylic Acid	6	5	1	6
Acetaminophen	4	4	2	1
Trimethoprim/Sulfa-methoxazole	3	12	5	3
Danazol	3	4	0	4
Methyldopa	3	3	0	1
Digoxin	3	0	0	2
Acyclovir	2	14	0	1
Carbamezapine	2	14	0	1
Vancomycin	2	3	1	0
Diclofenac	2	2	0	2
Aminoglutethimide	2	1	1	1
Aminosalicylic Acid	2	1	1	1
Amphoteracin B	2	1	0	0
Oxprenolol	2	1	0	1
Levamisole	2	0	0	0
Meclofenamate	2	0	0	0
Diatrizoate Meglu-mine/Diatrizoate Sodium	2	0	0	0
Amiodarone	2	0	0	0
Tamoxifen	2	0	0	0
Indinavir	2	0	0	0
Interferon	1	11	1	7
Cimetidine	1	6	0	1
Nalidixic Acid	1	5	0	1
Sulfisoxazole	1	4	2	2
Valproate	1	4	1	0
Ethambutol	1	2	1	0
Chlorothiazide	1	2	0	1
Diatrizoate Meglumine	1	2	0	2
Sulfasalazine	1	2	0	0
Sulfathiozole	1	1	1	1
Iopanoic Acid	1	1	0	1
Tolmetin	1	1	0	1
Diazoxide	1	1	0	0

(Continued)

Table 3 Drugs Causing Thrombocytopenia, Supported by Patient Case Reports with Level I (Definite) Evidence or Level II (Probable) Clinical Evidence (*Continued*)

	Patient case reports		Severity of bleeding	
Drug (Generic name)	Level I Evidence	Level II Evidence	Major	Minor
Isotretinoin	1	1	0	1
Thiothixene	1	0	0	0
Naphazoline	1	0	0	0
Amrinone	1	0	0	0
Lithium	1	0	0	0
Diazepam	1	0	0	0
Haloperidol	1	0	0	0
Alprenolol	1	0	0	1
Nitroglycerine	1	0	0	0
Minoxidil	1	0	0	1
Chlorpromazine	1	0	0	0
Isoniazid	1	0	0	0
Cephalothin	1	0	0	0
Diflouromethylornithine(Eflornithine)	1	0	0	0
Piperacillin	1	0	0	1
Diethylstilbestrol	1	0	0	0
Methicillin	1	0	0	1
Deferoxamine	1	0	0	0
Novobiocin	1	0	0	0
Atorvastatin	1	0	0	0
Mesalamine	1	0	0	0
Octreotide	1	0	0	0
Pentoxifylline	1	0	0	0
Tiagabine	1	0	0	0
Gold	0	11	3	3
Lotrafiban	0	5	1	2
Chlorpropamide	0	5	1	1
Hydrochlorothiazide	0	5	0	2
Ranitidine	0	4	0	0
Naproxen	0	4	0	0
Abciximab C7e3 Fab	0	3	1	0
Sulfamethoxypyridazine	0	3	0	3
Ticlopidine	0	3	0	1
Sulfapyridine	0	2	2	0
Acetazolamide	0	2	1	0
Ampicillin	0	2	1	1

(Continued)

Table 3 Drugs Causing Thrombocytopenia, Supported by Patient Case Reports with Level I (Definite) Evidence or Level II (Probable) Clinical Evidence (*Continued*)

	Patient case reports		Severity of bleeding	
Drug (Generic name)	Level I Evidence	Level II Evidence	Major	Minor
Oxyphenbutazone	0	2	0	2
Ibuprofen	0	2	0	2
Phenytoin	0	2	0	1
Oxtetracyline	0	2	0	0
Glibenclamide	0	2	0	1
Captopril	0	2	0	0
Procainamide	0	2	0	0
Sulindac	0	2	0	1
Fluconazole	0	2	0	0
Clidinium Bromide/Chlordiazepoxide	0	2	0	1
Roxifiban	0	2	0	0
Simvastatin	0	2	0	0

Drugs are listed for which the causal relation to thrombocytopenia is supported by the description of at least one patient case report with definite evidence (Level I) or two or more patient case reports with probable evidence (Level II). Data are adapted from references (3,148,149), last updated August 1, 2002. Drugs are listed in the order of the number of case reports describing definite or probable clinical evidence. Complete data, listing drugs in alphabetical order for easier searching and describing all citations and data from each individual patient case report, are available at the website http://moon.ouhsc.edu/jgeorge.

beverages (approximately 3–8 mg/100 mL) is sufficient to cause sensitization and also to induce severe thrombocytopenia in sensitized subjects (160–166).

Evidence from Demonstration of Drug-Dependent Antibodies

In addition to drugs that have been documented to cause thrombocytopenia by clinical evidence (3,148,149), other drugs have been documented to cause thrombocytopenia by the demonstration of drug-dependent antibodies in the laboratory of the Blood Center of Southeastern Wisconsin (BR Curtis, DA Bougie, RH Aster, unpublished observations).

Evidence from Case Reports of Individual Patients Describing Thrombocytopenia Caused by Herbal Remedies and Foods

These systematic reviews of case reports of drug-induced thrombocytopenia (3,148,149) excluded agents that are not currently in use, as documented in the United States by listing in the American Hospital Formulary Service and in other countries by listing in the Martindale Pharmacopoeia. However, the wide and steadily increasing use of herbal remedies and other alternative and complementary medicines (167) emphasizes the potential for drug-induced thrombocytopenia by these non-formulary agents. Publications documenting thrombocytopenia caused by herbal remedies are uncommon, and definite evidence for a causal relationship to a specific compound may be difficult because the composition of herbal remedies is often undocumented and uncertain (167). However, one clear example is the report of a patient with repeated, profound thrombocytopenia from a traditional Chinese herbal medicine, Jui (168), with level I evidence (Table 2). The difficulty of determining the exact etiology for the thrombocytopenia is illustrated by Jui, which is a commercial name for a product that contains five separate herbs (168). Foods may also cause acute and severe thrombocytopenia, and they also were not included in our systematic review. As with herbal remedies, published reports are few, but one clearly documented case report describes recurrent severe thrombocytopenia, with Level I evidence (Table 2), caused by tahini, the principal ingredient of the traditional Middle Eastern food, hummus (169). Another report describes a patient who had four episodes of acute, severe thrombocytopenia caused by the Lupinus termis bean (170).

CLINICAL COURSE OF DRUG-INDUCED THROMBOCYTOPENIA

The history of drug ingestion in a patient with drug-induced thrombocytopenia reveals that the sensitizing drug was almost always taken within one day of the onset of symptoms. Often, acute bleeding symptoms occur within hours of drug ingestion. Drug-induced thrombocytopenia, similar to other manifestations of drug hypersensitivity, is more common when the drug ingestion has been intermittent, or when a daily regimen of the drug has been used for only several weeks. The occurrence of acute thrombocytopenia caused by a drug that has been taken regularly for many months or years is uncommon. In the systematic review of case reports describing drug-induced thrombocytopenia (3), case reports that met the criteria for level I evidence showed that the time of drug ingestion before the initial occurrence of thrombocytopenia ranged from less than 1 day to 3 years, with a median of 14 days.

The onset of drug-induced thrombocytopenia is often accompanied by systemic symptoms of flushing, with a feeling of warmth, often also chills. Bleeding manifestations are the typical mucocutaneous symptoms characteristic of severe thrombocytopenia. Table 3 describes the frequency of major and minor bleeding in the case reports with level I or level II evidence for a causal association of the drug with thrombocytopenia. The definition of major bleeding used in these reviews was adapted from clinical trials of anti-thrombotic agents (171). Major bleeding was defined as intracranial or retroperitoneal bleeding, or overt bleeding (that is, visible or symptomatic bleeding) with a decrease of hemoglobin concentration by more than 2 gm/dL or the requirement of transfusion of two or more units of red cells. Minor bleeding was defined as overt bleeding that did not meet the criteria for major bleeding. The frequency of clinically important bleeding in these reports emphasizes the severity of drug-induced thrombocytopenia. Even though the more severe patients are more likely to be reported, the severity of drug-induced thrombocytopenia is apparent. Two reported patients died from hemorrhage caused by quinine-induced thrombocytopenia (172).

The key diagnostic feature is prompt spontaneous resolution of thrombocytopenia following discontinuation of the drug. In the systematic review of case reports (3), the time to recovery to a normal platelet count after discontinuation of the drug was 1 to 30 days with a median of 7 days. Upon rechallenge with a single administration of the offending drug, the time to the nadir of thrombocytopenia was a median of 3 days, although in some patients acute thrombocytopenia occurred within minutes or hours. The time to recovery following a rechallenge was similar to the time to recovery after the initial occurrence of thrombocytopenia, a median of 5 days.

Patients with drug-induced thrombocytopenia are often treated with glucocorticoids, since the distinction from acute ITP is not possible at the time of initial evaluation. However, glucocorticoid treatment appears to make no difference in the time to recovery from drug-induced thrombocytopenia (173). Platelet transfusions are appropriate for patients with severe thrombocytopenia and overt bleeding, especially if the suspected drug is a fibrinogen receptor antagonist that also inhibits the function of the platelets remaining in the circulation. Once established, sensitivity to drugs causing immune thrombocytopenia is usually permanent. Therefore, patients must be explicitly instructed to avoid all potential reexposures.

REFERENCES

1. Vipan WH. Quinine as a cause of purpura. Lancet 1865; 2:37.
2. Aster RH. Response of thrombocytes to toxic injury. In: Bloom JC, ed. Toxicology of the Hematopoietic System. St. Louis: Elsevier Science Publishers, 1997.
3. George JN, Raskob GE, Shah SR, et al. Drug-Induced Thrombocytopenia: a systematic review of published case reports. Ann Int Med 1998; 129:886–890.
4. Aster R. Drug-induced immune thrombocytopenia: an overview of pathogenesis. Semin Hematol 1999; 36:2–6.
5. Rizvi MA, Shah SR, Raskob GE, George JN. Drug-induced thrombocytopenia. Curr Opinion in Hematol 1999; 6:349–353.
6. Aster RH. Drug-induced thrombocytopenia. In: Michelson AD, ed. Platelets. Amsterdam: Academic Press, 2002:593–606.
7. Blay JY, Le Cesne A, Mermet C, et al. A risk model for thrombocytopenia requiring platelet transfusion after cytotoxic chemotherapy. Blood 1998; 92:405–410.
8. Kurzrock R, Cortes J, Thomas DA, Jeha S, Pilat S, Talpaz M. Pilot study of low-dose interleukin-11 in patients with bone marrow failure. J Clin Oncol 2001; 19:4165–4172.

9. Kaufam DW, Kelly JP, Jurgelon JM, et al. Drugs in the aetiology of agranulocytosis and aplastic anaemia. Eur J Haematol 1996; 60:23–30.
10. Wilholm BE, Emanuelsson S. Drug-related blood dyscrasias in Swedish reporting system. Eur J Haematol 1996; 60:42–46.
11. Young NS. Immune pathophysiology of acquired aplastic anaemia. Eur J Haematol 1996; 60:55–59.
12. Solberg LA, Tefferi A, Oles KJ, et al. The effects of anagrelide on human megakaryocytopoiesis. Br J Haematol 1997; 99:174–180.
13. Oertel MD. Anagrelide a selective thrombocytopenic agent. Am J Health-System Pharmacy 1998; 55:1979–1986.
14. Anonymous. Anagrelide a therapy for thrombocytopenia states: experience in 577 patients. Am J Med 1992; 92:69.
15. Silverstein MN, Tefferi A. Treatment of essential thrombocythemia with anagrelide. Semin Hematol 1999; 36:23–25.
16. McCune JS, Liles D, Lindley C. Precipitous fall in platelet count with anagrelide: case report and critique of dosing recommendations. Pharmacotherapy 1998; 17:822–826.
17. Trannel TJ, Ahmed I, Goebert D. Occurrence of thrombocytopenia in psychiatric patients taking valproate. Am J Psychiatry 2001; 158:128–130.
18. Kaufman KR, Gerner R. Dose-dependent valproic acid thrombocytopenia in bipolar disorder. Ann Clin Psychiatry 1998; 10:35–37.
19. Eastham RD, Jancar J. Sodium valproate and platelet counts. BMJ 1980; 280:186.
20. May RB, Sunder TR. Hematologic manifestations of long-term valproate therapy. Epilepsia 1993; 34:1098–1101.
21. Brichard B, Vermylen C, Scheiff JM, Ninane J, Cornu G. Harmatological disturbances during long-term valproate therapy. Eur J Pediatr 1994; 153:378–380.
22. Poisson L, Gutierrez-Ramos JC, Weich NS. Sodium valproate directly inhibits thrombopoietin induced megakaryocytopoiesis from human bone marrow $CD34^+$ cells invitro. Exp Hematol 2000; 28:1505.
23. Proulle V, Masnou P, Cartron J, et al. GPIa/IIa as a candiate target for anti-platelet autoantibody occurring during valproate therapy and associated with preoperative bleeding [letter]. Thromb Haemost 2000; 83:175–176.
24. Sleiman C, Raffy O, Roue C, Mal H. Fatal pulmonary hemorrhage during high-dose valproate monotherapy. Chest 2000; 117:613.
25. Girard DE, Kumar KL, McAfee JH. Hematologic effects of acute and chronic alcohol abuse. Hematol Oncol Clin North Am 1987; 1:321–334.
26. Gewirtz AM, Hoffman R. Transitory hypomegakaryocytic thrombocytopenia: etiological association with ethanol abuse and complications regarding regulation of human megakaryocytopoiesis. Br J Haematol 1986; 62:333.
27. Rakela J, Wood JR, Czaja AJeal. Long-term versus short-term treatment with recombinant interferon alfa-2a in patients with chronic hepatitis B: a prospective randomized treatment trial. Mayo Clin Proc 1990; 65:1330–1335.
28. Martin TG, Shuman MA. Interferon-induced thrombocytopenia: is it time for thrombopoietin? Hepatology 1998; 28:1430–1432.
29. Toccaceli F, Rosati S, Scuderi M, Iacomi F, Picconi R, Laghi V. Leukocyte and platelet lowering by some interferon types during viral hepatitis treatment. Hepatogastroenterology 1998; 45:1748–1752.

30. Ganser A, Carlo-Stella C, Greher Jeal. Effect of recombinant interferon alpha and gamma on human bone marrow-derived megakaryocytic progenitor cells. Blood 1987; 70:1173–1179.
31. Peck-Radosavljevic M, Wichlas M, Homoncik-Kraml M, Kreil M, et al. Rapid suppression of hematopoiesis by standard or pegylated interferon-alpha. Gastroenterology 2002; 123:141–151.
32. Khan HA, Khawaja FI, Mahrous AR. Life-threatening severe immune thrombocytopenia after alpha-interferon therapy for chronic hepatitis C infection. Am J Gastro 1996; 91:821–822.
33. Dourakis SP, Deutsch M, Hadziyannis SJ. Immune thrombocytopenia and alpha-interferon therapy. J Hepatol 1996; 25:972–975.
34. Sata M, Yano Y, Yoshiyama Y, et al. Mechanisms of thrombocytopenia induced by interferon therapy for chronic hepatitis B. J Gastroenterology 1997; 32:206–210.
35. Verma A, Deb DK, Sassano A, et al. Activation of the p38 mitogen-activated protein kinase mediates the suppressive effects of Type I interferons and transforming growth factor-beta on normal hematopoiesis. J Biol Chem 2002; 277:7726–7735.
36. Benci A, Caremani M, Tacconi D. Thrombocytopenia in patients with HCV-positive chronic hepatitis: efficacy of leucocyte interferon-alpha treatment. Int J Clin Pract 2003; 57:17–19.
37. Rajan S, Liebman HA. Treatment of hepatitis C related thrombocytopenia with interferon alpha. Am J Hematol 2001; 68:202–209.
38. Wakefield TW, Bouffard JA, Spauldin SA. Sequestration of platelets in the pulmonary circulation as a consequence of protamine reversal of the anticoagulant effects of heparin. J Vasc Surg 1987; 5:187.
39. Al-Mondhiry H, Pierce W, Basarab R. Protamine-induced thrombocytopenia and leukopenia. Thromb Haemost 1985; 53:60–64.
40. Barstad RM, Stephens RW, Hamers MJ, Sakariassen KS. Protamine sulphate inhibits platelet membrane glycoprotein Ib-von Willebrand factor activity. Thromb Haemost 2000; 83:334–337.
41. Griffin MJ, Rinder HM, Smith BR, et al. The effects of heparin, protamine, and heparin/protamine reversal on platelet function under conditions of arterial shear stress. Anesth Analg 2001; 93:20–27.
42. Bukowski RM, Murthy S, McLain D. Phase I trial of recombinant granulocyte-microphage colony-stimulating factor in patients with lung cancer: clinical and immunologic effects. J Immunother 1993; 13:267–274.
43. Tortajada C, Garcia F, Miro JM, Gatell JM. Severe thrombocytopenia related to granulocyte-macrophage colony-stimulating factor (rHUGM-CSF). Ann Med Intern 2000; 17:671.
44. Baker GR, Levin J. Transient thrombocytopenia produced by administration of macrophage colony-stimulating factor: investigations of the mechanism. Blood 1998; 91:89–99.
45. Michelmann I, Bockmann D, Nurnberger W, Eckhof-Donovan S, Gobel U. Thrombocytopenia and complement activation under recombinant TNF alpha/IFN gamma therapy in man. Ann Hematol 1987; 74:179–184.
46. Paciucci PA, Mandeli J, Oleksowicz L, Ameglio F, Holland JF. Thrombocytopenia during immunotherapy with interleukin-2 by constant infusion. Am J Med 1990; 89:308–312.

47. Fleischmann JD, Shingleton WB, Gallagher C, Ratnoff OD, Chahine A. Fibrinolysis, thrombocytopenia, and coagulation abnormalities complicating high-dose interleukin-2 immunotherapy. J Lab Clin Med 1991; 117:76–82.
48. Gringeri A, Santagostino E, Tradati Feal. Adverse effects of treatment with porcine factor VIII. Thromb Haemost 1991; 65:245–247.
49. Chang H, Mody M, Lazarus AH, et al. Platelet activation induced by porcine factor VIII (Hyate:C). Am J Hematol 1998; 57:200–205.
50. Holmberg L, Nilsson M, Borge L, Gunnarsson M, Sjorin E. Platelet aggregation induced by 1-desamino-Darginine vasopressin (DDAVP) in Type IIB von Willebrand's disease. New Engl J Med 1983; 309:816–821.
51. Casonato A, Pontara E, Dannhauser D, et al. Re-evaluation of the therapeutic efficacy of DDAVP in Type IIb von Willebrand's disease. Blood Coagul Fibrinolysis 1994; 5:959–964.
52. Sun HL, Chien CC. Thrombocytopenia and subdural hemorrhage after desmopressin administration. Anesthesiology 1998; 88:1115–1117.
53. Miller JL. Platelet-type von willebrand disease. Thromb Haemost 1996; 75:865–869.
54. Tait AS, Cranmer SL, Jackson SP, Dawes IW, Chong BH. Phenotype changes resulting in high-affinity binding of von Willebrand factor to recombinant glycoprotein Ib-IX: analysis of the platelet-type von Willebrand disease mutations. Blood 2001; 98:1812–1828.
55. Takahashi H, Okada K, Abe Seal, Wada K, Nagayama R, Tatewaki W, Hanano M, Takizawa S, Shibata A. Platelet aggregation induced by cryoprecipitate infusion in platelet-type von Willebrand's disease. Thromb Res 1987; 46:255–262.
56. Offerman SR, Barry JD, Schneir A, Clark RF. Biphasic rattlesnake venom-induced thrombocytopenia. J Emerg Med 2003; 24:289–293.
57. Rucavado A, Sota M, Kamiguti AS, et al. Characterization of aspercetin, a platelet aggregating component from the venom of the snake Bothrops asper which induces thrombocytopenia and potentiates metalloproteinase-induced hemorrhage. Thromb Haemost 2001; 85:710–715.
58. Chong BH. Drug-induced immune thrombocytopenia. Platelets 1991; 2:173.
59. Salama A, Mueller-Eckhardt C. Immune-mediated blood dyscrasias related to drugs. Semin Hematol 1992; 29:54.
60. Neylon AJ, Saunders PWG, Howard MR, Proctor SJ, Taylor PRA. Clinically significant newly presenting autoimmune thrombocytopenic purpura in adults: a prospective study of a population-based cohort of 245 patients. Br J Haematol 2003; 122:966–974.
61. Ackroyd JF. Allergic purpura, including purpura due to food, drugs and infection. Am J Med 1953; 14:605.
62. Ackroyd JF. The immunological basis of purpura due to drug hypersensitivity. Proc R Soc Med 1962; 55:30.
63. Garratty G. Immune cytopenia associated with antibiotics. Transfus Med Rev 1993; VII:255–267.
64. Levine B, Redmond A. Immunochemical mechanisms of penicillin induced Coombs positivity and hemolytic anemia in man. Int Arch Allergy 1967; 21:594–606.
65. Murphy MF, Riordan T, Minchinton RM. Demonstration of an immume-mediated mechanism of penicillin-induced neutropenia and thrombocytopenia. Br J Haematol 1983; 55:155.

66. Lang R, Lishner M, Ravid M. Adverse reactions to prolonged treatment with high doses of carbenicillin and ureidopenicillins. Rev Infect Dis 1992; 13:68–72.
67. Parker JD, Barrett DA, II. Microangiopathic hemolysis and thrombocytopenia related to penicillin drugs. Arch Intern Med 1971; 127:474–477.
68. Shulman NR, Reid DM. Mechanisms of drug-induced immunologically mediated cytopenias. Transfus Med Rev 1993; 7:215–229.
69. Mueller-Eckhardt C, Salama A. Drug-induced immune cytopenias: a unifying pathogenetic concept with special emphasis on the role of drug metabolites. Trans Med Rev 1990; 4:69.
70. Bougie D, Aster R. Immune thrombocytopenia resulting from sensitivity to metabolites of naproxen and acetaminophen. Blood 2001; 97:3846–3850.
71. Shulman NR. Immunoreactions involving platelets. I. A steric and kinetic model for formation of a complex from a human antibody, quinidine as a haptene, and platelets, and for fixation of complement by the complex. J Exp Med 1958; 107:665.
72. Shulman NR. Immunoreactions involving platelets. III. Quantitative aspects of platelet agglutination, in hibition of clot retraction, and other reactions caused by the antibody of quinidine purpura. J Exp Med 1958; 107:697.
73. Shulman NR. A mechanism of cell destruction in individuals sensitized to foreign antigens and its implications in autoimmunity. Ann Intern Med 1964; 60:506.
74. Christie DJ, Mullen PC, Aster RH. Fab-mediated binding of drug-dependent antibodies to platelets in quinidine- and quinine-induced thrombocytopenia. J Clin Invest 1985; 75:310.
75. Smith ME, Reid DM, Jones CE. Binding of quinine- and quinidine-dependent drug antibodies to platelets is mediated by the Fab domain of the immunoglobulin G and is not Fc dependent. J Clin Invest 1987; 79:912.
76. Koch-Weser J, Sellers EM. Binding of drugs to serum albumin (First of two parts). New Eng J Med 1976; 294:311–316.
77. Koch-Weser J, Sellers EM. Binding of drugs to serum albumin (Second of two parts). New Engl J Med 1976; 294:526–531.
78. Christie DJ, Aster RH. Drug-antibody-platelet interaction in quinine-and quinidine-induced thrombocytopenia. J Clin Invest 1982; 70:989–998.
79. Chong BH, Du X, Berndt MD, Horn S, Chesterman CN. Characterization of the binding domains on platelet glycoproteins Ib-IX and IIb/IIIa complexes for the quinine/quinidine-dependent antibodies. Blood 1991; 77:2190.
80. Visentin GP, Newman PJ, Aster RH. Characteristics of quinine- and quinidine-induced antibodies specific for platelet glycoproteins IIb and IIIa. Blood 1991; 77:2668.
81. Peterson JA, Nyree CE, Newman PJ, Aster RH. A site involving the "hybrid" and PSI homology domains of GPIIIa (ß-integrin subunit) is a common target for antibodies associated with quinine-induced immune thrombocytopenia. Blood 2003; 101:937–942.
82. Asvadi P, Ahmadi Z, Chong BH. Drug-induced thrombocytopenia: localization of the binding site of GOIX-specific quinine-dependent antibodies. Blood 2003; 102:1670–1677.
83. Curtis BR, McFarland JG, Wu G-G, Visentin GP, Aster RH. Antibodies in sulfonamide-induced immune thrombocytopenia recognize calcium-dependent epitopes on the glycoprotein IIb/IIIa Complex. Blood 1994; 84:176–183.

84. Pereira J, Hidalgo P, Ocqueteau M, et al. Glycoprotein Ib/IX complex is the target in rifampicin-induced immune thrombocytopenia. Br J Haematol 2000; 110:907–910.
85. Burgess JK, Lopez JA, Gaudry LE, Chong BH. Rifampicin-dependent antibodies bind a similar or identical epitope to glycoprotein IX-specific quinine-dependent antibodies. Blood 2000; 95:1988–1992.
86. Kroll H, Sun QH, Santoso S. Platelet endothelial cell adhesion molecule-1 (PECAM-1) is a target glycoprotein in drug-induced thrombocytopenia. Blood 2000; 96:1409–1414.
87. Merk HF, Baron J, Kawakubo Y, Hertl M, Jugert F. Metabolites and allergic drug reactions. Clin Exp Allergy 1998; 28:21–24.
88. Park BK, Kitteringham NR, Pirmohamed M. Metabolic activation in drug allergies. Toxicology 2001; 158:11–23.
89. Cohen SD, Pumford NR, Khairallah EA, et al. Contemporary issues in toxicology. Selective protein covalent binding and target organ toxicity. Toxicol Appl Pharmacol 1997; 143:1–12.
90. de Wildt SN, Kearns GL, Leeder JS, Van den Anker JN. Glucuronidation in humans. Clin Pharmacokinet 1999; 36:439–452.
91. Williams AM, Worrall S, DeJersey J, Dickinson RG. On the reactivity of acyl glucuronides. VIII. Generation of an antiserum for the detection of dlflunisal-modified proteins in diflunisal-dosed rats. Biochem Pharmacol 1995; 49:209–217.
92. Zia-Amirhosseinin P, Spahn-Langguth H, Benet LZ. Bioactivation by glucuronide-conjugate formation. Adv Phamracol 1994; 27:385–397.
93. Zia-Amirhosseinin P, Harris RZ, Brodsky FM, Benet LZ. Hypersensitivity to nonsteroidal anti-inflammatory drugs. Nature Med 1995; 1:2–4.
94. Pohl LR, Satoh H, Chris DD, Kenna JG. The immunologic and metabolic basis of drug hypersensitivies. Ann Rev Pharmacol Toxicol 1988; 28:367–387.
95. Pessayre D. Role of reactive metabolites in drug-induced hepatitis. J Hepatol 1995; 23:16–24.
96. Uetrecht JP. New concepts in immunology relevant to idiosyncratic drug reactions; the "danger hypothesis" and innate immune system. Chem Res Toxicol 1999; 12:387–395.
97. Roujeau JC, Stern RS. Severe adverse cutaneous reactions to drugs. New Engl J Med 1994; 331:1272–1285.
98. Roujeau JC, Kelly JP, Naldi L, Rzany B. Medication use and the risk of Stevens-Johnson syndrome or toxic epidermal necrolysis. New Eng J Med 1995; 333:1600–1607.
99. Meyer UA, Zanger UM. Molecular mechanisms of genetic polymorphisms of drug metabolism. Annu Rev Pharmacol Toxicol 1997; 37:269–296.
100. Pirmohamed M, Park BK. Genetic susceptibility to adverse drug reactions. Pharmacol Sci 2001; 22:298–305.
101. Bougie D, Johnson ST, Weitekamp LA, Aster RH. Sensitivity to a metabolite of diclofenac as a cause of acute immune hemolytic anemia. Blood 1997; 90:407–413.
102. Cines DB. Glycoprotein IIb/IIIa antagonists: potential induction and detection of drug-dependent antiplatelet antibodies. Am Heart J 1998; 135:S152–S159.
103. Bougie DW, Wilker PR, Wuitschick ED, et al. Acute thrombocytopenia after treatment with tirofiban or eptifibatide is associated with antibodies specific for ligand-occupied GPIIb/IIIa. Blood 2002; 100:2071–2076.

104. Billheimer JT, Dicker IB, Wynn R, et al. Evidence that thrombocytopenia observed in humans treated with orally bioavailable glycoprotein IIb/IIIa antagonists is immune mediated. Blood 2002; 99:3540–3546.
105. Brassard JA, Curtis BR, Cooper RA, et al. Acute thronmbocytopenia in patients treated with the oral glycoprotein IIb/IIIa inhibitors xemilofiban and orbofiban: evidence for an immune etiology. Thromb Haemost 2002; 88:892–897.
106. Frelinger AL, Du XP, Plow EF, et al. Monoclonal antibodies to ligand-occupied conformers of intgrin alpha IIb beta 3 (glycoprotein IIb/IIIa) alter receptor affinity specificity and function. J Biol Chem 1991; 266:17106–17111.
107. Jennings LK, White MM. Expression of ligand-induced binding sites on glycoprotein IIb/IIIa complexes and the effect of various inhibitors. Am Heart J 1998; 135:S179–S183.
108. Seiffert D, Stern AM, Ebling W, Rossi RJ, Barret YC, Wynn R, et al. Prospective testing for drug-dependent antibodies reduces the incidence of thrombocytopenia observed with the small molecule glycoprotein IIb/IIIa antagonist roxifiban: implications for the etiology of thrombocytopenia. Blood 2003; 101:58–63.
109. Coller BS, Platelet GP IIb/IIIa antagonists: the first anti-integrin receptor therapeutics. J Clin Invest 1997; 99:1467–1471.
110. Lincoff AM, Califf RM, Moliterno DJ, et al. Complementary clinical benefits of coronary-artery stenting and blockade of platelet glycoprotein IIb/IIIa receptors. New Eng J Med 1999; 341:319–327.
111. Tcheng JE. Clinical challenges of platelet glycoprotein IIb/IIIa receptor inhibitor therapy: bleeding reversal thrombocytopenia and retreatment. Am Heart J 2000; 139:S38–S45.
112. Berkowitz SD, Sane DC, Sigmon KN, et al. Occurrence and clinical significance of thrombocytopenia in a population undergoing high-risk percutaneous coronary revascularization. J Amer Coll Cardiol 1998; 32:311–319.
113. Jubelirer SJ, Koenig BA, Bates MC. Acute profound thrombocytopenia following C7E3 Fab (abciximab) therapy: case reports, review of the literature and implications for therapy. Amer J Hematol 1999; 61:205–208.
114. Curtis BR, Swyers J, Divgi A, McFarland JG, Aster RH. Thrombocytopenia after second exposure to abciximab is caused by antibodies that recognize abciximab-coated platelets. Blood 2002; 99:2054–2059.
115. Trivedi SM, Shani J, Hollander G. Bleeding complications of platelet glycoprotein IIb/IIIa inhibitor abciximam (ReoPro™). J Invasive Cardiol 2002; 14:423–425.
116. Iakovou Y, Manginas A, Melissari E, Cokkinos DV. Acute profound thrombocytopenia associated with anaphylactic reaction after abciximab therapy during percutaneous coronary angioplasty. Cardiology 2001; 95:215–216.
117. Peter K, Straub A, Kohler B, et al. Platelet activation as a potential mechanism of GP IIb/IIIa inhibitor-induced thrombocytopenia. Amer J Cardiol 1999; 84:519–524.
118. Worlledge SM. Immune drug-induced hemolytic anemias. Semin Haematol 1973; 4:327–344.
119. Petz LD. Drug-induced autoimmune hemolytic anemia. Transfus Med Rev 1993; 7:242–254.
120. Adachi JD, Bensen WG, Kassam Y. Gold induced thrombocytopenia: 12 cases and a review of the literature. Semin Arthritis Rheum 1987; 16:287.

121. von dem Borne AEGKr, Pegels JG, van der Stadt RJ. Thrombocytopenia associated with gold therapy: a drug-induced autoimmune disease? Br J Haematol 1986; 63:509.
122. Aster R. Can drugs cause autoimmune thrombocytopenic purpura? Semin Hematol 2000; 37:229–238.
123. Lerner W, Caruso R, Faig D, Karpatkin S. Drug-dependent and non-drug-dependent antiplatelet antibody in drug-induced immunologic thrombocytopenic purpura. Blood 1985; 66:306.
124. Eisner EV, Shaidi NT. Immune thrombocytopenia due to a drug metabolite. N Engl J Med 1972; 287:376.
125. Eisner EV, Kasper K. Immune thrombocytopenia due to a metabolite of para-aminosalicylic acid. Am J Med 1972; 53:709.
126. Kiefel V, Santoso S, Schmidt S. Metabolite-specific (IgG) and drug-specific antibodies (IgG, IgM) in two cases of trimethoprim-sulfamethoxazole-induced immune thrombocytopenia. Transfusion 1989; 27:262.
127. Salamon DJ, Nusbacher J, Stroupe T. Red cell and platelet-bound IgG penicillin antibodies in a patient with thrombocytopenia. Transfusion 1984; 24:395.
128. Christie DJ, Lennon SS, Drew RL, Swinehart CD. Cefotetan-induced immunologic thrombocytopenia. Br J Haematol 1988; 70:423–426.
129. Aljitawi O, Krishnan K, Curtis B, Bougie D, Aster R. Serologically documented loracarbef (Lorabid)—induced immune thrombocytopenia. Am J Hematol 2003; 73:41–43.
130. Arndt PA, Leger R, Garratty G. Serology of antibodies to second-and third-generation cephalosporins associated with immune hemolytic anemia and/or positive direct antiblodbulin tests. Transfusion 1999;(1999):1239–1246.
131. Arndt P, Garratty G. Cross-reactivity of cefotetan and ceftriaxone antibodies, associated with hemolytic anemia. Am J Clin Pathol 2002; 118:256–262.
132. Salama A, Mueller-Eckhardt C. Cianidanol and its metabolites bind tightly to red cells and are responsible for the production of auto and/or drug-dependent antibodies against these cells. Br J Haematol 1987; 66:263–266.
133. Habibi B. Drug induced red blood cell autoantibodies co-developed with drug specific antibodies causing haemolytic anaemias. Br J Haematol 1985; 61:139–143.
134. Cimo PL, Pisciotta AV, Desai RG. Detection of drug-dependent antibodies by the ^{51}Cr platelet lysis test: documentation of immune thrombocytopenia induced by diphenylhydantoin, diazepam, and sulfisoxazole. Am J Hematol 1977; 2:65.
135. Visentin GP, Wolfmeyer K, Newman PJ, Aster RH. Detection of drug-dependent, platelet-reactive antibodies by antigen-capture ELISA and flow cytometry. Transfusion 1990; 30:694–700.
136. Peterson JA, Visentin GP, Newman PJ, Aster RH. A recombinant soluble form of the integrin $\alpha_{IIb}\beta_3$ (GPIIb-IIIa) assumes an active, ligand-binding conformation and is recognized by GPIIb-IIIa specific monoclonal, allo-, auto-, and drug-dependent platelet antibodies. Blood 1998; 92:2053–2063.
137. Leach MF, Cooper LK, AuBuchon JP. Detection of drug-dependent, platelet-reactive antibodies by solid-phase red cell adherence assays. Br J Haematol 1997; 97:755–761.

138. Burgess JK, Lopez JA, Berndt MC, Dawes I, Chesterman CN, Chong BH. Quinine-dependent antibodies bind a restricted set of epitopes on the glycoprotein Ib-IX complex: characterization of the epitopes. Blood 1998; 92:2366–2373.
139. Salama A, Mueller-Eckhardt C, Kissel K, Pralle H, Seeger W. Ex vivo antigen preparation for the serological detection of drug-dependent antibodies in immune hemolytic anemias. Br J Haematol 1984; 58:525.
140. Salama A, Santoso S, Mueller-Eckhardt C. Antigenic determinants responsible for the reactions of drug-dependent antibodies with blood cells. Br J Haematol 1991; 78:535.
141. D'Cunha P, Lord RS, Johnson ST, Wilker PR, Aster RH, Bougie DW. Immune hemolytic anemia caused by sensitivity to a metabolite of the nonsteroidal anti-inflammatory drug etodolac. Transfusion 2000; 40:663–668.
142. Bednar B, Cook JJ, Holahan MA, Cunningham ME, Jumes PA, Bednar RA, et al. Fibrinogen receptor antagonist-induced thrombocytopenia in chimpanzee and rhesus monkey associated with preexisting drug-dependent antibodies to platelet glycoprotein IIb/IIIa. Blood 1999;94.
143. Knight DM, Wagner C, Jordan R, McAleer MF, DeRita R, Fass DN. The immunogenicity of the 7E3 murine monoclonal Fab antibody fragment variable region is dramatically reduced in humans by substitution of human for murine constant regions. Mol Immunol 1995; 32:1271–1281.
144. Kelton JG. The serological investigation of patients with autoimmune thrombocytopenia. Thromb Haemost 1995; 74:228–233.
145. McMillan R. The pathogenesis of chronic immune (idiopathic) thrombocytopenic purpura. Semin Hematol 2000; 37:5–9.
146. Chong BH, Keng TB. Advances in the diagnosis of idiopathic thrombocytopenic purpura. Semin Hematol 2000; 37:249–260.
147. Warner MN, Moore JC, Warkentin TE, Santos AV, Kelton JG. A prospective study of protein-specific assays used to investigate idiopathic thrombocytopenic purpura. Br J Haematol 1999; 104:442–447.
148. Hibbard AB, Medina PJ, Vesely SK. Reports of drug-induced thrombocytopenia. Ann Int Med 2003; 138:239.
149. Rizvi MA, Kojouri K, George JN. Drug-induced thrombocytopenia: an updated systematic review. Ann Int Med 2001; 134:346.
150. Gurwitz JH, Field TS, Harrold LR, et al. Incidence and preventability of adverse drug events among older persons in the ambulatory setting. JAMA 2003; 289:1107–1116.
151. Cook DJ, Mulrow CD, Haynes RB. Systematic reviews: synthesis of best evidence for clinical decisions. Ann Int Med 1997; 126:376–380.
152. Sorbye H, Bruserud Y, Dahl O. Oxaliplatin-induced haematological emergency with an immediate severe thrombocytopenia and haemolysis. Acta Oncol 2001; 40:882–883.
153. Dold FG, Mitchell EP. Sudden-onset thrombocytopenia with oxaliplatin. Ann Int Med 2003; 139:E156.
154. Curtis BR, Kaliszewski J, Blank J, McFarland J, Aster RH. Severe thrombocytopenia caused by high titer IgG oxaliplatin-dependent platelet antibodies. Blood 2003; 102:538a.
155. Oboler SK, Prochazka AV, Meyer TJ. Leg symptoms in outpatient veterans. West J Med 1991; 155:256–259.

156. Naylor JR, Young JB. A general population survey of rest cramps. Age and Aging 1994; 23:418–420.
157. Moss HK, Herrmann LG. The use of quinine for the relief of "night cramps" in the extremeties. JAMA 1940; 115:1358–1359.
158. Brinker AD, Beitz J. Spontaneous reports of thrombocytopenia in association with quinine: Clinical attributes and timing related to regulatory action. Am J Hematol 2002; 70:313–317.
159. Kojouri K, Perdue JJ, Medina PJ, George JN. Occult quinine-induced thrombocytopenia. Oklahoma State Med J 2000; 93:519–521.
160. Belkin GA. Cocktail purpura: an unusual case of quinine sensitivity. Ann Intern Med 1967; 66:583.
161. Korbitz BC, Eisner E. Cocktail purpura. Quinine-dependent thrombocytopenia. Rocky Mt Med J 1973; 70:38–41.
162. Barrett AP, Tversky J, Griffiths CJ. Thrombocytopenia induced by quinine. Oral Surg Med Oral Path 1983; 55:351–354.
163. Wagner GH, Diffey BL, Ive FA. "I'll have mine with a twist of lemon." Quinine photosensitivity from excessive intake of tonic water. Br J Dermatol 1994; 131:734–735.
164. Brasic JR. Quinine-induced thrombocytopenia in a 64-year-old man who consumed tonic water to relieve nocturnal leg cramps. Mayo Clin Proc 2001; 76:863–864.
165. Barr E, Douglas JF, Hill CM. Recurrent acute hypersensitivity to quinine. Brit Med J 1990; 301:323.
166. Gottschall JL, Elliot W, Lianos E, McFarland JG, Wolfmeyer K, Aster RH. Quinine-induced immune thrombocytopenia associated with hemolytic uremic syndrome: a new clinical entity. Blood 1991; 77:306–310.
167. De Smet PAGM. Herbal remedies. New Eng J Med 2002; 347:2046–2056.
168. Azuno Y, Yaga K, Sasayama T, Kimoto K. Thrombocytopenia induced by Jui, a traditional Chinese herbal medicine. Lancet 1999; 354:304–305.
169. Arnold J, Ouwehand WH, Smith G, Cohen H. A young women with petechiae. Lancet 1998; 352:618.
170. Lavy R. Thrombocytopenic purpura due to lupinus termis bean. J Allergy 1964; 35:386–388.
171. Graafsma YP, Prins MH, Lensing AWA, de Haan RJ, Huisman MV, Buller HR. Bleeding classification in clinical trials: observer variability and clinical relevance. Thromb Haemost 1997; 78:1189–1192.
172. Freiman JP. Fatal quinine-induced thrombocytopenia. Ann Intern Med 1990; 112:308–309.
173. Pedersen-Bjergaard U, Andersen M, Hansen PB. Drug-induced thrombocytopenia: clinical data on 309 cases and the effect of corticosteroid therapy. Eur J Clin Pharmacol 1997; 52:183–189.

8

Heparin-Induced Thrombocytopenia

Theodore E. Warkentin

Department of Pathology and Molecular Medicine and Department of Medicine, McMaster University, and Hamilton Regional Laboratory Medicine Program, Hamilton Health Sciences, General Site, Hamilton, Ontario, Canada

OVERVIEW

Immune heparin-induced thrombocytopenia (HIT) is a common adverse event in certain patient populations who receive standard, unfractionated heparin (UFH) for one week or more, such as postoperative patients (1). Describing this reaction as "common" or "frequent" is not an exaggeration: according to the Council for International Organization of Medical Sciences (2), an adverse drug effect seen in 1% or more patients is common (or frequent). In contrast, reactions that occur in 0.1 to 1% of patients are termed "uncommon" or "infrequent," and those affecting 0.01–0.1% and <0.01% are "rare" and "very rare," respectively.

HIT is caused by immune mechanisms and paradoxically is associated with thrombosis. The unusual prothrombotic character of HIT results from in vivo thrombin generation that results when antibodies are generated against a "self" molecule [platelet factor 4 (PF4)] that has undergone conformational modification in the presence of heparin. In recent years, emphasis has shifted towards treatment and prevention of HIT-associated thrombosis by non-heparin anticoagulants, and also to delaying therapy with oral anticoagulants because of the risk of warfarin-induced microvascular thrombosis. Recently, interest in preventing HIT or its complications has increased, using strategies such as targeted platelet count monitoring and considering use of heparin (and related) preparations that are less likely to cause this immune reaction. Recent reviews highlight these and other aspects of HIT (3–5).

Definition

HIT can be defined as an unexpected clinical event, most often thrombocytopenia with or without thrombosis, in which the presence of platelet-activating, PF4/heparin-dependent IgG antibodies can be implicated. Thus, HIT can be considered a *clinicopathologic syndrome*, since both clinical and laboratory features are important (5,6). As discussed later, defining thrombocytopenia is not as simple as using the lower limit of the normal range (150×10^9/L) (7).

History

The key features of the HIT syndrome were first recognized by a third-year Duke University medical student (Glen Rhodes) working with a hematology resident (Richard Dixon) and the vascular surgeon, Donald Silver [(8), Rhodes, personal communication, November, 2003]. Later, these investigators (9) remarked that previous vascular surgeons had likely observed this syndrome, given previous reports of patients who had developed arterial occlusion by pale, platelet-rich thrombi beginning a week or more after starting heparin (although platelet counts had not been measured) (10,11). Subsequently, Towne and colleagues (12) used the term "white clot syndrome," a term which became popular. This designation has somewhat obscured the relationship between HIT and venous thrombosis, including its link with warfarin-induced venous limb gangrene, which was not recognized until the mid-1990s. The history of HIT is reviewed elsewhere (13).

PATHOGENESIS

The central concept is heparin-induced generation of pathogenic antibodies of IgG class that recognize multimolecular complexes of PF4 and heparin on platelet surfaces, leading to platelet activation in vivo and associated thrombin generation (5). There is evidence that endothelial cells and monocytes also can be activated by HIT antibodies. The concurrence of thrombin generation and increased risk of venous and arterial thrombosis classifies HIT as an acquired hypercoagulability disorder (6). Figure 1 summarizes the pathogenesis of HIT (14).

Immune Disorder

Rhodes and colleagues (8) first suspected an immune pathogenesis of HIT based upon the typical delay of several days between starting heparin and the development of thrombocytopenia, as well as their observation that a circulating platelet-activating substance in patients' blood resulted in aggregation of normal donor platelets in the presence of heparin. Work by other investigators subsequently established that heparin-dependent IgG antibodies effect platelet activation (13).

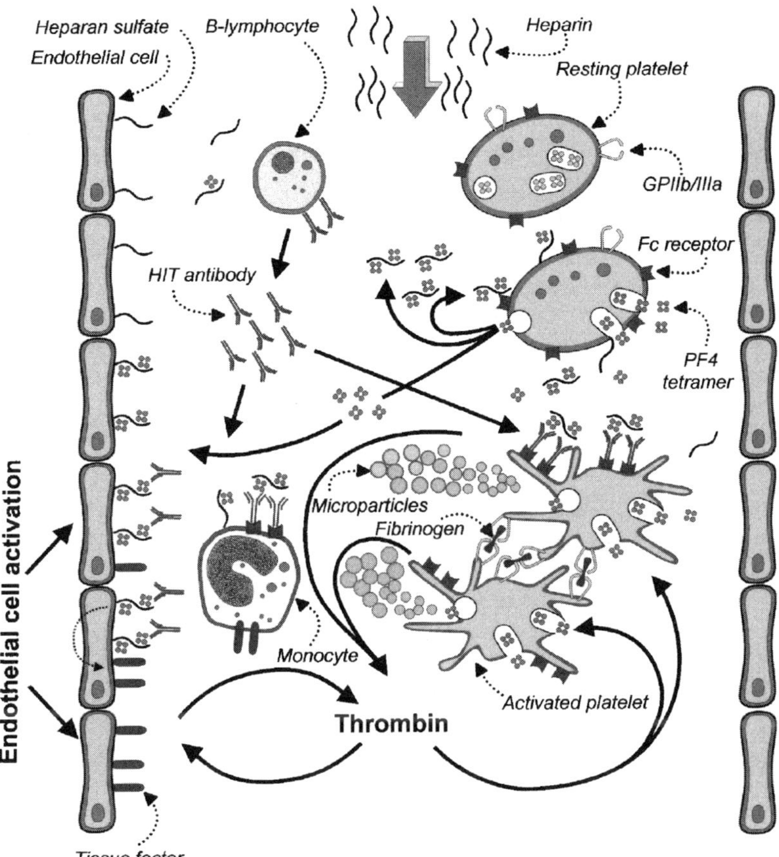

Figure 1 Pathogenesis of HIT: a central role for thrombin generation. PF4–heparin complexes that can express multiple neoepitope sites bind to platelet surfaces (binding via the heparin moiety). HIT-IgG antibodies recognize neoepitope sites on PF4, leading to formation of multimolecular PF4–heparin–IgG complexes on the platelet surface. The IgG Fc regions bind and cross-link the platelet FcγIIa receptors, resulting in platelet activation, including formation of procoagulant, platelet-derived microparticles, which provide altered membrane surfaces that support coagulation reactions. Activated platelets release additional PF4 from α-granules, leading to a vicious cycle of progressive platelet and coagulation activation. PF4 also can bind to endothelial heparan sulfate, leading to endothelial cell immunoinjury, with tissue factor expression. Monocytes also can bind PF4–heparin–IgG immune complexes, potentially leading to tissue factor expression on these cells. Ultimately, these results marked thrombin generation in vivo, which helps explain the strong association between HIT and thrombotic events. *Source*: From Ref. 14.

PF4-Dependent Neoepitope(s)

Amiral and colleagues (15) made the key discovery that HIT antibodies recognize PF4 bound to heparin. PF4 is a 70-amino acid (7780 Da), platelet-specific member of the C-X-C subfamily of chemokines. Four PF4 molecules self-associate to form compact tetramers of globular structure (~31,000 Da). PF4 is rich in the basic amino acids, lysine and arginine, which form a "ring of positive charge" to which heparin binds. Stored in platelet α-granules and on endothelial cells, PF4 levels increase 15- to 30-fold for several hours during heparin treatment as PF4 is displaced from endothelium.

The immune response against PF4–heparin complexes is polyspecific, i.e., at least three neoepitope sites are formed (16–18). Only a minority of sera from heparin-treated patients contain such IgG antibodies in sufficient titer (19) and with sufficient affinity for PF4–heparin (or PF4 alone) (20) to cause platelet activation. The role of the polyanion (heparin) in producing neoepitopes on PF4 is surprisingly nonspecific; indeed, certain non-heparin polyanions (e.g., pentosan polysulfate, polysulfated chondroitin sulfate, PI-88 [experimental anti-angiogenic agent]) can trigger a syndrome that mimics HIT (21–23). Moreover, a non-heparin polyanion (polyvinyl sulfonate) is used in one commercially-available assay to detect HIT antibodies (24).

There is evidence that in occasional patients with clinical evidence of HIT but without detectable PF4-dependent antibodies, other heparin-dependent neoepitopes such as interleukin-8 or neutrophil-activating peptide-2 can be implicated (25,26). It is possible that such antibodies may even predate the heparin exposure. However, HIT caused by antibodies directed against non-PF4-dependent neoepitopes is not well-established.

HIT as an Autoimmune Syndrome

Since HIT neoepitopes are on PF4 (not heparin), HIT can be considered an autoimmune disorder. This concept is particularly apropos given that some HIT-IgG recognize PF4 bound to a solid phase in the absence of heparin (20,27), and activate platelets in vitro without added heparin (20,28). These unusual properties may help explain the rare patient who develops HIT several days after discontinuation of heparin, so-called delayed-onset HIT (28–30).

IgG-Induced Platelet Activation

PF4–heparin complexes bind to platelets (at undetermined sites) by the negative charge of the sulfated heparin (31). Maximal binding of PF4–heparin complexes (and thus optimal platelet activation by HIT-IgG) occurs when the molar ratio of PF4 to heparin is about 1:1 to 2:1 (27,32,33).

Newman and Chong (34) have found that addition of heparin to citrated platelet-rich plasma from patients with HIT leads to release of small amounts of PF4 that bind to platelet surfaces. Subsequently, increasing amounts of HIT-IgG bind to platelets over time, in parallel with progressive platelet aggregation.

Interestingly, platelet activation occurs even though heparin remains in considerable molar excess to PF4, thus suggesting the platelet surface microenvironment provides the conditions to permit formation of PF4–heparin complexes in the appropriate stoichiometric relationship.

The PF4–heparin–IgG immune complexes that are formed occupy platelet FcγIIa receptors, leading to FcγIIa receptor clustering, phosphorylation, signaling events, and strong platelet activation [for review: (35)]. A consequence of platelet activation by HIT-IgG is the formation of procoagulant, platelet-derived microparticles (36–38). Warkentin and Sheppard (39) have shown that HIT-IgG and other platelet IgG agonists (heat-aggregated IgG, platelet-activating monoclonal IgG) cause an even greater platelet procoagulant response than physiologic platelet agonists such as collagen and thrombin. Evidence that platelet activation occurs in vivo in patients with HIT includes increased numbers of circulating platelet-derived microparticles (36).

Only HIT antibodies of IgG class activate platelets. Nevertheless, HIT antibodies of IgA and IgM class are frequently generated in patients who receive heparin (even without thrombocytopenia) and are also often found (together with HIT-IgG) in patients with HIT. There is controversy as to whether non-IgG antibodies cause HIT. Although anecdotal evidence has been presented (40), insufficient clinical details have been presented to support this claim. In prospective studies of HIT antibody formation, we found platelet-activating IgG antibodies in all 15 patients identified with HIT (41).

Any of the four HIT-IgG subclasses can be found in sera from HIT patients, some more often than others (IgG1 > IgG3 > IgG2 > IgG4), with more than one subclass often seen in individual patients (19,42). To date, no difference in clinical profile of HIT in relation to particular IgG subclasses or the added presence of IgM or IgA class antibodies has been identified. Although, in theory, the his_{131}/arg_{131} polymorphism found in human FcγIIa receptors could influence risk of HIT (because human IgG2 preferentially activates FcγRIIa bearing his_{131}), evidence suggests this has a minor (if any) effect (35). Indeed, the largest study (43) noted over-representation of the arg_{131} receptor among patients with HIT-associated thrombosis, leading the authors to suggest that less efficient clearance of immune complexes by the reticuloendothelial system might predispose to greater in vivo platelet activation, and thereby risk of thrombosis.

Transience of HIT Antibodies

The immunopathogenesis of HIT remains largely obscure. Bacsi and colleagues (44,45) found that PF4–heparin complexes stimulate T cells isolated from patients with HIT. Despite this observation, there exists little evidence for immune memory in HIT. First, HIT antibodies usually become undetectable within a few weeks after an episode of HIT (46). Second, HIT antibodies are usually not restimulated when such a patient with previous HIT is reexposed to heparin (47) and, if antibodies are regenerated, they are not formed more quickly than 5 days following reexposure (46,48).

Hypercoagulability Disorder

Thrombin Generation

Thrombin is irreversibly inhibited by covalent binding to its major physiologic inhibitor, antithrombin. The resulting thrombin-antithrombin (TAT) complexes have a short half-life (20 min) and thus quantify recent in vivo thrombin generation. Greatly elevated TAT complex levels exist in most HIT patients (49,50). Increased in vivo thrombin generation is a general feature of hypercoagulability disorders.

Procoagulant Effects of Cellular Activation

In vivo activation of platelets, endothelium, and perhaps even monocytes, helps to explain the prothrombotic effects of HIT (51). In particular, activation of platelets via FcγRIIa leads to formation of procoagulant, platelet-derived microparticles.

There is evidence that HIT antibodies can activate endothelium, perhaps because immunoinjury results from binding of PF4 to heparan sulfate glycosaminoglycan on endothelium (27,32,52). Tissue factor expression by injured endothelium could contribute to the prothrombotic effect of HIT. Kwaan and Sakurai (53) observed hyperplastic, proliferative endothelial cells, together with immunoglobulin deposition within platelet thrombi, in ischemic tissues obtained from patients with HIT. However, whether HIT-IgG antibodies activate endothelium directly (52) or via the consequences of platelet activation (54) remains unclear (51).

Two reports suggest HIT-IgG can activate monocytes in the presence of PF4 (55,56). Moreover, these activated monocytes expressed tissue factor and generated procoagulant activity. Heparin is not required for PF4 binding to monocytes, which is mediated by surface proteoglycans such as chondroitin sulfate.

Animal Models

Various animal models have been described for HIT (for review, see Ref. 57). Only one model recapitulates several key clinical and laboratory features of HIT (58). These investigators developed a novel murine model employing double-transgenic FcγRIIA/hPF4 mice, i.e., mice with platelets bearing human FcγRIIa and human PF4 (mice lack platelet Fcγ receptors and murine PF4 is not recognized by HIT antibodies). When these mice were treated with a HIT-mimicking murine monoclonal antibody that recognizes hPF4/heparin, and then given heparin, the mice developed severe thrombocytopenia and fibrin-rich thrombi in multiple organs, including the lungs.

LABORATORY TESTING FOR HIT ANTIBODIES

Viewed as a clinicopathologic syndrome, laboratory testing for HIT antibodies takes on an important diagnostic role. In general, there are two classes of assays: (a) platelet activation assays and (b) PF4-dependent antigen assays (6,59).

Platelet Activation Assays

Platelets in Citrated Plasma

The inherent platelet-activating properties of pathogenic HIT-IgG antibodies led to the development in the 1970s of standard platelet aggregometry to detect their presence (13). In this method, normal donor platelets [prepared as citrated platelet-rich plasma (c-PRP)] are studied for aggregation after the addition of patient (platelet-poor) plasma and heparin (60). However, this method is relatively insensitive for clinical HIT (sensitivity, 35 to 85%) (61), in part because of variable reactivity among donor platelets from different normal donors to be activated by HIT plasma (62). However, these assays remained popular for many years, owing in part to the wide availability of platelet aggregometers and standardized methods for preparing c-PRP. Unfortunately, these assays suffer from two limitations besides low sensitivity: false-positive reactions (low specificity) especially using c-PRP from critically ill patients (59), and technical limitations that allow only a few tests to be performed at any one time, meaning that relatively few control conditions can be studied. Thus, this group of assays has largely been supplanted by superior, more recent tests.

Washed Platelets

Compared with conventional aggregometry, platelets that are washed and resuspended in divalent cation-containing buffer have increased sensitivity and specificity for detecting platelet-activating HIT antibodies. Donor selection is important, as platelet responsiveness to HIT-IgG varies among normal donors (62). A variety of platelet activation endpoints can be used, including release of radioactive serotonin (62,63), visual assessment of platelet aggregation (64), or generation of platelet-derived microparticles detected by flow cytometry (37). The assays are performed in microtitre wells, so hundreds of reactions can be assessed simultaneously. This permits study of many reaction conditions, for example, various heparin concentrations or the effects of platelet Fc receptor-blocking monoclonal antibody, thus optimizing specificity. HIT antibodies produce a characteristic reaction profile: maximal platelet activation at 0.1 to 0.3 IU/mL heparin that exceeds that caused by the buffer control; greatly reduced activation at 100 U/mL heparin; and inhibition by Fc receptor-blocking monoclonal antibody. Unfortunately, washed platelet activation assays are technically demanding, and performance varies widely among laboratories (65). Another limitation of these assays is that about 2–3% of patient samples contain immune complexes or platelet-activating HLA alloantibodies and thus yield indeterminate results, i.e., platelet activation occurs at all heparin concentrations tested.

PF4-Dependent Antigen Assays

Several PF4-dependent antigen assays are available (for review, see Refs. 6,59).

Solid-Phase Enzyme-Immunoassay

Two solid-phase enzyme-immunoassays (EIAs) are commercially available to detect antibodies of the three major immunoglobulin classes (IgG, IgM, IgA) against PF4 bound either to heparin (Asserachrom, Stago, France) (15) or polyvinyl sulfonate (GTI, Brookfield, WI) (24). The former assay utilizes recombinant PF4, whereas the latter obtains PF4 from outdated platelets. One manufacturer (GTI) recommends a "confirmatory" step assessing whether adding high heparin concentrations inhibits the reaction; only minimal improvement in test specificity results, however (66). Research laboratories that perform in-house PF4/heparin-EIAs have the option to detect antibodies of just the IgG class, which increases specificity for clinical HIT by avoiding detection of non-pathogenic IgA and IgM antibodies (67).

Rapid Particle Gel Immunoassay

Recently, a rapid antigen assay has been developed (68) that appears to have operating characteristics (sensitivity–specificity tradeoffs) intermediate between the commercial EIAs and a washed platelet activation assay (69). The manufacturer's instructions indicate that using neat (undiluted) serum, the assay is to be read as "positive" (any agglutination within the gel), "negative" (no agglutination), or "borderline." However, Alberio and colleagues (70) modified this approach: when they obtained a positive or borderline test result, the assay was repeated using progressively diluted plasma (up to 1 in 1024) until the result was negative. The reported titer was the last positive result followed by either borderline or negative results. Patients judged clinically to have had "probable" or "highly probable/definite" HIT had antibody titers of 4 or more in 39 of 54 (72%) cases, compared with only 2 of 85 (2%) judged "unlikely" to have had HIT. Further, all 19 of the patient samples that tested positive in a c-PRP aggregation assay tested positive in the particle gel immunoassay (generally, in a titer of 8 or higher). Among all patients studied, the percentage with associated thrombotic complications increased from 8% (negative or low titer) to 55% (positive titer 4–16) to 74% (positive titer 32–256). This study suggests the potential diagnostic utility of reporting quantitatively the results of this assay, as a titer of 4 or more appears to be clinically significant. Currently, the particle gel immunoassay is available in Europe and Canada.

Fluid-Phase EIA

Newman and colleagues (71) developed a fluid-phase antigen assay that avoids problems of protein (antigen) denaturation inherent in solid-phase assays. This assay may give a lower rate of false-positive reactions, and unlike solid-phase EIAs is useful for assessing in vitro cross-reactivity of HIT-IgG against LMWH, danaparoid, and fondaparinux (72).

Iceberg Model

The "iceberg model" (1) provides a useful conceptual framework for understanding the relationship between seroconversion and clinical events (Fig. 2). Three such points: (a) only a subset of anti-PF4/heparin IgG antibodies have platelet-activating properties, but (b) those with platelet-activating properties tend to develop thrombocytopenia (i.e., clinical HIT), and (c) the increased risk of HIT-associated thrombosis is seen among patients who develop thrombocytopenia, not those who develop HIT antibody formation without a major platelet count fall (41,73).

Diagnostic Interpretation

Tests vary in their sensitivity and specificity for detecting clinically significant HIT antibodies (Table 1). In general, platelet activation assays using washed platelets have high sensitivity and moderate to high specificity. PF4-dependent antigen assays have high sensitivity and corresponding low to high specificity. For both classes of test, diagnostic specificity is higher when there is a "strong" positive test result, e.g., serotonin release > 80% (platelet activation assay) or > 1.5 absorbance

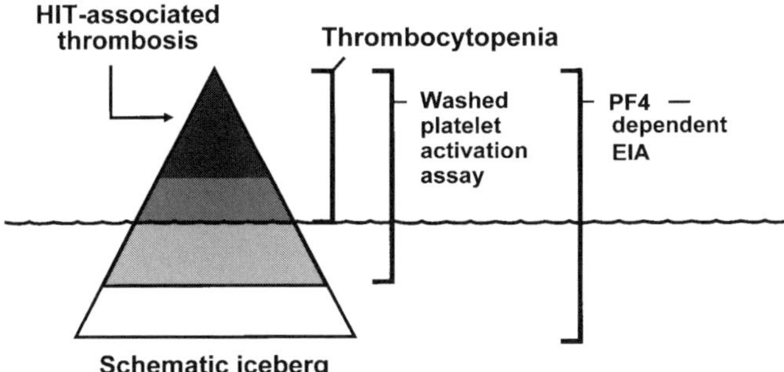

Figure 2 Iceberg model of HIT. Schematic "iceberg" model showing the relationship between HIT antibodies detected by antigen assay [PF4-dependent enzyme-immunoassay (EIA)], washed platelet activation assay [serotonin release assay (SRA)], thrombocytopenia, and HIT-associated thrombosis. Although the antigen assay is more sensitive for detecting HIT antibodies, it is less specific for clinical HIT than the washed platelet activation assay. *Source*: From Ref. 1.

Table 1 HIT Is a "Clinicopathologic" Syndrome

Clinical (percent of patients who exhibit the clinical feature)	Pathologic (tests for HIT antibodies)	Sensitivity	Specificity (0–4 days)[a]	Specificity (≥5 days)[a]
Thrombocytopenia (>95%)	Washed platelet activation assays	>95%	>95%	80–95%
Thrombosis (50–75%)	Serotonin release assay (SRA)			
Heparin-induced skin lesions (at injection sites) (5–10%)	Heparin-induced platelet activation assay (HIPA)			
Acute systemic reactions (post-iv heparin bolus) (5–10%)	PF4-dependent EIA (solid-phase)	>95%	>95%	50–80%
	PF4/polyvinyl sulfonate			
	PF4/heparin			
DIC (decompensated) (5–15%)	PF4/heparin particle-gel immunoassay	?	?	?

Abbreviation: DIC, disseminated intravascular coagulation; iv, intravenous; PF4, platelet factor 4.
[a] The specificity decreases in a patient who has received heparin 5–30 days ago, since subclinical HIT antibody seroconversion may have occurred.

units (PF4-dependent antigen assay) (74–76). In my view, the combination of two negative complementary assays, e.g., washed platelet activation assay and antigen assay, essentially rules out HIT. The diagnostic features of the rapid antigen assay require further study, but this assay appeared clinically useful when antibody titer was assessed (70).

FREQUENCY

Variable Frequency

A remarkable feature of HIT is that its frequency varies considerably in different clinical settings, depending primarily upon: (a) type of heparin (bovine UFH > porcine UFH > LMWH); (b) type of patient population (surgical > medical > obstetrical), and (c) duration of heparin treatment (risk increases progressively from day 5–14, and then decreases abruptly) (1,77). The apparent range in frequency thus ranges from common (> 1%), e.g., postoperative orthopedic and cardiac surgery patients receiving heparin for 1–2 wk, to infrequent (0.1–1%), e.g., medical patients receiving UFH or surgical patients receiving LMWH, to rare (< 0.1%), e.g., medical and obstetrical patients receiving LMWH (1). Within the infrequent category, it is possible that the frequency is closer to 1% among medical patients receiving UFH and closer to 0.1% among surgical patients receiving LMWH. If this is true, then a simpler classification would simply be to regard HIT during UFH treatment as common, and HIT during LMWH therapy as rare.

Definition of Thrombocytopenia

HIT usually produces a dramatic decline in platelet counts, with a decrease of more than 50% from baseline observed in more than 95% of patients (5,7). Because platelet counts fall frequently in hospitalized patients, often because of perioperative hemodilution or other acute illnesses, it is crucial to look for an otherwise unexpected platelet count decline that begins 5 to 10 days after starting heparin, as this is the typical temporal hallmark of HIT. For postoperative patients, the postoperative peak platelet count (on or after postoperative day), not the preoperative platelet count, is the appropriate platelet count baseline, and a decrease in the platelet count of 50% or greater from this value is suggestive of HIT (7).

A relevant consideration is that some exposures to heparin are more immunogenic than others. Thus, if a patient receives small doses of UFH during heart catheterization and then undergoes cardiac surgery 4 days later, it is far more likely for HIT to begin 5 to 10 days after the surgery, not 5 to 10 days after the heart catheterization, simply because heparin used at cardiac surgery is more likely to lead to formation of strong, platelet-activating HIT antibodies.

Type of Heparin

UFH derived from bovine lung has longer and more-sulfated polysaccharide chains, which may contribute to greater immunogenicity and risk of HIT, compared with UFH obtained from porcine intestinal mucosa. Bovine UFH appears to cause more HIT (when used to treat thrombosis) (1) and greater seroconversion when used for anticoagulation during cardiac surgery (78). In contrast, (porcine-derived) LMWH is less immunogenic than porcine UFH in surgical (7,73) and medical settings (80), and has been proven to result in a lower frequency of HIT and HIT-associated thrombosis in postoperative orthopedic surgery patients (7,73), including in a recent meta-analysis (79).

Patient Population

HIT antibody formation is particularly common in postoperative patients, particularly after cardiac surgery (35–65%), vascular surgery (35%), and orthopedic surgery (15%) (1,7,41,66,81,82). The highest risk of clinical HIT, i.e., HIT with thrombocytopenia, is about 5%, which has been found in two post-orthopedic surgery patient populations treated with UFH (7,83). HIT also appears to be more common in women than men (odds ratio, about 1.5–2.0) (84).

Treatment Duration

Because HIT antibody seroconversion begins about 5 days after starting heparin, with increase in antibody titer and reactivity that peaks at about day 10 to 14, it is logical that the risk of HIT increases each day that heparin is continued beyond day 5, with subsequent risk rapidly declining after day 14 (77). Indeed, by time-to-event analysis, the risk reached almost 6% among postorthopedic surgery patients who received UFH until postoperative day 14.

CLINICAL PICTURE

The clinical picture of HIT is dominated by two features: thrombocytopenia and thrombosis (Fig. 3).

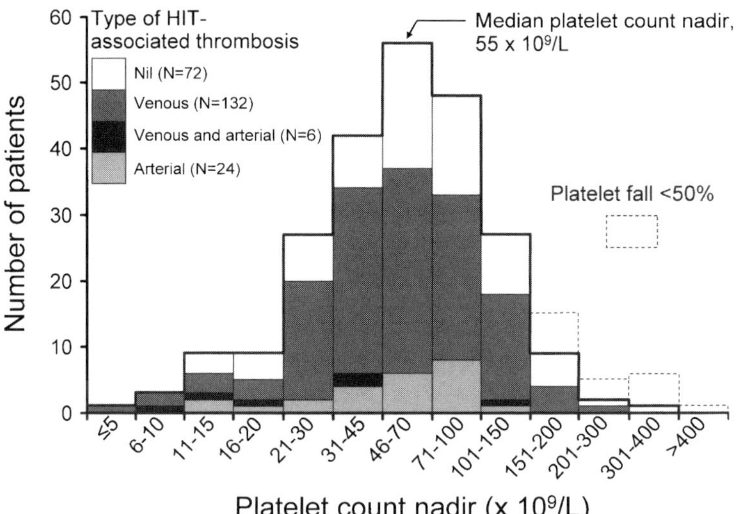

Figure 3 Platelet counts and thrombosis in HIT. All patients tested positive for HIT antibodies by washed platelet activation assay (serotonin release assay). All patients had a 50% or greater fall in the platelet count, except those indicated by dotted lines, who were suspected as having HIT (despite their lesser degree of platelet count fall) because of thrombotic events, heparin-induced skin lesions, or acute systemic reactions post-heparin bolus. The data used to prepare this figure have been published (46). The median platelet count nadir is approximately 55×10^9/L, and about 90% of patients have a platelet count nadir between 15 and 150×10^9/L. Further, venous thrombosis predominates over arterial thrombosis in HIT. *Source*: From Ref. 5.

Thrombocytopenia

Severity of Thrombocytopenia

Thrombocytopenia (defined as a 50% or greater fall in the platelet count) is the most common clinical manifestation of HIT and occurs in more than 95% of patients; in 90% of patients, the platelet count nadir is less than 150×10^9/L. Figure 3 illustrates the platelet count nadirs among a large series of patients with HIT: the median platelet count nadir is about 55×10^9/L, and for 90% of patients, the platelet count fell to a nadir between 15 and 150×10^9/L (5).

Timing of Thrombocytopenia

In 70% of patients, HIT is recognized based upon a fall in platelet count that typically occurs 5 to 10 days after starting heparin (first day of heparin = day 0) (46). This is called typical-onset HIT. In about 25 to 30% of patients, HIT is recognized because the platelet count fall occurs abruptly within 24 hr of starting heparin or giving a larger dose of heparin, e.g., UFH bolus plus therapeutic infusion after preceding course of prophylactic-dose heparin. This is termed rapid-onset HIT (46). This syndrome results from a recent immunizing exposure to heparin, generally within the past few weeks. Rarely (<5%), HIT is only recognized by a fall in the platelet count that begins several days after heparin has been stopped (delayed-onset HIT) (28–30). This last syndrome is often clinically severe, as it is associated with high-titer, platelet-activating HIT antibodies that do not require ongoing heparin administration for their prothrombotic effects (Fig. 4).

Thrombosis and Other Sequelae of HIT

Many, if not most, patients recognized with HIT develop thrombotic complications associated with their episode of HIT (whether or not treatment of thrombosis was the initial reason for giving heparin) (1,85,86). In one series, thrombosis was the presenting feature of HIT in about half of all patients recognized with HIT (85). Of the remaining patients who were recognized with "isolated HIT" (i.e., HIT not accompanied by clinically-evident thrombosis), 50% developed thrombosis during the subsequent four-week observation period. Prospective and case-controlled studies suggest that the risk (by odds ratio) of thrombosis in HIT is about 20 to 40 (for review, see Ref. 87).

Venous Thrombosis

The most common thrombotic event is venous thromboembolism: DVT (50% of patients), PE (25%), upper-limb DVT (10% if central venous catheter used), and sometimes (<5%) unusual events such as cerebral venous thrombosis (5,77,85,86). Venous thrombosis is particularly common in postoperative patients (7,73) (Fig. 5). Recent or concurrent use of a central venous catheter is strongly linked to developing upper-limb DVT (88).

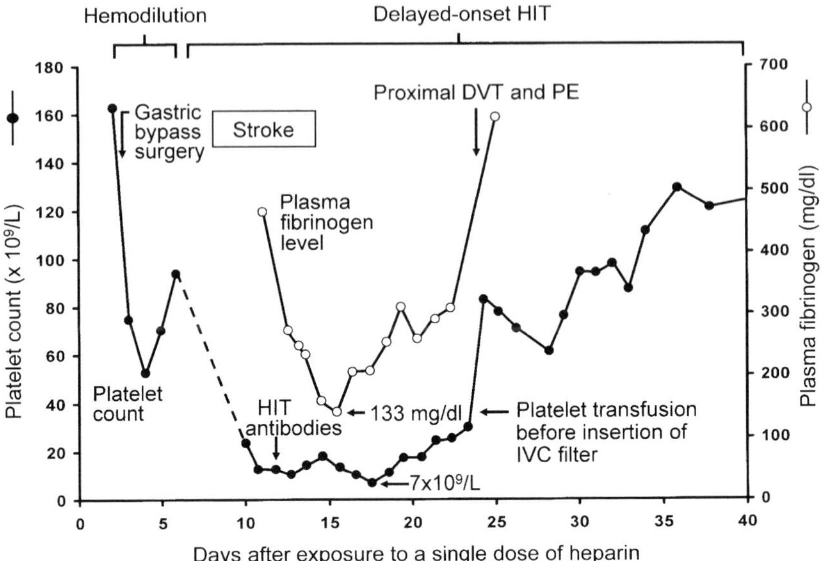

Figure 4 Delayed-onset HIT with disseminated intravascular coagulation (DIC) following a single injection of heparin. The initial perioperative platelet count fall was caused by hemodilution. The later platelet count fall (platelet count nadir, 7×10^9/L) resulted from delayed-onset HIT. The HIT-associated stroke, which progressed over one week to hemiplegia, was caused by cerebral venous thrombosis. The patient tested strongly positive for PF4-dependent antibodies by enzyme-immunoassay (EIA) (3.57 absorbance units; normal, <0.50). *Source*: From Ref. 30.

Adrenal Hemorrhagic Necrosis: Adrenal hemorrhage occurs in 3 to 5% of patients with HIT, and results from adrenal vein thrombosis, with resulting adrenal gland infarction (77,89). If adrenal necrosis is bilateral, shock can result, with adrenal corticosteroids being life-saving in this situation (90). Unilateral adrenal necrosis typically presents with flank or abdominal pain.

Arterial Thrombosis

Arterial thrombosis most often manifests as an ischemic lower limb, acute stroke, or acute myocardial infarction. Interestingly, this order of frequency (aorto-ileofemoral > cerebrovascular > coronary arteries) is the opposite of that seen with typical atherothrombosis. Platelet-rich "white clots" can be removed during thromboembolectomy by the vascular surgeon.

Limb Ischemic Syndromes, Including Venous Limb Gangrene

Severe thrombosis of limb arteries or veins sufficient to cause limb amputation occurs in about 10 to 20% of patients. Both arterial and venous thrombosis can

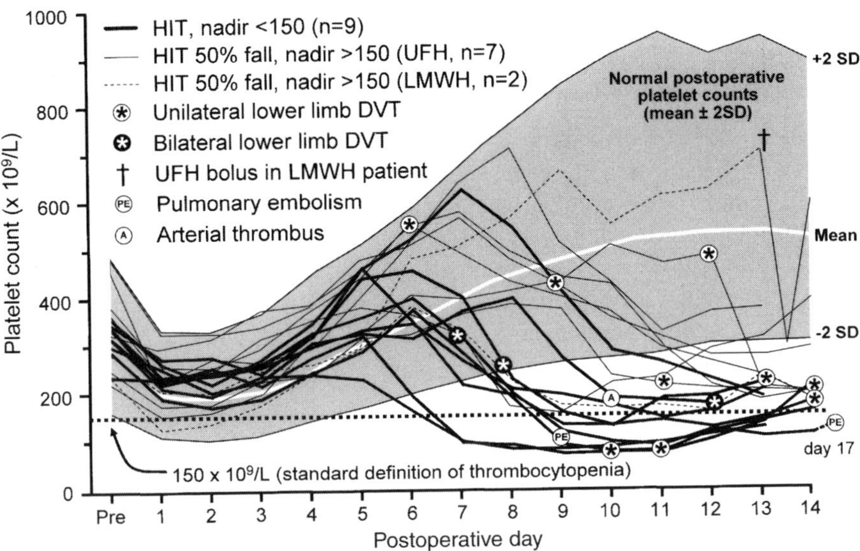

Figure 5 HIT and HIT-associated thrombosis in a post-orthopedic surgery population. The shaded area indicates the median (∀2 SD) platelet count range in patients who tested negative for HIT antibodies. Eighteen patients developed HIT (definition of thrombocytopenia: ≥50% fall in the platelet count between postoperative days 4–14): 9 with platelet count nadir <150 H 10^9/L, 9 with platelet count nadir >150 H 10^9/L. Overall, 18 thrombotic events occurred in 13 of the 18 patients with HIT. Note: bilateral deep vein thrombosis (DVT) is counted as two thrombotic events, and pulmonary embolism (PE) is also counted as a thrombotic event. *Source*: Modified from Refs. 7,73.

cause limb loss. Occlusion of large arteries by platelet-rich "white clots" is the classic explanation for limb loss (limb ischemia with absent pulses). However, in recent years, increasing recognition of venous limb gangrene as a cause of limb loss has been appreciated (limb ischemia with palpable pulses usually in the setting of DVT) (49,77,91–94). Most often, venous limb gangrene can be explained by use of coumarin anticoagulation. This is explained by microvascular thrombosis resulting from warfarin-induced depletion of the vitamin K-dependent natural anticoagulant factor, protein C, together with persisting thrombin generation. The syndrome is characterized by a supratherapeutic INR (>3.5) during warfarin therapy, accompanied by progression to acral (distal extremity) limb ischemia/necrosis in the limb(s) affected by DVT, while the patient remains thrombocytopenic from HIT. In less than 1% of HIT patients, microvascular thrombosis leading to limb loss occurs in the absence of warfarin treatment (77), presumably because of severe activation of coagulation associated with HIT. It is likely that acquired natural anticoagulant depletion (antithrombin, protein C) occurs in most of these cases, and some might also have associated hereditary risk factors, such as factor V Leiden. However, factor V Leiden is not a major factor in explaining thrombosis in HIT (95,96).

Heparin-Induced Skin Lesions

About 10 to 20% of patients who develop HIT while receiving subcutaneous injections of heparin manifest skin lesions at the heparin injection sites (77). These can range from painful, erythematous plaques to frank skin necrosis (97). Not all patients who develop heparin-induced skin lesions evince thrombocytopenia. Among those who do develop platelet count falls, there is evidence that arterial, rather than venous, thrombosis is most likely to occur (98). It is possible that FcγIIa receptors present on dermal vascular plexus endothelial cells play a role in pathogenesis (99).

Acute System Reactions

Table 2 lists signs and symptoms which, if they occur 5 to 30 minutes after an intravenous heparin bolus, strongly suggest the presence of HIT (77,100,101). In such a patient, measuring a post-bolus platelet count will reveal an abrupt decrease from a recent pre-bolus level. These acute systemic reactions will be the presenting feature of HIT in about 5 to 10% of patients. In a patient who develops dyspnea and tachypnea following a heparin bolus, acute pulmonary embolism may be mistakenly diagnosed (pseudo-PE) (102).

Disseminated Intravascular Coagulation

Although disseminated intravascular coagulation (DIC), as defined by increased markers of thrombin generation (e.g., thrombin–antithrombin complexes) and fibrin formation [e.g., cross-linked fibrin degradation products (fibrin D-dimers)], occurs in virtually all patients with HIT, overt DIC, as defined by low fibrinogen or elevated PT/INR levels, is seen only in about 10 to 15% of patients (77). The presence of nucleated and fragmented red blood cells is another clinical feature. The presence of overt DIC likely corresponds to more severe HIT

Table 2 Clinical Features of Acute Systemic Reactions Following Intravenous Heparin Bolus

Timing: onset 5–30 min after intravenous heparin bolus
Previous heparin use: recent use of heparin (past 5–100 days)
Laboratory features: abrupt (partially) reversible fall in the platelet count
Signs and symptoms (only some are observed in any one patient):
Inflammatory: chills, rigors, fever, flushing
Cardiorespiratory: tachycardia, hypertension (not hypotension), tachypnea, dyspnea, chest pain or tightness, cardiac or pulmonary arrest (rare)
Gastrointestinal: nausea, vomiting, diarrhea
Neurological: headache, transient global amnesia (rare)

Source: From Ref. 77.

(by platelet count nadirs) and may reflect greater risk for microvascular thrombosis, e.g., venous limb gangrene.

Differential Diagnosis

Both heparin use and thrombocytopenia are common in hospitalized patients, and by no means does the concurrence of these two events indicate HIT. Indeed, concurrence of heparin anticoagulation and perioperative hemodilution is probably the most common basis for consulting a hematologist with the question: "Does the patient have HIT?" Other common reasons for thrombocytopenia in hospitalized patients include septicemia, multi-organ system failure, and DIC (of multiple etiologies). Many drugs can cause thrombocytopenia; however, drugs that cause immune thrombocytopenia (e.g., quinine, quinidine, rifampin, vancomycin, sulfa antibiotics, etc.) usually cause the platelet count to fall to less than 20×10^9/L, whereas such severe thrombocytopenia occurs in less than 10% of patients with HIT. Abciximab (or another platelet gpIIb/IIIa antagonist) is more likely than heparin to be the cause of an abrupt drop in platelet count to less than 20×10^9/L following heart catheterization, even if the patient has previously received heparin but not the gpIIb/IIIa antagonist; this is because preexisting gpIIb/IIIa antagonist-dependent antibodies are a relatively common explanation for abrupt-onset of severe thrombocytopenia in this patient population.

Pseudo-HIT

Some disorders, such as PE or adenocarcinoma-associated DIC, can strongly mimic HIT on clinical grounds (103,104). Posttransfusion purpura (PTP) also can mimic HIT, as it typically occurs 5 to 10 days after surgery in which blood products were given. In contrast to HIT, however, patients with PTP evince mucocutaneous hemorrhage (105). Table 3 lists such "pseudo-HIT" disorders. Despite their occasional strong resemblance to clinical HIT, negative testing for HIT antibodies using one or more reliable assays excludes the diagnosis of HIT.

TREATMENT

Treatment of HIT generally involves discontinuing heparin, initiating nonheparin alternative parenteral anticoagulation, avoiding coumarin, and, sometimes, special adjunctive measures (e.g., surgical thromboembolectomy).

Treatment Overview: Thrombin Generation

As mentioned, HIT is a profound prothrombotic situation with greatly increased thrombin generation in vivo (49,50). This concept helps explain the increased risk of venous and arterial thrombosis, warfarin-associated venous limb gangrene,

Table 3 Pseudo-HIT Disorders Characterized by Thrombocytopenia and Thrombosis

Pseudo-HIT disorder	Pathogenesis of thrombocytopenia and thrombosis	Timing
Adenocarcinoma	DIC secondary to procoagulant material(s) produced by neoplastic cells	Late
Pulmonary embolism	Platelet activation via clot-bound thrombin	Early or late
Diabetic ketoacidosis	Hyperaggregable platelets in ketoacidosis (?)	Early
Antiphospholipid antibody syndrome	Multiple mechanisms described, including platelet activation by antiphospholipid antibodies (?)	Early
Thrombolytic therapy	Platelet activation by thrombin bound to fibrin degradation products (?)	Early
Septicemia-associated purpura fulminans	Symmetrical peripheral gangrene secondary to DIC with depletion of protein C and/or antithrombin	Early
Infective endocarditis	Infection-associated thrombocytopenia; ischemic events secondary to septic emboli	Early
Paroxysmal nocturnal hemoglobinuria (PNH)	Platelets susceptible to complement-mediated damage; platelet hypoproduction	Early
Post-transfusion purpura (PTP)	'Pseudospecific' alloantibody-mediated platelet destruction (bleeding, not thrombosis)	Late

These 'pseudo-HIT' disorders can mimic HIT by causing thrombocytopenia and thrombosis in association with heparin treatment. An exception is PTP, which causes bleeding but not thrombosis; however, PTP can resemble HIT because both disorders usually occur about a week after major surgery requiring blood and postoperative heparin. The pseudo-HIT disorders can be categorized based on whether the onset of thrombocytopenia is typically "early" (<5 days) or "late" (≥ 5 days) in relation to the heparin. *Source*: From Warkentin, 2004 (103).

decompensated DIC, and the ongoing risk of thrombosis despite cessation of heparin. Once this severe procoagulant process is initiated, simply stopping heparin will not interrupt the process (85,86).

Treatment Paradoxes

Table 4 lists several treatment paradoxes observed in HIT (14). Ironically, although heparin initiates HIT, it also may help to control thrombin in this syndrome. Indeed, simply discontinuing heparin does not decrease risk of subsequent thrombosis (5,85,86). Thus, an alternative, non-heparin anticoagulant should be substituted for heparin in patients strongly suspected of having HIT. Indeed, the Food and Drug Administration has approved an anticoagulant (argatroban) for prophylaxis against thrombosis in HIT (106), and off-label use of lepirudin for this indication has also been reported (107).

Table 4 Treatment Paradoxes in HIT Management

Paradox	Comment
Discontinuation of heparin fails to prevent thrombosis	Hypercoagulability state of HIT generally requires an alternative, non-heparin anticoagulant to reduce risk of thrombosis
Coumarins such as warfarin predispose to venous limb gangrene and/or skin necrosis syndromes	Await substantial resolution of thrombocytopenia in HIT (preferably, $>150 \times 10^9$/L) before cautiously introducing coumarin for longer-term antithrombotic treatment
LMWH is contraindicated in HIT because of the high risk of thrombocytopenia and/or thrombosis	Benefit of LMWH in reducing risk of HIT (vis-a-vis UFH) does not mean that LMWH should be used to treat HIT
Low (prophylactic) dose danaparoid often fails to prevent thrombosis in HIT[a]	High (therapeutic) dose danaparoid recommended for treating HIT, even in patients with isolated HIT
Platelet transfusions for preventing bleeding are (relatively) contraindicated despite thrombocytopenia	Spontaneous bleeding is uncommon even in severe HIT; theoretically, platelet transfusions might increase risk of thrombosis
Vena cava filters are (relatively) contraindicated in patients with HIT	Vena cava filters may be more harmful than beneficial in HIT patients because they could predispose to massive IVC and lower-limb venous thrombosis

[a] Low-dose danaparoid (750 U two or three times a day by subcutaneous injection) is approved for prevention of thrombosis in acute HIT in some jurisdictions.

Evaluating Pretest Probability of HIT

Treatment decisions depend in large part on the physician's assessment of the probability of a patient actually having this disorder (5,74,108). For example, if the pretest probability of HIT is considered to be high, then the appropriate treatment response is to stop heparin and to initiate an alternative (non-heparin) anticoagulant, generally in therapeutic doses. On the other hand, if the pretest probability of HIT is judged to be low, then it may well be appropriate to continue heparin. In patients in whom the diagnosis is unclear (e.g., intermediate or 50–50 probability), other factors become important. For example, if the patient is judged to be at high bleeding risk or has certain clinical features that make treatment with alternative anticoagulants problematic [e.g., renal/hepatic failure, baseline elevation in the activated partial thromboplastin time (APTT)], then approaches other than high-dose anticoagulation might be more appropriate. For example, in

Canada, low-dose danaparoid (750 U bid or tid) is appropriate in many such patients (danaparoid is not available in the U.S.). In a patient who has good renal function, low-dose lepirudin (15 mg bid sc) or fondaparinux (2.5 mg od sc) might be appropriate as an off-label approach when the risk of HIT is not considered sufficiently great to justify therapeutic-dose anticoagulation, but at the same time is not judged to be so low so as to allow continued treatment with heparin.

Table 5 lists one approach by which pretest probability for HIT can be assessed (5,74,77,108). Known as the "4 Ts," the physician determines the likelihood of HIT based on the (a) magnitude of *T*hrombocytopenia, (b) the *T*iming of thrombocytopenia, (c) the presence of *T*hrombosis or other sequelae of HIT, and (d) whether o*T*her plausible explanations for thrombocytopenia are present. Further work is required to validate this (or any other) pretest scoring system, although preliminary evidence suggests that a low score makes HIT unlikely (<5%) (109). Also, the 4 Ts appeared useful in evaluating thrombocytopenic patients post-cardiac surgery (110).

Diagnostic Investigations

Generally speaking, patients with clinically suspected HIT should undergo laboratory testing for HIT antibodies. Particularly if clinical suspicion is moderate or high, I recommend that patients also undergo routine investigation for lower-limb DVT, e.g., using ultrasonography. Even if treatment decisions are made prior to receiving the results of HIT antibody tests, these tests may well influence subsequent treatment decisions. For example, if a patient tests negative for HIT antibodies using a sensitive test, then it may be appropriate to resume heparin, especially if the evolving clinical picture also suggests an alternative explanation for the thrombocytopenia.

Further, other issues raised by the clinical evaluation will determine whether other tests should be performed. For example, blood cultures may be crucial for determining whether bacteremia, rather than HIT, is the explanation for thrombocytopenia. Alternatively, clinical evidence of unilateral neurologic deficit, limb or abdominal pain, and so forth, will further direct the evaluations.

Direct Thrombin Inhibitors

Direct thrombin inhibitors (DTIs) inhibit thrombin without requiring a cofactor. (In contrast, heparin only indirectly inhibits thrombin by catalyzing its inhibition via antithrombin.) Two DTIs, lepirudin and argatroban, are approved in the U.S. and Canada for treating HIT (87,111,112). Lepirudin is additionally approved in Europe and Australia, whereas argatroban is also approved for treatment of HIT in Japan and certain countries in Europe. These agents have considerable differences (Table 6). A third DTI, bivalirudin, recently received U.S. approval for anticoagulation during percutaneous coronary intervention (PCI) in patients with (or at risk of) HIT.

Table 5 Estimating the Pretest Probability of HIT: The "Four Ts"

	Points (0, 1, or 2 for each of 4 categories: maximum possible score=8)		
	2	1	0
Thrombocytopenia (acute)	Platelet fall >50% (nadir <20)	Nadir, 10–19 × 10^9/L; or any 30–50% fall; or, >50% fall associated with surgery	Nadir, <10 × 10^9/L; or any <30% fall
Timing[a] of platelet count fall, thrombosis, or other sequelae first day of heparin course=day zero)	Clear onset between days 5–10; or ≤1 day (if heparin exposure within past 30 days)	Consistent with day 5–10 fall, but not clear (e.g., missing platelet counts); or, ≤1 day (heparin exposure within past 31–100 days); or, platelet fall after day 10	Platelet count fall ≤4 days without recent heparin exposure
Thrombosis or other sequelae (e.g., skin lesions, ASR)	New thrombosis; skin necrosis; ASR after iv heparin bolus	Progressive or recurrent thrombosis; erythematous skin lesions; suspected thrombosis (not yet proven); asymptomatic upper-limb DVT	None
Other cause for thrombocytopenia not evident	No explanation for platelet count fall is evident	Possible other cause is evident	Definite other cause is present

Pretest probability score: 6–8, high; 4–5, intermediate; 0–3, low. *Abbreviation*: ASR, acute systemic reaction; DVT, deep venous thrombosis. The scoring system shown here has undergone minor modifications from previously published scoring systems (5,74,77).

[a] First day of immunizing heparin exposure considered day zero (the most immunizing exposure should be considered first, e.g., UFH received during cardiac surgery is more immunogenic than UFH or LMWH given for acute coronary syndrome); the day the platelet count begins to fall is considered the day of onset of thrombocytopenia (it generally takes 1 to 3 more days until an arbitrary threshold that defines thrombocytopenia is passed).

Table 6 Pharmacologic Comparison of Two Direct Thrombin Inhibitors Approved for Management of HIT

Drug	Structure (molecular mass, Da)	Thrombin affinity, specificity, and reversibility of binding	Dosing for HIT-thrombosis	Half-life (organ site of clearance)	Comments
Lepirudin	Leu^1-Thr^2-desulfato-hirudin, 65-amino acid polypeptide (6980)	High affinity (Ki = 60 pmol/l); high specificity; irreversible, non-covalent binding	(±0.4 mg/kg i.v. bolus[a]); initial IV infusion rate, 0.15 mg/kg/h[b]	80 min[b] (renal clearance)	Immunogenic; fatal anaphylaxis post-IV bolus has been reported
Argatroban	Arginine derivative that binds to thrombin active site (527)	Moderate affinity (Ki = 40 nmol/l); moderate specificity;[c] reversible binding	Initial IV infusion rate, 2 g/kg/min[d]	40–50 min[d] (hepatobiliary excretion)	Non-immunogenic; Raises the PT (INR) more than lepirudin
Bivali-rudin	20–amino acid derivative of hirudin	Moderate affinity (Ki = 2 nmol/l); high specificity; reversible binding (via proteolysis)	Dosing not established for treatment of HIT–thrombosis (only for PCI)	25–35 min; enzymic (80%); renal (20%)	Approved for PCI (± HIT)

Abbreviation: CrCl, creatinine clearance; IV, intravenous; INR, international normalized ratio; PCI, percutaneous coronary intervention; PT, prothrombin time; sCr, serum creatinine.

[a] Consider omitting the IV bolus in patients without life- or limb-threatening thrombosis (minimize overdosing, anaphylaxis).

[b] Reduce initial lepirudin infusion rate in patients with renal failure, as follows (subsequent dose-adjustments by APTT): (a) normal renal function: 0.10 (isolated HIT) to 0.15 (HIT-associated thrombosis) mg/kg/h; (b) est. CrCl, 45–60 mL/min (sCr, ~1.6–2.0 mg/dL [~141–177 mol/L]): 50% of usual infusion rate; (c) est. CrCl, 30–44 mL/min (sCr, ~2.1–3.0 mg/dL [~178–265 mol/L]): 25% of usual infusion rate; (d) est. CrCl, 15–29 mL/min (sCr, ~3.1–6.0 mg/dL [266–530 mol/L]): 10% of usual infusion rate; (e) dialysis-dependent renal failure; <15 mL/min (sCr, >6.0 mg/dL (>530 mol/L): 0.005 mg/kg/h, i.e., either 0.005 mg/kg/h or intermittent boluses of 0.005 mg/kg.

[c] Argatroban can be considered thrombin-*selective*, rather than thrombin-*specific*, as it may inhibit other serine proteases.

[d] Reduce argatroban to 25% of the usual infusion dose if significant hepatic (or hepatobiliary) dysfunction is present.

Lepirudin

Lepirudin (Refludan) is a 65-amino acid protein manufactured using recombinant technology (113,114). It resembles closely the structure of hirudin, the natural anticoagulant produced by the medicinal leech, a hematophagous invertebrate. It is a bivalent DTI, since it binds both to thrombin's fibrinogen-binding site (exosite 1), as well as the apolar binding site, thereby blocking access to thrombin's active (catalytic) site (Fig. 6) (111). Affinity of lepirudin for thrombin is extremely high (Ki = 60 pmol/l) and irreversible. Specificity for thrombin also is extremely high, and there is minimal prolongation of the prothrombin time (PT) (usually expressed as the INR) (cf. argatroban) (115).

Some features of this drug:

(1) *Pharmacokinetics*. Clearance of hirudin (and hirudin–thrombin complexes) occurs primarily by the kidneys. In individuals with normal renal function, the elimination half-life is about 80 min. However, as clearance critically depends on renal function, the half-life increases greatly in patients with significant renal dysfunction. The volume of distribution is 0.24 to 0.33 L/kg. Thus, most lepirudin distributes into the extravascular space. The practical consequence is that during extended high dosing (e.g., cardiac surgery), the drug accumulates in the extravascular space, which provides a pool from which ongoing redistribution back into the intravascular compartment occurs for some time, leading to continuing high blood levels for several hours even after stopping the drug (116).

(2) *Dosing*. Lepirudin is usually given by intravenous infusion, beginning at 0.15 mg/kg/h in patients with thrombosis and normal renal function (0.10 mg/kg/h if the patient has isolated HIT) (50,107,117–120). In prospective studies evaluating lepirudin for treatment of HIT, an initial intravenous bolus (0.40 mg/kg) was generally given. However, to avoid overdosing and post-bolus anaphylaxis, it is reasonable to start therapy without an initial bolus, unless life- or limb-threatening thrombosis is present (113). The initial infusion rate is greatly reduced in patients with renal failure (Table 6, Footnote b).

(3) *Monitoring*. Lepirudin is usually monitored using the activated partial thromboplastin time (APTT). The usual target range is 1.5 to 2.5 times the baseline APTT value (generally, the mean of the laboratory normal range). Depending upon the thromboplastin reagent used, however, this target range is not optimal. For example, the APTT–lepirudin concentration relationship is not linear at high-therapeutic APTT levels. Thus, it is recommended that the laboratory perform an APTT–lepirudin standard curve by "spiking" normal pooled plasma with various concentrations of lepirudin (113). Appropriate lepirudin plasma levels range from 0.2 to 0.4 mg/L (antithrombotic prophylaxis in non-HIT situations), to 0.5 to 0.8 mg/L (isolated HIT), to 0.6 to

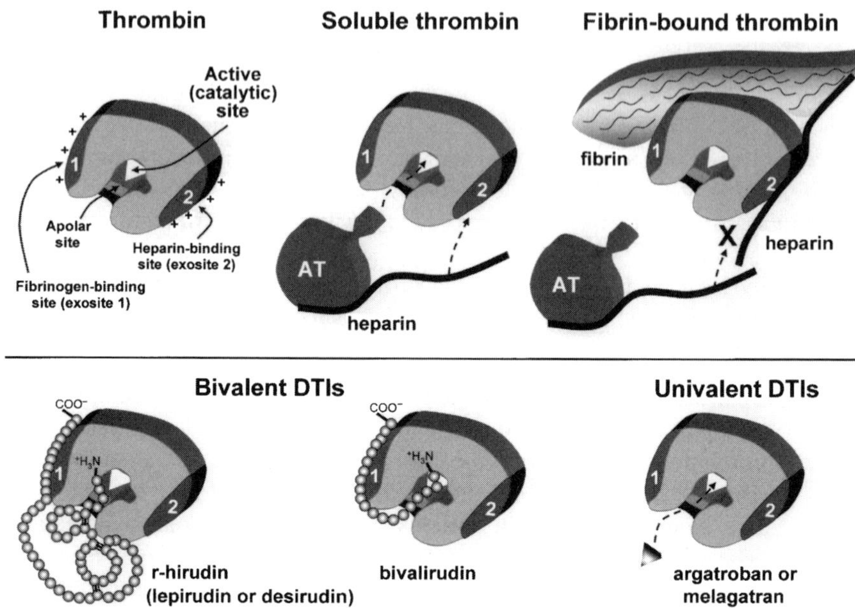

Figure 6 Schematic representation of thrombin and its inhibition. (*top left*) Structure of thrombin. Two positively-charged regions on thrombin (exosites) are shown: exosite 1 (fibrinogen recognition site) and exosite 2 (heparin-binding site). The apolar binding site is a non-charged region to which hirudin binds. The active (catalytic) site resides within the "canyon" of thrombin, and near the apolar site. (*top middle*) Inhibition of soluble thrombin by antithrombin. Heparin of 18 or greater saccharide units catalyzes the interaction of antithrombin and thrombin, leading to formation of covalently-linked thrombin–antithrombin complexes. Thrombin inhibition by heparin is therefore *indirect*, i.e., it is mediated by antithrombin. (*top right*) Inhibition of fibrin-bound (clot-bound) thrombin. Since heparin binds simultaneously to fibrin and fibrin-bound thrombin, forming a ternary complex that enhances affinity of the heparin for exosite 2 on thrombin, it is difficult for other heparin molecules to displace the fibrin–thrombin-bound heparin, and so antithrombin–heparin is a poor inhibitor of fibrin-bound thrombin. (*bottom left*) Hirudin (e.g., lepirudin, desirudin) binds to both exosite 1 as well as to the apolar region of thrombin, with its N-terminal moiety blocking access to thrombin's active site. Thus, hirudin is a *bivalent* direct thrombin inhibitor (DTI). Although hirudin also inhibits fibrin-bound thrombin (not shown), the large size of hirudin, as well as the competition of its C-terminal region with fibrin for exosite 1, means that it inhibits fibrin-bound thrombin less efficiently than the univalent DTIs. (*bottom middle*) Bivalirudin binds to both exosite 1 of thrombin, as well as to its active site (bivalent DTI). Inhibition of fibrin-bound thrombin (not shown) is intermediate between that of hirudin and univalent DTIs. (*bottom right*) Argatroban and melagatran bind noncovalently and reversibly only to the active site of thrombin, i.e., they are *univalent* DTIs. They also inhibit fibrin-bound thrombin efficiently (not shown). *Source*: From Ref. 111.

1.4 mg/L (HIT plus thrombosis) (113). A more accurate monitoring method that is usually used in situations in which high lepirudin concentrations are required (e.g., during cardiac surgery) is the ecarin clotting time (ECT) (121,122).

(4) *Bleeding*. Bleeding is the most important adverse effect of hirudin. Major bleeding occurred in 18.8 to 20.4% of patients receiving lepirudin during therapy of HIT, with five hemorrhagic deaths (2.4%) in the most recent prospective study (50,117–119). As no antidote exists, attention should focus on careful dose selection and monitoring.

(5) *Immunization and anaphylaxis*. Lepirudin is immunogenic: antihirudin antibodies typically form between 1 to 4 weeks after beginning treatment, with immunization rates similar between lepirudin and desirudin (123,124). Another study (125) found that some antihirudin antibodies generated during lepirudin treatment cross-react in vitro against bivalirudin. (Bivalirudin itself rarely, if at all, results in formation of antibivalirudin antibodies.) (126) Whether patients who form antihirudin antibodies during lepirudin treatment could develop immunologically mediated adverse reactions during subsequent treatment with bivalirudin is unknown. Anaphylaxis (including fatal outcomes) has been reported in patients receiving intravenous bolus lepirudin for treatment of HIT (127,128). The frequency is estimated at 1 in 625 during readministration to a patient who received lepirudin within the previous three months. Since fatal anaphylaxis to date invariably has followed intravenous bolus use, this provides a rationale to begin lepirudin by intravenous infusion (without bolus), unless the clinical situation justifies rapid anticoagulation (113).

Outcomes of HIT patients treated with lepirudin are discussed later.

Argatroban

Argatroban (marketed under the name Argatroban in the U.S. and Novastan elsewhere) is a small-molecule arginine derivative (106). Pharmacological features of argatroban includes its reversible thrombin inhibition, short half-life (40–50 min), hepatobiliary excretion, lack of immunogenicity, and prolongation of the PT (INR) (Fig. 7) (111,115,129–131).

Argatroban is a univalent DTI, since it binds reversibly only to thrombin's active (catalytic) site (cf. lepirudin) (106,111,132). Affinity of argatroban to thrombin (Ki = 40 nmol/l) is less than that for lepirudin, and lower specificity for thrombin suggests that argatroban should be termed thrombin-*selective*, rather than thrombin-*specific*. The relatively high molar concentrations of argatroban required for anticoagulant effect (compared with lepirudin and bivalirudin) likely explains its disproportionate prolongation of the INR (115).

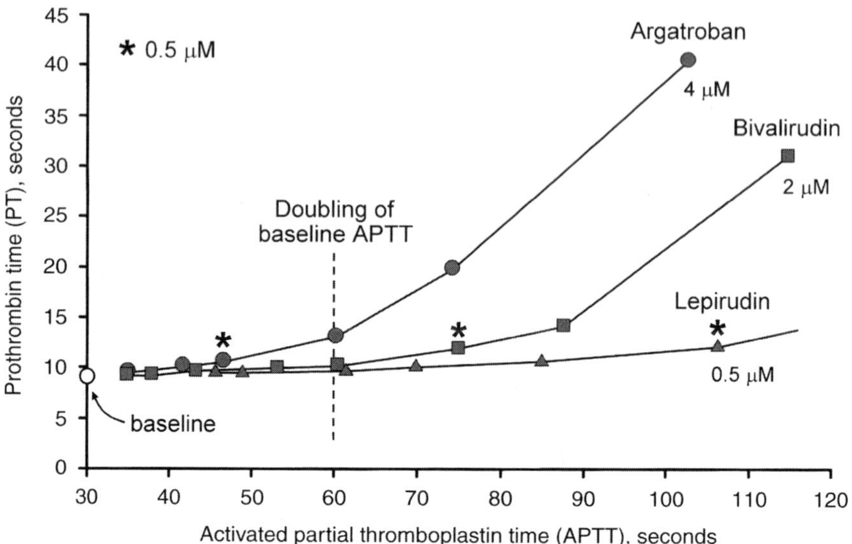

Figure 7 PT–APTT relationship for three DTIs. Data points shown are for serial two-fold dilutions of DTI. The increase in PT (for a given APTT) depends upon the DTI, and is greatest for argatroban, intermediate for bivalirudin, and least for lepirudin. The asterisk (*) indicates 0.5 μM concentration (final) of the DTI. [The international normalized ratio INR corresponding to the highest plotted PT–APTT data point for each DTI is: argatroban, INR = 4.40; bivalirudin, INR = 3.38; lepirudin, INR = 1.32.] The data were obtained using: (a) a recombinant human tissue factor [Innovin, Dade Behring, Mississauga, ON; instrument-specific international sensitivity index (ISI) = 1.0]; (b) Hemoliance Thrombosil IL (Instrumentation Laboratories, Lexington, MA); (c) an STA Compact (Diagnostica Stago, Asnieres, France); and (d) pooled normal human plasma. *Source*: From Ref. 111.

(1) *Pharmacokinetics*. Argatroban and its metabolites undergo hepatobiliary excretion. In normal individuals, the elimination half-life is about 40 to 50 min. The volume of distribution is 0.17 L/kg. Thus, like lepirudin, it distributes mostly in the extravascular space. It is about 50% serum protein-bound.

(2) *Dosing*. Argatroban is given by intravenous infusion, usually beginning at 2 μg/kg/min for patients treated for HIT (133,134). The dose is reduced by 75% in patients with liver insufficiency. Although in theory dose reduction is not required for patients with renal failure, clinical experience suggests that target aPTT is often attained with lower doses (e.g., 1 μg/kg/min) in patients with renal failure (135). For patients undergoing percutaneous coronary intervention for whom argatroban is given because of acute or previous HIT, the dose is substantially higher (350 μg/kg initial bolus, intravenous infusion 25 μg/kg/min to maintain the activated clotting time between 300–450 s) (136).

(3) *Monitoring*. Argatroban is usually monitored using the APTT, with the usual target range being 1.5 to 3.0 times the baseline APTT value (maximum, 100 s) (133,134).

(4) *Bleeding*. Bleeding is the most important adverse effect of argatroban. Major bleeding occurred in about 5% of patients enrolled in the clinical trials evaluating argatroban for HIT (106,133,134). Minor bleeding was reported in about 40% of patients. As with lepirudin, no antidote exists.

(5) *Other adverse events*. Unlike hirudin, argatroban does not appear to be immunogenic (129). Common adverse events reported in the trials were diarrhea (11%) and pain (9%) (106).

Bivalirudin

Bivalirudin (Angiomax™) is a "hirulog," i.e., an analogue of hirudin (111,137). It combines a 12-amino acid sequence that binds to the exosite 1 on thrombin with a tetrapeptide sequence that recognizes thrombin's active site (both moieties are linked by "spacer" of four glycine residues) (Fig. 6). Despite its bivalent binding characteristics, it exhibits much lower affinity for thrombin (Ki= 2 nmol/l) than lepirudin (138,139). Further, its inhibition of thrombin reverses over time, as thrombin cleaves bivalirudin at its Arg^3–Pro^4 bond. On account of such enzymic metabolism, only about 20% of bivalirudin clearance is renal (although some dose-reduction is still required with moderate or greater renal dysfunction) (140). These differences from lepirudin probably explain the generally lower rates of bleeding observed with bivalirudin, compared with lepirudin, in studies of patients with acute coronary syndrome.

To date, minimal off-label experience with bivalirudin for HIT has been reported (141,142). The largest experience is by Francis and colleagues (142 and unpublished data), who used bivalirudin in 40 patients with clinically suspected HIT, with favorable results. Only two patients were given intravenous boluses. Initial infusion rates generally ranged from 0.15 to 0.20 mg/kg/h; the overall mean infusion rate was 0.165 mg/kg/h. The target APTT was a 1.5- to 2.5-fold prolongation of the baseline value. Thus, a reasonable regimen suggested by the experience of these authors is to initiate therapy at 0.15 mg/kg/h (no initial bolus), with subsequent adjustments according to APTT.

Results of Direct Thrombin Inhibitor Therapy of HIT

Table 7 summarizes the efficacy outcomes in the clinical evaluation of lepirudin and argatroban for HIT. Both programs used historical controls and used as the primary endpoint a composite of all-cause mortality, all-cause limb amputation, and new thrombosis (each patient could contribute only once to the endpoint). In my view, the secondary endpoint of new thrombosis best reflects drug efficacy, since death and amputation are influenced by comorbidities and severity of limb ischemia prior to initiating treatment. For the treatment of thrombosis complicating HIT, the relative risk reduction (RRR) for new thrombosis ranged

Table 7 Direct Thrombin Inhibitor Therapy of HIT Complicated by Thrombosis: Efficacy Endpoints

Study drug and trial	New thrombosis	Limb amputation	Composite endpoint[a]
Lepirudin			
Meta-analysis of HAT-1 and HAT-2 (N=113, n=75[b]) (50,113)	10.1% vs 27.2%[c] RRR=0.63 (p=0.005)	6.5% vs 10.4%[c] RRR=0.38; (p=NS)	21.3 vs 47.8%[c] RRR=0.55 (p=0.004)
HAT-3 study, including both isolated HIT and HIT complicated by thrombosis (113) (N=191, n=120)	9.9% vs 32.1%[c] RRR=0.69, p=0.0002	5.5% vs 8.2%[c] RRR=0.29; p=0.71	26.2% vs 52.1%[c] RRR=0.50 (p=0.0015)
HAT-3 study, subgroup with HIT and thrombosis treated with lepirudin (but not thrombolysis) (N=98)[d] (119)	6.1%	5.1%	21.4%
Drug monitoring program (N=496)[d] (113,120)	5.2%	5.8%	21.9%

Argatroban			
Arg-911 (N=144, n=46) (133)	19.4% vs 34.8%[c] RRR=0.44 (p=0.044)	11.1%[e] vs 8.7%[c] RRR=−0.28 (p=0.79)	43.8% vs 56.5%[c] RRR=0.22 (p=0.13[f])
Arg-915 (N=229, n=46) (134)	13.1% vs 34.8%[c] RRR=0.62 (p<0.001)	14.8% vs 10.9%[c] RRR=−0.36 (p=0.64)	41.5% vs 56.5%[c] RRR=0.27 (p=0.07[f])

N, number of patients receiving DTI; n, number of control patients. For the HAT-1/2 meta-analysis and the HAT-3 study, the data are shown from diagnosis of HIT (positive laboratory testing) to day 35, whereas for the drug monitoring program, the data are shown from beginning of treatment to end of treatment (plus one day) (time-to-event analyses). However, for the HAT-3 study subgroup with HIT and thrombosis, the data represent categorical analysis, and show the events from start of lepirudin to end of study. For the argatroban trials, the data represent categorical analysis (37-day follow-up). From Warkentin, 2004 (111).

[a] The composite endpoint is defined as: all-cause mortality, all-cause limb amputation, and new thrombotic events (each patient could contribute only once to the endpoint).

[b] 75 historical controls received danaparoid (n=24), phenprocoumon (n=21), and other treatment (n=30).

[c] Historical controls were used.

[d] No control group data presented.

[e] The amputation rate in the argatroban-treated patients in the Arg-911 study could have been underestimated because patients who both died and developed limb amputation were not included in the limb amputation results. (This explains why the limb amputation rates differ in the identical 46-patient control group between the Arg-911 and Arg-915 studies.).

[f] The P value was <0.05 when argatroban-treated patients were compared with historical controls using time-to-event analysis.

from 0.63 to 0.69 for lepirudin, and ranged from 0.44 to 0.62 for argatroban. For the treatment of isolated HIT, the RRR ranged from 0.64 to 0.75 for argatroban. Absolute thrombotic rates (no historical control) for patients with isolated HIT treated with lepirudin were low (<5%).

Despite overall similarities in study design, important differences also were present (87). Perhaps most importantly, patients only entered lepirudin studies if the HIT assay was positive, whereas patients were entered into the argatroban trials on clinical suspicion of HIT. Since many patients therefore might not have had HIT in the argatroban trials (65% tested positive in the Arg-911 study), this has the potential to overestimate the RRR for new thrombosis, and to underestimate the RRR for the composite endpoint, for reasons that many non-HIT thrombocytopenic disorders (multiorgan dysfunction syndrome, sepsis) have a high mortality but low thrombosis rate. More patients received coumarin anticoagulation in the lepirudin than in the argatroban trials (at least 83% vs 62%). The mean treatment duration ranged from 12 to 14 days in the lepirudin trials (50,119,120), but only 5.9 and 7.1 days in the two argatroban studies (133,134). Theoretically, a short treatment duration could contribute to higher thrombotic event rates and, possibly, higher risk of warfarin-induced venous limb ischemia/necrosis.

Overlapping DTI–Coumarin

Coumarins, such as warfarin (Coumadin®, used in the U.S., Canada, and the U.K.) and phenprocoumon (continental Europe) can contribute to microvascular thrombosis in patients with acute HIT, and have been implicated in the pathogenesis of venous limb gangrene (49,91–94). Accordingly, caution is required in managing the overlap between DTI therapy and subsequent long-term coumarin anticoagulation (92,93). In particular, the tendency for cotherapy with argatroban and warfarin to lead to a supratherapeutic INR (111,130,131) might lead to premature discontinuation of the DTI, and thus create the circumstances favoring venous limb gangrene, particularly given the short elimination half-lives of the DTIs. Thus, postponing coumarin until the platelet count has substantially recovered is important (14,111,112). Table 8 lists recommendations for managing DTI–warfarin overlap.

Indirect Factor Xa Inhibitors

This section will discuss two agents with predominant (danaparoid) or exclusive (fondaparinux) anti-factor Xa activity. Danaparoid is no longer marketed in the U.S., but remains available in Canada and Europe (143).

Danaparoid (Orgaran®) is a mixture of anticoagulant glycosaminoglycans, predominantly (low-sulfated) heparan sulfate and dermatan sulfate, with anti-Xa/anti-IIa ratio of about 22. It is the only anticoagulant evaluated by randomized clinical trial for treatment of HIT, proving more effective than dextran-70 (144). When used in therapeutic doses (usually, 200 U/h IV after a loading dose that

Table 8 Recommendations for Managing Direct Thrombin Inhibitor–Warfarin Overlap in HIT

1. If a patient has already received warfarin when acute HIT is recognized, administer vitamin K (up to 10 mg i.v. or p.o., depending upon the INR) to reverse the effects of warfarin[a].
2. Use the DTI alone, without initiating warfarin, until HIT has substantially recovered, i.e., the platelet count has attained *at least* 100×10^9/L (preferably $>150 \times 10^9$/L).
3. Begin with maintenance doses of warfarin ($\leq$5 mg of warfarin as the initial dose).
4. Maintain the overlap of DTI and warfarin for *at least* 4 or 5 days, and with the INR in the target therapeutic INR range for at least the last 2 days[b].
5. Do not stop the DTI unless criteria 2 to 4 (above) are met, and the platelet count has recovered to a stable plateau, and clinical symptoms and signs of thrombosis have improved.
6. After stopping the DTI, subsequent INR values should be in the usual therapeutic range (generally, 2.0–3.0).

Abbreviations: APTT, activated partial thromboplastin time; DTI, direct thrombin inhibitor; i.v., intravenous; p.o., per os (orally). Modified from Warkentin, 2004 (111).

[a] Reversal of warfarin with vitamin K is suggested for two reasons: first, to reduce the risk of developing warfarin-associated venous limb gangrene or skin necrosis, and second, to prevent inappropriate underdosing of DTI therapy (because of APTT prolongation from warfarin).

[b] For combined therapy with argatroban and warfarin, the target INR during overlapping therapy is generally above the usual therapeutic range of 2.0–3.0, and varies depending upon the thromboplastin reagent used to measure the INR, the dose of argatroban, and, possibly, patient-dependent factors. (e.g., for a patient receiving argatroban at 2 μg/kg/min, the target INR using a sensitive thromboplastin (e.g., international sensitivity index [ISI] = 0.9) is about 3.0–5.0, whereas the target INR is about 4.0–6.0 if the thromboplastin is less sensitive (e.g., ISI = 2.1) (106,130).

depends upon patient weight), it was as effective as lepirudin in a non-randomized comparison, with less bleeding (145). Danaparoid is less effective in HIT when used in prophylactic doses (e.g., 750 U bid or tid), which ironically is its approved dose for HIT in some jurisdictions (145,146). In my view, the low-dose protocol is useful in non-HIT clinical situations in which an alternative to heparin for antithrombotic prophylaxis is desired. However, when HIT is strongly suspected, I recommend it be given in therapeutic dosing (14,146,147). Although 15 to 40% of HIT sera exhibit weak cross-reactivity with danaparoid in vitro, this is rarely clinically significant, thus justifying use without prior cross-reactivity testing (14).

Fondaparinux (Arixtra®) is a synthetic, antithrombin-binding pentasaccharide anticoagulant with anti-Xa (and anti-IXa) activity, but no anti-IIa (antithrombin) activity. HIT-IgG do not cross-react with fondaparinux (72), and thus it theoretically should be effective in patients with HIT. However, minimal experience (148) and uncertainty regarding optimal dosing in patients with HIT are relevant issues. Interestingly, fondaparinux appears to interact with PF4 in such a way as to promote formation of anti-PF4/heparin antibodies that, ironically, react poorly if at all with PF4/fondaparinux (72,149).

Since both danaparoid and fondaparinux have long anti-Xa half-lives (25 and 17 hr, respectively), and since neither prolongs the PT, this facilitates a smooth transition to warfarin therapy. No antidote exists for either.

Adjunctive Therapies

Besides anticoagulation with one of the agents discussed above, there are situations in which various adjunctive therapies might be appropriate (14). Surgical thromboembolectomy may be limb-saving in situations of acute large artery occlusion by platelet-rich "white clots" (150). Thrombolysis (combined with anticoagulation) may be helpful in patients with severe pulmonary embolism. Plasmapheresis (replacing with fresh frozen plasma) or high-dose intravenous gammaglobulin are unproven but potentially useful treatment adjuncts to anticoagulation in patients with very severe HIT. Although inferior vena cava filters are sometimes used to manage patients with severe HIT, in my view these do not obviate the need for anticoagulation in HIT and may contribute to lower limb thrombosis and possibly even limb ischemia/necrosis. I do not advocate their use in patients with HIT. In my experience, severe venous limb ischemia complicating HIT is sometimes diagnosed clinically to represent "compartment syndrome" leading to treatment with fasciotomy. However, reversal of warfarin anticoagulation and aggressive anticoagulation are more likely to benefit such a patient than performing fasciotomy when the underlying pathologic process is progressive macro- and microvascular thrombosis in veins and venules.

Renal Failure and HIT

Drug pharmacokinetics are important considerations in patients with HIT who have renal failure (151). For example, if lepirudin is used, the dose must be greatly reduced, e.g., 0.005 to 0.010 mg/kg/h (about 3–10% of the usual infusion rate), and monitoring should ideally be repeated at 4–6 hr intervals until the patient is stably anticoagulated. As an alternative to low intravenous infusion, intermittent low-dose boluses (e.g., 0.08–0.15 mg/kg) can be given, e.g., immediately predialysis for patients requiring anticoagulation for hemodialysis. Argatroban can be given without initial dose-reduction; thus, for patients undergoing intermittent hemodialysis, a bolus of 250 μg/kg can be given predialysis, with an infusion rate of 2 μg/kg/min (152). Protocols for use of danaparoid (143,151) or argatroban (106,152) in uremic patients with HIT are available.

Cardiac Surgery and HIT

The topic of managing cardiac surgery in a patient with previous, subacute, or acute HIT has been reviewed recently (112,116,121). For patients with previous HIT (fully recovered, with HIT antibodies no longer detectable) who require cardiac surgery, it is recommended that UFH be given in usual doses for cardiac surgery (112,116,121). This is based on the following rationale: (a) repeat formation of HIT antibodies does not appear to occur more often in patients with a previous history of HIT; (b) if antibodies are regenerated, these will take at least five days following cardiac surgery to reach significant levels (at a time when alternative, non-heparin anticoagulation can be given); (c) heparin remains the standard anticoagulant of choice for cardiac surgery, at least until suitable alternatives are proven to be routinely safe (46,47,112,116,121). Heparin is a reasonable option also for a patient with a weak-positive PF4-dependent EIA (absorbance <0.75 units) and a negative washed platelet activation assay (116).

For patients with acute HIT, or whose platelets have recovered but who still have detectable HIT antibodies (subacute HIT), many different treatment options are available (for review, see Ref. 116). No one recommendation is applicable to all situations, however, especially given jurisdictional differences in drug availability, patient-dependent factors (e.g., renal function), availability of specialized anticoagulant monitoring assays, and physician experience and preference. Three general approaches are available: (a) await disappearance of HIT antibodies and use heparin; (b) give a non-heparin anticoagulant (e.g., bivalirudin, lepirudin, danaparoid) (143,153–158); or (c) combine heparin with an antiplatelet agent (e.g., prostacyclin analogue, glycoprotein IIb/IIIa inhibitor) for intraoperative anticoagulation (159–161).

ACKNOWLEDGMENTS

Studies described in this chapter (7,28,30,36–39,41,42,46,49,51,57,62,67, 72–75,84,85,87,88,91,92,94,95,97,98,100,104,109,111,112,115,116,147) were supported by operating grants from the Heart and Stroke Foundation of Ontario from 1993 to 2005 (A2449, T2967, B3763, T4502, and T5207). I thank Jo-Ann I. Sheppard for preparing the figures.

REFERENCES

1. Lee DH, Warkentin TE. Frequency of heparin-induced thrombocytopenia. In: Warkentin TE, Greinacher A, eds. In: Heparin-induced Thrombocytopenia, 3rd ed. New York: Marcel Dekker, Inc., 2004:107–148.
2. Council for International Organization of Medical Sciences (CIOMS Working Group IV), Geneva, Switzerland, 1998.
3. Alving BM. How I treat heparin-induced thrombocytopenia and thrombosis. Blood 2003; 101:31–37.
4. Chong BH. Heparin-induced thrombocytopenia. J Thromb Haemost 2003; 1:1471–1478.
5. Warkentin TE. Heparin-induced thrombocytopenia: pathogenesis and management. Br J Haematol 2003; 121:535–555.

6. Warkentin TE. Platelet count monitoring and laboratory testing for heparin-induced thrombocytopenia: recommendations of the College of American Pathologists. Arch Pathol Lab Med 2002; 126:1415–1423.
7. Warkentin TE, Roberts RS, Hirsh J, Kelton JG. An improved definition of immune heparin-induced thrombocytopenia in postoperative orthopedic patients. Arch Intern Med 2003; 163:2518–2524.
8. Rhodes GR, Dixon RH, Silver D. Heparin induced thrombocytopenia with thrombotic and hemorrhagic manifestations. Surg Gynecol Obstet 1973; 136:409–416.
9. Rhodes GR, Dixon RH, Silver D. Heparin induced thrombocytopenia: eight cases with thrombotic-hemorrhagic complications. Ann Surg 1977; 186:752–758.
10. Weismann RE, Tobin RW. Arterial embolism occurring during systemic heparin therapy. Arch Surg 1958; 76:219–227.
11. Roberts B, Rosato FE, Rosato EF. Heparin—a cause of arterial emboli? Surgery 1964; 55:803–808.
12. Towne JB, Bernhard VM, Hussey C, Garancis JC. White clot syndrome. Peripheral vascular complications of heparin therapy. Arch Surg 1979; 114:372–377.
13. Warkentin TE. History of heparin-induced thrombocytopenia. In: Warkentin TE, Greinacher A, eds. In: Heparin-Induced Thrombocytopenia, 3rd ed. New York: Marcel Dekker, Inc., 2004:1–23.
14. Greinacher A, Warkentin TE. Treatment of heparin-induced thrombocytopenia: an overview. In: Warkentin TE, Greinacher A, eds. In: Heparin-Induced Thrombocytopenia, 3rd ed. New York: Marcel Dekker, Inc., 2004:355–370.
15. Amiral J, Bridey F, Dreyfus M, et al. Platelet factor 4 complexed to heparin is the target for antibodies generated in heparin-induced thrombocytopenia [letter]. Thromb Haemost 1992; 68:95–96.
16. Suh JS, Aster RH, Visentin GP. Antibodies from patients with heparin-induced thrombocytopenia/thrombosis recognize different epitopes on heparin:platelet factor 4. Blood 1998; 91:916–922.
17. Ziporen L, Li ZQ, Park KS, et al. Defining an antigenic epitope on platelet factor 4 associated with heparin-induced thrombocytopenia. Blood 1998; 92:3250–3259.
18. Li ZQ, Liu W, Park KS, et al. Defining a second epitope for heparin-induced thrombocytopenia/thrombosis antibodies using KKO, a murine HIT-like monoclonal antibody. Blood 2002; 99:1230–1236.
19. Suh JS, Malik MI, Aster RH, Visentin GP. Characterization of the humoral immune response in heparin-induced thrombocytopenia. Am J Hematol 1997; 54:196–201.
20. Amiral J, Pouplard C, Vissac AM, Walenga JM, Jeske W, Gruel Y. Affinity purification of heparin-dependent antibodies to platelet factor 4 developed in heparin-induced thrombocytopenia: biological characteristics and effects on platelet activation. Br J Haematol 2000; 109:336–341.
21. Greinacher A, Michels I, Schafer M, Kiefel V, Mueller-Eckhardt C. Heparin-associated thrombocytopenia in a patient treated with polysulphated chondroitin sulphate: evidence for immunological crossreactivity between heparin and polysulphated glycosaminoglycan. Br J Haematol 1992; 81:252–254.
22. Goad KE, Horne MK, III, Gralnick HR. Pentosan-induced thrombocytopenia: support for an immune complex mechanism. Br J Haematol 1994; 88:803–808.
23. Rosenthal MA, Rischin D, McArthur G, et al. Treatment with the novel anti-angiogenic agent PI-88 is associated with immune-mediated thrombocytopenia. Ann Oncol 2002; 13:770–776.

24. Visentin GP, Moghaddam M, Beery SE, McFarland JG, Aster RH. Heparin is not required for detection of antibodies associated with heparin-induced thrombocytopenia/thrombosis. J Lab Clin Med 2001; 138:22–31.
25. Amiral J, Marfaing-Koka A, Wolf M, et al. Presence of autoantibodies to interleukin-8 or neutrophil-activating peptide-2 in patients with heparin-associated thrombocytopenia. Blood 1996; 88:410–416.
26. Regnault V, de Maistre E, Carteaux JP, et al. Platelet activation induced by human antibodies to interleukin-8. Blood 2003; 101:1419–1421.
27. Greinacher A, Pötzsch B, Amiral J, Dummel V, Eichner A, Mueller-Eckhardt C. Heparin-associated thrombocytopenia: isolation of the antibody and characterization of a multimolecular PF4–heparin complex as the major antigen. Thromb Haemost 1994; 71:247–251.
28. Warkentin TE, Kelton JG. Delayed-onset heparin-induced thrombocytopenia and thrombosis. Ann Intern Med 2001; 135:502–506.
29. Rice L, Attisha WK, Drexler A, Francis JL. Delayed-onset heparin-induced thrombocytopenia. Ann Intern Med 2002; 136:210–215.
30. Warkentin TE, Bernstein RA. Delayed-onset heparin-induced thrombocytopenia and cerebral thrombosis after a single administration of unfractionated heparin (letter). N Engl J Med 2003; 348:1067–1069.
31. Greinacher A, Michels I, Liebenhoff U, Presek P, Mueller-Eckhardt C. Heparin-associated thrombocytopenia: immune complexes are attached to the platelet membrane by the negative charge of highly sulfated oligosaccharides. Br J Haematol 1993; 84:711–716.
32. Visentin GP, Ford SE, Scott JP, Aster RH. Antibodies from patients with heparin-induced thrombocytopenia/thrombosis are specific for platelet factor 4 complexed with heparin or bound to endothelial cells. J Clin Invest 1994; 93:81–88.
33. Horne MK, III, Hutchison KJ. Simultaneous binding of heparin and platelet factor-4 to platelets: further insights into the mechanism of heparin-induced thrombocytopenia. Am J Hematol 1998; 58:24–30.
34. Newman PM, Chong BH. Heparin-induced thrombocytopenia: new evidence for the dynamic binding of purified anti-PF4–heparin antibodies to platelets and the resultant platelet activation. Blood 2000; 96:182–187.
35. Denomme GA. The platelet Fc receptor in heparin-induced thrombocytopenia. In: Warkentin TE, Greinacher A, eds. In: Heparin-Induced Thrombocytopenia, 3rd ed, 2004:223–250.
36. Warkentin TE, Hayward CPM, Boshkov LK, et al. Sera from patients with heparin-induced thrombocytopenia generate platelet-derived microparticles with procoagulant activity: an explanation for the thrombotic complications of heparin-induced thrombocytopenia. Blood 1994; 84:3691–3699.
37. Lee DH, Warkentin TE, Denomme GA, Hayward CPM, Kelton JG. A diagnostic test for heparin-induced thrombocytopenia: detection of platelet microparticles using flow cytometry. Br J Haematol 1996; 95:724–731.
38. Hughes M, Hayward CPM, Warkentin TE, Horsewood P, Chorneyko KA, Kelton JG. Morphological analysis of microparticle generation in heparin-induced thrombocytopenia. Blood 2000; 96:188–194.
39. Warkentin TE, Sheppard JI. Generation of platelet-derived microparticles and procoagulant activity by heparin-induced thrombocytopenia IgG/serum and other

IgG platelet agonists: a comparison with standard platelet agonists. Platelets 1999; 10:319–326.
40. Amiral J, Wolf M, Fischer AM, Boyer-Neumann C, Vissac AM, Meyer D. Pathogenicity of IgA and/or IgM antibodies to heparin–PF4 complexes in patients with heparin-induced thrombocytopenia. Br J Haematol 1996; 92:954–959.
41. Warkentin TE, Sheppard JI, Horsewood P, Simpson PJ, Moore JC, Kelton JG. Impact of the patient population on the risk for heparin-induced thrombocytopenia. Blood 2000; 96:1703–1708.
42. Denomme GA, Warkentin TE, Horsewood P, Sheppard JI, Warner MN, Kelton JG. Activation of platelets by sera containing IgG1 heparin-dependent antibodies: an explanation for the predominance of the FcγRIIa "low responder" (His_{131}) gene in patients with heparin-induced thrombocytopenia. J Lab Clin Med 1997; 130:278–284.
43. Carlsson LE, Santoso S, Baurichter G, et al. Heparin-induced thrombocytopenia: new insights into the impact of the FcγRIIa-R-H_{131} polymorphism. Blood 1998; 92:1526–1531.
44. Bacsi S, De Palma R, Visentin GP, Gorski J, Aster RH. Complexes of heparin and platelet factor 4 specifically stimulate T cells from patients with heparin-induced thrombocytopenia/thrombosis. Blood 1999; 94:208–215.
45. Bacsi S, Geoffrey R, Visentin GP, De Palma R, Aster RH, Gorski J. Identification of T cells responding to a self-protein modified by an external agent. Hum Immunol 2001; 62:113–124.
46. Warkentin TE, Kelton JG. Temporal aspects of heparin-induced thrombocytopenia. N Engl J Med 2001; 344:1286–1292.
47. Pötzsch B, Klövekorn WP, Madlener K. Use of heparin during cardiopulmonary bypass in patients with a history of heparin-induced thrombocytopenia [letter]. N Engl J Med 2000; 343:515.
48. Lubenow N, Kempf R, Eichner A, Eichler P, Carlsson LE, Greinacher A. Heparin-induced thrombocytopenia: temporal pattern of thrombocytopenia in relation to initial use or reexposure to heparin. Chest 2002; 122:37–42.
49. Warkentin TE, Elavathil LJ, Hayward CPM, Johnston MA, Russett JI, Kelton JG. The pathogenesis of venous limb gangrene associated with heparin-induced thrombocytopenia. Ann Intern Med 1997; 127:804–812.
50. Greinacher A, Eichler P, Lubenow N, Kwasny H, Luz M. Heparin-induced thrombocytopenia with thromboembolic complications: meta-analysis of two prospective trials to assess the value of parenteral treatment with lepirudin and its therapeutic aPTT range. Blood 2000; 96:846–851.
51. Warkentin TE. An overview of the heparin-induced thrombocytopenia syndrome. Semin Thromb Hemost 2004; 30:273–283.
52. Cines DB, Tomaski A, Tannenbaum S. Immune endothelial-cell injury in heparin-associated thrombocytopenia. N Engl J Med 1987; 316:581–589.
53. Kwaan HC, Sakurai S. Endothelial cell hyperplasia contributes to thrombosis in heparin-induced thrombocytopenia. Semin Thromb Hemost 1999; 25:23–27.
54. Herbert JM, Savi P, Jeske WP, Walenga JM. Effect of SR121566A, a potent GP IIb-IIIa antagonist, on the HIT serum/heparin-induced platelet mediated activation of human endothelial cells. Thromb Haemost 1998; 80:326–331.
55. Pouplard C, Iochmann S, Renard B, et al. Induction of monocyte tissue factor expression by antibodies to heparin-platelet factor 4 complexes developed in heparin-induced thrombocytopenia. Blood 2001; 97:3300–3302.

56. Arepally GM, Mayer IM. Antibodies from patients with heparin-induced thrombocytopenia stimulate monocytic cells to express cells to express tissue factor and secrete interleukin-8. Blood 2001; 98:1252–1254.
57. Warkentin TE. Heparin-induced thrombocytopenia. Curr Hematol Rep 2002; 1:63–72.
58. Reilly MP, Taylor SM, Hartman NK, et al. Heparin-induced thrombocytopenia/-thrombosis in a transgenic mouse model requires human platelet factor 4 and platelet activation through FcγRIIA. Blood 2001; 98:2442–2447.
59. Warkentin TE, Greinacher A. Laboratory testing for heparin-induced thrombocytopenia. In: Warkentin TE, Greinacher A, eds. In: Heparin-induced Thrombocytopenia, 3rd ed. New York: Marcel Dekker, Inc., 2004:271–311.
60. Chong BH, Burgess J, Ismail F. The clinical usefulness of the platelet aggregation test for the diagnosis of heparin-induced thrombocytopenia. Thromb Haemost 1993; 69:344–350.
61. Greinacher A, Amiral J, Dummel V, Vissac A, Kiefel V, Mueller-Eckhardt C. Laboratory diagnosis of heparin-associated thrombocytopenia and comparison of platelet aggregation test, heparin-induced platelet activation test, and platelet factor 4/heparin enzyme-linked immunosorbent assay. Transfusion 1996; 34:381–385.
62. Warkentin TE, Hayward CPM, Smith CA, Kelly PM, Kelton JG. Determinants of donor platelet variability when testing for heparin-induced thrombocytopenia. J Lab Clin Med 1992; 120:371–379.
63. Sheridan D, Carter C, Kelton JG. A diagnostic test for heparin-induced thrombocytopenia. Blood 1986; 67:27–30.
64. Greinacher A, Michels I, Kiefel V, Mueller-Eckhardt C. A rapid and sensitive test for diagnosing heparin-associated thrombocytopenia. Thromb Haemost 1991; 66:734–736.
65. Eichler P, Budde U, Haas S, et al. First Workshop for detection of heparin-induced antibodies: validation of the heparin-induced platelet activation (HIPA) test in comparison with a PF4/heparin ELISA. Thromb Haemost 1999; 81:625–629.
66. Warkentin TE, Sheppard JI. No significant improvement in diagnostic specificity of an anti-PF4/polyanion immunoassay with use of high heparin confirmatory procedure [letter]. J Thiomb Haemost 2006; 4:281–282.
67. Warkentin TE, Sheppard JI, Moore JC, Moore KM, Sigouin CS, Kelton JG. Laboratory testing for HIT antibodies: how much class do we need? J Lab Clin Med 2005; 146:341–346.
68. Meyer O, Salama A, Pittet N, Schwind P. Rapid detection of heparin-induced platelet antibodies with particle gel immunoassay (ID-HPF4). Lancet 1999; 354:1525–1526.
69. Eichler P, Raschke R, Lubenow N, Meyer O, Schwind P, Greinacher A. The new ID-heparin/PF4 antibody test for rapid detection of heparin-induced antibodies in comparison with functional and antigenic assays. Br J Haematol 2002; 116:887–891.
70. Alberio L, Kimmerle S, Baumann A, Taleghani BM, Biasiutti FD, Lämmle B. Rapid determination of anti-heparin/platelet factor 4 antibody titers in the diagnosis of heparin-induced thrombocytopenia. Am J Med 2003; 114:528–536.
71. Newman PM, Swanson RL, Chong BH. Heparin-induced thrombocytopenia: IgG binding to PF4-heparin complexes in the fluid phase and cross-reactivity with low molecular weight heparin and heparinoid. Thromb Haemost 1998; 80:292–297.

72. Warkentin TE, Cook RJ, Marder VJ, et al. Anti-platelet factor 4/heparin antibodies in orthopedic surgery patients receiving antithrombotic prophylaxis with fondaparinux of enoxaparin. Blood 2005; 106:3791–3796.
73. Warkentin TE, Levine MN, Hirsh J, et al. Heparin-induced thrombocytopenia in patients treated with low-molecular-weight heparin or unfractionated heparin. N Engl J Med 1995; 332:1330–1335.
74. Warkentin TE, Heddle NM. Laboratory diagnosis of immune heparin-induced thrombocytopenia. Curr Hematol Rep 2003; 2:148–157.
75. Warkentin TE. New approaches to the diagnosis of heparin-induced thrombocytopenia. Chest 2005; 27 (Suppl.):35S–45S
76. Zwicker JI, Uhl L, Huang WY, Shaz BH, Bauer KA. Thrombosis and ELISA optical density values in hospitalized patients with heparin-induced thrombocytopenia. J Thromb Haemost 2004; 2:2133–2137.
77. Warkentin TE. Clinical picture of heparin-induced thrombocytopenia. In: Warkentin TE, Greinacher A, eds. In: Heparin-induced Thrombocytopenia, 3rd ed. New York: Marcel Dekker, Inc., 2004:53–106.
78. Francis JL, Palmer GJ, III, Moroose R, Drexler A. Comparison of bovine and porcine heparin in heparin antibody formation after cardiac surgery. Ann Thorac Surg 2003; 75:17–22.
79. Martel N, Lee J, Wells PS. Risk for heparin-induced thrombocytopenia with unfractionated and low-molecular weight heparin thromboprophylaxis: a meta-analysis. Blood 2005; 106:2710–2715.
80. Lindhoff-Last E, Nakov R, Misselwitz F, Breddin HK, Bauersachs R. Incidence and clinical relevance of heparin-induced antibodies in patients with deep vein thrombosis treated with unfractionated heparin or low-molecular-weight heparin. Br J Haematol 2002; 118:1137–1142.
81. Visentin GP, Malik M, Cyganiak KA, Aster RH. Patients treated with unfractionated heparin during open heart surgery are at high risk to form antibodies reactive with heparin:platelet factor 4 complexes. J Lab Clin Med 1996; 128:376–383.
82. Lindhoff-Last E, Eichler P, Stein M, et al. A prospective study on the incidence and clinical relevance of heparin-induced antibodies in patients after vascular surgery. Thromb Res 2000; 97:387–393.
83. Greinacher A, Eichler P, Lietz T, Warkentin TE. Replacement of unfractionated heparin by low-molecular-weight heparin for postorthopedic surgery antithrombotic prophylaxis lowers the overall risk of symptomatic thrombosis because of a lower frequency of heparin-induced thrombocytopenia [letter]. Blood 2005; 106:2921–2922.
84. Warkentin TE, Sigouin CS. Gender and risk of immune heparin-induced thrombocytopenia [abstr]. Blood 2002; 100:17a.
85. Warkentin TE, Kelton JG. A 14-year study of heparin-induced thrombocytopenia. Am J Med 1996; 101:502–507.
86. Wallis DE, Workman DL, Lewis BE, Steen L, Pifarre R, Moran JF. Failure of early heparin cessation as treatment for heparin-induced thrombocytopenia. Am J Med 1999; 106:629–635.
87. Warkentin TE. Management of heparin-induced thrombocytopenia: a critical comparison of lepirudin and argatroban. Thromb Res 2003; 110:73–82.

88. Hong AP, Cook DJ, Sigouin CS, Warkentin TE. Central venous catheters and upper-extremity deep-vein thrombosis complicating immune heparin-induced thrombocytopenia. Blood 2003; 101:3049–3051.
89. Arthur CK, Grant SJB, Murray WK, Isbister JP, Stiel N, Lauer CS. Heparin-associated acute adrenal insufficiency. Aust NZ J Med 1985; 15:454–455.
90. Ernest D, Fisher MM. Heparin-induced thrombocytopaenia complicated by bilateral adrenal haemorrhage. Intensive Care Med 1991; 17:238–240.
91. Warkentin TE, Sikov WM, Lillicrap DP. Multicentric warfarin-induced skin necrosis complicating heparin-induced thrombocytopenia. Am J Hematol 1999; 62:44–48.
92. Smythe MA, Warkentin TE, Stephens JL, Zakalik D, Mattson JC. Venous limb gangrene during overlapping therapy with warfarin and a direct thrombin inhibitor for immune heparin-induced thrombocytopenia. Am J Hematol 2002; 71:50–52.
93. Srinivasan AF, Rice L, Bartholomew JR, et al. Warfarin-induced skin necrosis and venous limb gangrene in the setting of heparin-induced thrombocytopenia. Arch Intern Med 2004; 164:66–70.
94. Warkentin TE, Whitlock RP, Teoh KHT. Warfarin-associated multiple digital necrosis complicating heparin-induced thrombocytopenia and Raynaud's phenomenon after aortic valve replacement for adenocarcinoma-associated thrombotic endocarditis. Am J Hematol 2004; 75:56–62.
95. Lee DH, Warkentin TE, Denomme GA, Lagrotteria DD, Kelton JG. Factor V Leiden and thrombotic complications in heparin-induced thrombocytopenia. Thromb Haemost 1998; 79:50–53.
96. Carlsson LE, Lubenow N, Blumentritt C, et al. Platelet receptor and clotting factor polymorphisms as genetic risk factors for thromboembolic complications in heparin-induced thrombocytopenia. Pharmacogenetics 2003; 13:253–258.
97. Warkentin TE. Heparin-induced skin lesions. Br J Haematol 1996; 92:494–497.
98. Warkentin TE. Heparin-induced thrombocytopenia, skin lesions, and arterial thrombosis: a new clinical syndrome [abstr]. Can J Cardiol 1996; 12:151E.
99. Gröger M, Sarmay G, Fiebiger E, Wolff K, Petzelbauer P. Dermal microvascular endothelial cells express CD32 receptors in vivo and in vitro. J Immunol 1996; 156:1549–1556.
100. Warkentin TE, Hirte HW, Anderson DR, Wilson WEC, O'Connell GJ, Lo RC. Transient global amnesia associated with acute heparin-induced thrombocytopenia. Am J Med 1994; 97:489–491.
101. Mims MP, Manian P, Rice L. Acute cardiorespiratory collapse from heparin: a consequence of heparin-induced thrombocytopenia. Eur J Haematol 2004; 72:366–369.
102. Popov D, Zarrabi MH, Foda H, Graber M. Pseudopulmonary embolism: acute respiratory distress in the syndrome of heparin-induced thrombocytopenia. Am J Kidney Dis 1997; 29:449–452.
103. Warkentin TE. Pseudo-heparin-induced thrombocytopenia. In: Warkentin TE, Greinacher A, eds. In: Heparin-induced Thrombocytopenia, 3rd ed. New York: Marcel Dekker, Inc., 2004:313–334.
104. Warkentin TE. Venous limb gangrene during warfarin treatment of cancer-associated deep venous thrombosis. Ann Intern Med 2001; 135:589–593.
105. Lubenow N, Eichler P, Albrecht D, et al. Very low platelet counts in post-transfusion purpura falsely diagnosed as heparin-induced thrombocytopenia. Report of four cases and review of literature. Thromb Res 2000; 100:115–125.

106. Lewis BE, Hursting MJ. Agratroban therapy in heparin-induced thrombocytopenia. In: Warkentin TE, Greinacher A, eds. In: Heparin-induced Thrombocytopenia, 3rd ed. New York: Marcel Dekker, Inc., 2004:437–444.
107. Lubenow N, Eichler P, Lietz T, Farner B, Greinacher A. Lepirudin for prophylaxis of thrombosis in patients with isolated heparin-induced thrombocytopenia: an analysis of 3 prospective studies. Blood 2004; 104:3072–3077.
108. Warkentin TE, Aird WC, Rand JH. Platelet-endothelial interactions: sepsis, HIT, and antiphospholipid syndrome. Hematology (Am Soc Hematol Educ Program) 2003;497–519.
109. Lo GK, Juhl A, Warkentin TE, Sigouin CS, Eichler P, Greinacher A. Evaluation of the pretest clinical score (4 T's) for the diagnosis of heparin-induced thrombocytopenia in two clinical settings. J Thromb Haemost 2006; in press.
110. Lillo-Le Louet A, Boutouyrie P, Alhenc-Gelas M, et al. Diagnostic score for heparin-induced thrombocytopenia after cardiopulmonary bypass. J Thromb Haemost 2004; 2:1882–1888.
111. Warkentin TE. Bivalent direct thrombin inhibitors: hirudin and bivalirudin. Best Pract Res Clin Haematol 2004; 17:105–125.
112. Warkentin TE, Greinacher A. Heparin-induced thrombocytopenia: recognition, treatment, and prevention: The Seventh ACCP Conference on Antithrombotic and Thrombolytic Therapy. Chest 2004; 126:311S–337S.
113. Greinacher A. Lepirudin for the treatment of heparin-induced thrombocytopenia. In: Warkentin TE, Greinacher A, eds. In: Heparin-Induced Thrombocytopenia, 3rd ed. New York: Marcel Dekker, Inc., 2004:397–436.
114. Salzet M. Leech thrombin inhibitors. Curr Pharm Des 2002; 8:125–133.
115. Warkentin TE, Greinacher A, Craven S, Dewar L, Sheppard JI, Ofosu FA. Differences in the clinically effective molar concentrations of four direct thrombin inhibitors explain their variable prothrombin time prolongation. Thromb Haemost 2005; 94:958–964.
116. Warkentin TE, Greinacher A. Heparin-induced thrombocytopenia and cardiac surgery. Ann Thorac Surg 2003; 76:2121–2131.
117. Greinacher A, Völpel H, Janssens U, et al. Recombinant hirudin (lepirudin) provides safe and effective anticoagulation in patients with heparin-induced thrombocytopenia. A prospective study. Circulation 1999; 99:73–80.
118. Greinacher A, Janssens U, Berg G, et al. Lepirudin (recombinant hirudin) for parenteral anticoagulation in patients with heparin-induced thrombocytopenia. Circulation 1999; 100:587–593.
119. Lubenow N, Eichler P, Lietz T, Greinacher A. Lepirudin in patients with heparin-induced thrombocytopenia–results of the third prospective study (HAT-3) and a combined analysis of HAT-1, HAT-2, and HAT-3. J Thromb Haemost 2005; 3:2428–2436.
120. Lubenow N, Eichler P, Greinacher A. Results of a large drug monitoring program confirms the safety and efficacy of Refludan (lepirudin) in patients with immune-mediated heparin-induced thrombocytopenia [abstr]. Blood 2002; 100:502a.
121. Poetzsch B, Madlener K. Management of cardiopulmonary bypass anticoagulation in patients with heparin-induced thrombocytopenia. In: Warkentin TE, Greinacher A, eds. In: Heparin-Induced Thrombocytopenia, 3rd ed. New York: Marcel Dekker, Inc., 2004:531–551.

122. Pötzsch B, Madlener K, Seelig C, Riess CF, Greinacher A, Müller-Berghaus G. Monitoring of r-hirudin anticoagulation during cardiopulmonary bypass—assessment of the whole blood ecarin clotting time. Thromb Haemost 1997; 77:920–925.
123. Eichler P, Friesen HJ, Lubenow N, Jaeger B, Greinacher A. Antihirudin antibodies in patients with heparin-induced thrombocytopenia treated with lepirudin: incidence, effects on aPTT, and clinical relevance. Blood 2000; 96:2373–2378.
124. Greinacher A, Eichler P, Albrecht D, Strobel U, Pötzsch B, Eriksson BI. Antihirudin antibodies following low-dose subcutaneous treatment with desirudin for thrombosis prophylaxis after hip-replacement surgery: incidence and clinical relevance. Blood 2003; 101:2617–2619.
125. Eichler P, Lubenow N, Strobel U, Greinacher A. Antibodies against lepirudin are polyspecific and recognize epitopes on bivalirudin. Blood 2004; 103:613–616.
126. Berkowitz SD. Antigenic potential of bivalirudin [abstr]. Blood 1999; 94:102b.
127. Greinacher A, Eichler P, Lubenow N. Anaphylactic and anaphylactoid reactions associated with lepirudin in patients with heparin-induced thrombocytopenia. Circulation 2003; 108:2062–2065.
128. Badger NO, Butler K, Hallman LC. Excessive anticoagulation and anaphylactic reaction after rechallenge with lepirudin in a patient with heparin-induced thrombocytopenia. Pharmacotherapy 2004; 24:1800–1803.
129. Walenga JM, Ahmad S, Hoppensteadt DA, Iqbal O, Hursting MJ, Lewis BE. Argatroban therapy does not generate antibodies that alter its anticoagulant activity in patients with heparin-induced thrombocytopenia. Thromb Res 2002; 105:401–405.
130. Sheth SB, DiCicco RA, Hursting MJ, Montague T, Jorkasky DK. Interpreting the International Normalized Ratio (INR) in individuals receiving argatroban and warfarin. Thromb Haemost 2001; 85:435–440.
131. Hursting MJ, Lewis BE, Macfarlane DE. Transitioning from argatroban to warfarin therapy in patients with heparin-induced thrombocytopenia. Clin Appl Thromb Haemost 2005; 11:279–287.
132. Kikumoto R, Tamao Y, Tezeka T, et al. Selective inhibition of thrombin by (2*R*, 4*R*)-4-methyl-1-[N^2-[(3-methyl-1,2,3,4-tetrahydro-8-quinolinyl)sulfonyl]-L-arginyl)]-2-piperidinecarboxylic acid. Biochemistry 1984; 23:85–90.
133. Lewis BE, Wallis DE, Berkowitz SD, et al, The ARG-911 Study Investigators. Argatroban anticoagulant therapy in patients with heparin-induced thrombocytopenia. Circulation 2001; 103:1838–1843.
134. Lewis BE, Wallis DE, Leya F, Hursting MJ, Kelton JG. Argatroban anticoagulation in patients with heparin-induced thrombocytopenia. Arch Intern Med 2003; 163:1849–1856.
135. Arpino PA, Hallisey RK. Effect of renal function on the pharmacodynamics of argatroban. Ann Pharmacother 2004; 38:25–29.
136. Lewis B, Matthai WH, Cohen M, Moses JW, Hursting MJ, Leya F, for the ARG-216/310/311 investigators. Argatroban anticoagulation during percutaneous coronary intervention in patients with heparin-induced thrombocytopenia. Cathet Cardiovasc Intervent 2002; 57:177–184.
137. Bartholomew JR. Bivalirudin for the treatment of heparin-induced thrombocytopenia. In: Warkentin TE, Greinacher A, eds. In: Heparin-Induced Thrombocytopenia, 3rd ed. New York: Marcel Dekker, Inc., 2004:475–507.

138. Maraganore JM, Bourdon P, Jablonski J, Ramachandran KL, Fenton JW, II. Design and characterization of hirulogs: a novel class of bivalent peptide inhibitors of thrombin. Biochemistry 1990; 29:7095–7101.
139. Parry MA, Maraganore JM, Stone SR. Kinetic mechanism for the interaction of Hirulog with thrombin. Biochemistry 1994; 33:14807–14814.
140. Robson R, White H, Aylward P, Frampton C. Bivalirudin pharmacokinetics and pharmacodynamics: effect of renal function, dose, and gender. Clin Pharmacol Ther 2002; 71:433–439.
141. Chamberlin JR, Lewis B, Leya F, et al. Successful treatment of heparin-associated thrombocytopenia and thrombosis using Hirulog. Can J Cardiol 1994; 11:511–514.
142. Francis JL, Drexler A, Gwyn G, Moroose R. Bivalirudin, a direct thrombin inhibitor, is a safe and effective treatment for heparin-induced thrombocytopenia [abstr]. Blood 2003; 102:164a.
143. Chong BH, Magnani HN. Danaparoid for the treatment of heparin-induced thrombocytopenia. In: Warkentin TE, Greinacher A, eds. In: Heparin-Induced Thrombocytopenia, 3rd ed. New York: Marcel Dekker, Inc., 2004:371–396.
144. Chong BH, Gallus AS, Cade JF, et al. Prospective randomised open-label comparison of danaparoid with dextran 70 in the treatment of heparin-induced thrombocytopaenia with thrombosis: a clinical outcome study. Thromb Haemost 2001; 86:1170–1175.
145. Farner B, Eichler P, Kroll H, Greinacher A. A comparison of danaparoid and lepirudin in heparin-induced thrombocytopenia. Thromb Haemost 2001; 85:950–957.
146. Warkentin TE. Heparin-induced thrombocytopenia: yet another treatment paradox? Thromb Haemost 2001; 85:947–949.
147. Lubenow N, Warkentin TE, Greinacher A, et al. Results of a systematic evaluation of treatment outcomes for heparin-induced thrombocytopenia in patients receiving danaparoid, ancrod, and/or coumarin explain the rapid shift in clinical practice during the 1990s. Throm Res 2005 May 19; [Epub ahead of print].
148. Kuo KHM, Kovacs MJ. Fondaparinux: a potential new therapy for HIT. Hematology 2005; 10:271–275.
149. Greinacher A, Gopinadhan M, Guenther JU, et al. The molecular structure of the antigen in heparin-induced thrombocytopenia [abstr]. J Thromb Haemost 2005; 3 (1 Suppl): OR 217.
150. Sobel M, Adelman B, Szentpeterey S, Hofmann M, Posner MP, Jenvey W. Surgical management of heparin-associated thrombocytopenia. Strategies in the treatment of venous and arterial thromboembolism. J Vasc Surg 1988; 8:395–401.
151. Fischer KG. Hemodialysis in heparin-induced thrombocytopenia. In: Warkentin TE, Greinacher A, eds. In: Heparin-Induced Thrombocytopenia, 3rd ed. New York: Marcel Dekker, Inc., 2004:509–530.
152. Murray PT, Reddy BV, Grossman EJ, et al. A prospective comparison of three argatroban treatment during hemodialysis in end-stage renal disease. Kidney Int 2004; 66:2446–2453.
153. Bott JN, Reddy K, Krick S. Bivalirudin in off-pump myocardial revascularization in patients with heparin-induced thrombocytopenia. Ann Thorac Surg 2003; 76:273–275.
154. Vasquez JC, Vichiendilokkul A, Mahmood S, Baciewicz FA, Jr. Anticoagulation with bivalirudin during cardiopulmonary bypass in cardiac surgery. Ann Thorac Surg 2002; 74:2177–2179.

155. Davis Z, Anderson R, Short D, Garber D, Valgiusti A. Favorable outcome with bivalirudin anticoagulation during cardiopulmonary bypass. Ann Thorac Surg 2003; 75:264–265.
156. Merry AF, Raudkivi PJ, Middleton NG, et al. Bivalirudin versus heparin and protamine in off-pump coronary artery bypass surgery. Ann Thorac Surg 2004; 77:925–931.
157. Riess FC, Löwer C, Seelig C, et al. Recombinant hirudin as a new anticoagulant during cardiac operations instread of heparin: successful for aortic valve replacement in man. Thorac Cardiovasc Surg 1995; 110:265–267.
158. Riess FC, Pötzsch B, Bader K, et al. A case report on the use of recombinant hirudin as an anticoagulant for cardiopulmonary bypass in open heart surgery. Eur J Cardiothorac Surg 1996; 10:386–388.
159. Mertzlufft F, Kuppe H, Koster A. Management of urgent high-risk cardiopulmonary bypass in patients with heparin-induced thrombocytopenia type II and coexisting disorders of renal function: use of heparin and epoprostenol combined with on-line monitoring of platelet function. J Cardiothorac Vasc Anesth 2000; 14:304–308.
160. Aouifi A, Blanc P, Piriou V, et al. Cardiac surgery with cardiopulmonary bypass in patients with type II heparin-induced thrombocytopenia. Ann Thorac Surg 2001; 71:678–683.
161. Koster A, Meyer O, Fischer T, et al. One-year experience with the platelet glycoprotein IIb/IIIa antagonist tirofiban and heparin during cardiopulmonary bypass in patients with heparin-induced thrombocytopenia type II. J Thorac Cardiovasc Surg 2001; 122:1254–1255.

9

Neonatal Alloimmune Thrombocytopenia

Cecile Kaplan
Platelet Immunology Unit, Institut National de la Transfusion Sanguine, Paris, France

Neonatal alloimmune thrombocytopenia (NAIT), regarded as the platelet counterpart of hemolytic disease of the newborn (HDN), is the most common cause of severe thrombocytopenia in the neonatal period. During pregnancy, maternal alloantibodies are elicited against paternal specific platelet alloantigens on fetal platelets. The fetal thrombocytopenia is due to destruction by the macrophage system of fetal platelets coated with maternal alloantibodies which have crossed the placental barrier (1–3). Considering the pathogenesis, a more appropriate term for this condition is feto-maternal alloimmune thrombocytopenia (FMAIT).

Prospective studies have shown that FMAIT is frequent (1/800–1/1000 live births in Caucasians), but nevertheless still underdiagnosed (4). Although it is a transient passive disease which usually resolves in a few days, the major complication in cases of severe thrombocytopenia is the occurrence of intracranial hemorrhage (ICH) leading to death (in up to 10% of reported cases) or neurological sequelae (in 20% of the cases). Since the first description of this condition by Harrington (1), there has been remarkable progress in platelet immunology and better understanding of the natural history and clinical management of FMAIT. However, there are still questions to be answered and controversies in this area.

PATHOPHYSIOLOGY

Platelet Antigens

FMAIT is mainly caused by alloantibodies made against certain platelet-specific alloantigens. Although platelets also express HLA Class I and ABH blood group antigens on their surface, controversies still exist concerning their pathogenic relevance to FMAIT. Studies have shown that HLA antibodies do not cause neonatal thrombocytopenia (5–7). However, the possible relevance of such antibodies in low birth weight infants cannot be ruled out, especially when neutropenia is associated with FMAIT (8). It has also been reported that rare cases of NAIT could be observed in infants whose mothers were treated by allogenic leukocyte immunization for unexplained recurrent abortions (9). There is no consensus concerning the implication of ABO incompatibility in FMAIT (10). Although blood group A and B antigens are expressed on platelets (11), there are no data concerning their expression on fetal platelets.

Since the description of the first relevant platelet antigen (12), 24 platelet-specific alloantigens have been described to date and 12 of them have a bi-allelic polymorphism (Table 1). The molecular basis of these antigens is known in 22/24

Table 1 Platelet Alloantigens

System	Antigen	Original name	Glyco-protein	Amino acid polymorph-ism	References
HPA-1	HPA-1a	Pl^{A1}, Zw^a	GPIIIa	Leu/Pro^{33}	(12,104)
	HPA-1b	Pl^{A2}, Zw^b			
HPA-2	HPA-2a	Ko^a Ko^b,	GP1bα	Thr/Met^{145}	(105,106)
	HPA-2b	Sib^a			
HPA-3	HPA-3a	Bak^a, Lek^a	GPIIb	Ile/Ser^{843}	(107–109)
	HPA-3b	Bak^b			
HPA-4	HPA-4a	Yuk^b, Pen^a	GPIIIa	Arg/Gln^{143}	(53,110,111)
	HPA-4b	Yuk^a, Pen^b			
HPA-5	HPA-5a	Br^b,Zav^b	GPIa	Glu/Lys^{505}	(112,113)
	HPA-5b	Br^a, Zav^a			
	HPA-6bw	Ca^a, Tu^a	GPIIIa	Arg/Gln^{489}	(114–116)
	HPA-7bw	Mo^a	GPIIIa	Pro/Ala^{407}	(117)
	HPA-8bw	Sr^a	GPIIIa	Arg/Cys^{636}	(118,119)
	HPA-9bw	Max^a	GPIIb	Val/Met^{837}	(120)
	HPA-10bw	La^a	GPIIIa	Arg/Gln^{62}	(121,122)
	HPA-11bw	Gro^a	GPIIIa	Arg/His^{633}	(123,124)
	HPA-12bw	Hy^a	GPIbβ	Gly/Glu^{15}	(125,126)
	HPA-13bw	Sit^a	GPIa	Thr/Met^{799}	(127)
	HPA-14bw	Oe^a	$GPIII^a$	Lys^{611}/deletion	(26)
HPA-15	HPA-15a	Gov^b Gov^a	CD109	Tyr/Ser^{703}	(128,129)
	$HPA-15^b$				
	HPA-16wb	Duv^a	GPIIIa	Thr/Ile^{140}	(25)

[a] High incidence allele.
[b] Low incidence allele.

and a single nucleotide polymorphism in the gene encoding the membrane protein has been found in 21/22. The human platelet antigen (HPA) nomenclature has been adopted since 1990 to replace the personalized nomenclature that existed before. The antigenic systems are numbered in order of the date of discovery; the high incidence allele is called "a" and the low incidence "b" in the index population (13). Progress in molecular biology has led to discussion of a further nomenclature since 1994 (14,15). Recently under the auspices of the International Society of Blood Transfusion (ISBT) and the International Society of Thrombosis and Haemostasis (ISTH), a Platelet Nomenclature Committee (PNC) has published three linked tables which will be maintained: the HPA antigens, the genetic basis, and the platelet antigen alleles. The HPA nomenclature will continue to be used for clinical and scientific purposes (16).

Frequencies of platelet antigens vary among different populations (17–19). In Caucasians, HPA-1a is by far the most common antigen implicated in FMAIT (20), followed at much lower frequency by HPA-5b (21), then HPA-3 (22). In Orientals, FMAIT is essentially linked with HPA-4. A number of antigens described in recent years and implicated in FMAIT are either rare or private antigens (16,23–26)

Fetal and Neonatal Thrombocytopenia: Maternal Immunization, the Epitopes, the Antibodies

Platelets are present in the fetal circulation as early as 5 weeks of gestation (27). Studies have reported that the mean fetal platelet count is above 150×10^9/L by the end of the first trimester of pregnancy (28) and ranges from $241 \pm 45 \times 10^9$/L at 18–23 weeks of gestation to $265 \pm 59 \times 10^9$/L at 30–35 weeks of gestation (29); thus, thrombocytopenia has been defined in the fetus, as in the neonate, as a platelet count less than 150×10^9/L whatever the gestational age. Fetal alloimmune thrombocytopenia results from platelet destruction caused by the transplacental passage of maternal immunoglobulin G alloantibodies directed against specific platelet alloantigens. This transfer can occur from 14 weeks of pregnancy and the fetal platelet alloantigens are fully expressed as early as 18 weeks; thus, thrombocytopenia can exist very early during pregnancy and such cases have been documented.

To date there are few data concerning the mechanisms implicated in maternal immunization, development of alloantibodies and cellular interactions leading to fetal platelet destruction.

Maternal Immunization

In retrospective studies there is a frequent occurrence of affected infants in the first pregnancy (20). It has been shown by prospective studies that primiparous primigravida women are able to become immunized during the first pregnancy. Specific alloantibodies were detectable at 16 weeks gestation and led to fetal thrombocytopenia. However, among the four immunized women studied, only two fetuses were found to be thrombocytopenic despite feto-maternal incompatibility (30), so that immunization is not synonymous with fetal thrombocytopenia. It is not known yet if the fetus itself plays a role in the occurrence of alloimmune thrombocytopenia.

Retrospective and prospective studies draw attention to the importance of immunogenetic factors in platelet alloimmunization.

Alloimmunization to HPA-1a antigen appears to be associated with HLA class II alleles: DRB3*0101 and/or DQB1*0201 (odds ratio 24.9 and 39.7 respectively) (31–33). An anti HPA-1b response was not associated with either DRB3*0101 or any known HLA class II molecules (34). This finding implies the Leu^{33}/Pro^{33} substitution on the platelet glycoprotein IIIa plays a role in the antigen presentation. Data have shown that the binding of peptides from the Leu^{33}/Pro^{33} dimorphic region to HLA-DR3*0101 is allele-specific with stimulation of specific T cells providing help to B cells for generating alloantibodies (35,36).

The immune response to HPA-5b antigen was strongly associated with a particular DRB1 gene sequence encoding residue Glu-Asp at position 69–70 of the DRβ chain. Three patients with anti HPA-5a antibody had the same DRβ1-chain residue Glu-Asp 69–70 (37). Resistance to anti HPA-5b alloimmunization could be conferred by DRB1*0301 allele which has a very low frequency in the immunized population.

An identical DRB1*1501, DQA1*0102, DQB1*0602 haplotype was shared by mothers immunized against HPA-6b who gave birth to thrombocytopenic infants, but the association was not statistically significant when compared to the general population (38).

All these results suggest that the genetic background of alloimmunization against HPA antigens clearly differs one from another, with a difference in the responder genetic background varying according to the molecular polymorphism of the platelet antigens.

Alloantigens and Alloantibodies

Studies have been conducted using recombinant fragments or synthetic peptides that mimic the antigens better to define the structures involved in the binding of alloantibodies to their epitopes.

The Leu^{33}/Pro^{33} polymorphism of GPIIIa is necessary for the expression of the HPA-1a epitope. The disruption of disulfide bonds located at or near the N-terminal part of GPIIIa abolishes the antibody binding. Two categories of anti-HPA-1a antibodies have thus been defined: those for which the binding requires only an intact amino-acid terminus and those for which the binding depends on other structural requirements within the entire glycoprotein (39). In vitro experiments with the construction of human platelet antigen HPA-1a epitopes within murine glycoprotein IIIa have led to the identification of amino acids critical for alloantibody binding (40). An Arg^{93}/Gln substitution on GPIIIa has been shown to play a role in the binding of anti-HPA-1a alloantibodies (41). For Duv^{a+} antigen located on GPIIIa, the disruption of disulfide bonds of GPIIIa impaired the binding of the alloantibody. The Thr^{140}/Ile dimorphism localized three amino-acids upstream from Arg^{143} (involved in the expression of HPA-4a) did not interfere with the binding of an anti-HPA-4a antibody in flow cytometry (25).

All these data have shown that the amino acid polymorphism is necessary, but not sufficient to express the epitope recognized by the alloantibody.

Studies with murine monoclonal antibodies during investigation of alloimmunity have shown that recognition of the HPA-1a epitope is not uniform and further investigations are needed to clarify whether this heterogeneity plays a role in clinical conditions (42).

CLINICAL DATA

Most of the data come from retrospective studies of cases diagnosed after birth and concern anti HPA-1a immunization which is the major cause of FMAIT in Caucasians. With the progress in platelet immunology and in fetal medicine and with the results of prospective studies, more precise diagnosis of this condition is now possible. The incidence of FMAIT has been estimated by large prospective studies to be about 1/800–1/1500 births (30,43,44). However, most of the cases had no evidence of clinical bleeding and would be overlooked in the absence of routine screening to detect thrombocytopenia in the newborn or immunization in pregnant women (4). Therefore, it is important to know when to suspect FMAIT in order to plan the optimal management for the index case and for subsequent pregnancies (Table 2).

Fetal Thrombocytopenia

Progress in fetal imaging and fetal medicine has led to a better knowledge of this condition. Some years ago, a retrospective survey of 5194 fetal blood samplings

Table 2 When to Suspect FMAIT

In the fetus	(a) Severe thrombocytopenia discovered incidentally (b) Intracranial hemorrhage (c) Hydrops fetalis (d) Unexplained fetal anemia (e) Recurrent late miscarriages (f) History of affected sibling with FMAIT
In the neonate	(a) Early onset severe neonatal thrombocytopenia and exclusion of infection, congenital anomalies, increased platelet consumption (57,130) (b) Unexplained thrombocytopenia (c) Asymptomatic thrombocytopenia (d) History of affected sibling with FMAIT

(FBS) showed that the fetal thrombocytopenia resulting from maternal alloimmunization was the most severe thrombocytopenia observed among the different disorders encountered including chromosomal malformations, infections, or maternal autoimmune thrombocytopenia (45). It was thus suggested that investigation for alloimmunization is warranted when an isolated incidental thrombocytopenia is discovered by FBS even though another cause appears to be present, especially if thrombocytopenia is more severe than might be expected for that cause. When serial platelet counts have been available, a fall in the platelet count has been observed as gestation progresses without any spontaneous correction of thrombocytopenia (46).

The most deleterious consequence of severe fetal thrombocytopenia is the occurrence of ICH (47–49). In cases where the timing of ICH was recorded, 80.5% (29/36) occurred antenatally, 13.8% of them before 20 weeks of gestation, 27.6% before 30 weeks gestation (50–52). In utero ICH has been observed whatever the platelet alloantigens implicated (20–22,52,53), but with a lower incidence in FMAIT linked to HPA-5b (21,52).

In utero ICH may be diagnosed by ultrasound and magnetic resonance imaging, which are reliable and safe methods. Recent reports have suggested Doppler flow velocimetry and color Doppler imaging as additional tools in detecting fetal cranial hemorrhage.

The nature of the brain lesion in fetuses with FMAIT was studied some years ago and a sequence of events proposed: subarachnoid hemorrhage seems to be the first event, then extension of the bleeding leads to subarachnoid hematoma (47,54). When intraventricular hemorrhage is present, primarily or as a secondary event, this may result in arachnoiditis with or without cerebrospinal obstruction leading to hydrocephalus. Porencephalic cysts resulting either from ischemic or hemorrhagic lesions have been described (49). FMAIT should be considered among other etiological factors in the setting of ICH as it is an important cause of severe bleeding and poor outcome.

Clinical changes, such as reduced fetal activity especially when dramatic or persistent or fetal heart rate change, may alert the clinician to the existence of ICH.

Recurrent miscarriages, unexplained fetal anemia, or hydrops fetalis have also been reported as complications of feto-maternal platelet alloimmunization which should be considered for specific investigation in these conditions (55,56).

Neonatal Thrombocytopenia

The usual presentation is a full-term neonate born to a first time pregnant healthy mother, and who exhibits widespread purpura at birth or a few hours afterwards. Otherwise this infant is well, with no clinical signs of infection (hepatosplenomegaly) or malformation (hemangioma, absence of radii). Visceral hemorrhages such as gastrointestinal bleeding or hematuria are less common than purpura or hematoma. Anti-HPA-1a and anti-HPA-3a immunization induce severe neonatal thrombocytopenia (20,22). However NAIT linked to HPA-5b incompatibility seems to be less severe than HPA-1a NAIT (21). The most serious complication is ICH (25,5% of cases for HPA-1a, 24% for HPA-3a, 15% for HPA-5b) (52) leading to death in up to 10% or neurological sequelae in up to 20% of the reported cases. ICH may be present at birth or can occur as long as the newborn is thrombocytopenic. The risk of life-threatening hemorrhage necessitates prompt diagnosis and effective therapy.

On the other hand, thrombocytopenia may be asymptomatic and pass unnoticed unless there is a routine platelet count performed. Therefore, unexpected or unexplained neonatal thrombocytopenia or severe early onset thrombocytopenia in both pre-term and term babies should raise the possibility of NAIT and guide investigations accordingly.

The diagnosis of NAIT is usually made initially on clinical grounds and depends upon exclusion of other causes of neonatal thrombocytopenia (57). Nevertheless NAIT may be associated also with other causes of neonatal thrombocytopenia, especially with maternal autoimmune thrombocytopenic purpura (44).

LABORATORY DIAGNOSIS

Severe, confirmed, isolated thrombocytopenia is present in the majority of cases from birth ($<50\times10^9$/L in 69% of cases (52)), and anemia is seen only when secondary to bleeding. The fetal bleeding observed in FMAIT, mostly in anti-HPA-1a maternal alloimmunization, is not associated with inhibition of fibrinogen binding to its receptor as has been postulated (58).

Testing in an experienced laboratory is mandatory to confirm the diagnosis. The testing involves the detection of circulating maternal antibody directed against a paternal platelet antigen present in the fetus/neonate. Knowledge of the ethnic origin of the family may be helpful because it has been shown that phenotype frequencies of the platelet antigens differ among ethnic groups (17–19).

Detection of the maternal antibody and platelet phenotype includes assays using whole platelets as in the platelet immunofluorescence test (flow cytometry) or ELISA techniques. These tests are usually combined with a specific antigen capture ELISA, such as the monoclonal antibody specific immobilization of platelet antigen (MAIPA) test allowing detection of weak antibodies or mixtures of antibodies (59,60). The identification of the maternal alloantibody relies on testing the sera against phenotyped donor O platelets and a cross-match against paternal platelets. The combination of these two techniques ensures the detection of a low-frequency antigen and could be helpful for paternity exclusion.

Different molecular biology techniques are used for platelet genotyping allowing typing not only for the most frequent antigens, but also for the rare or private antigens (23,61,62). Fetal genotyping can be performed either on chorionic villi or amniotic cells (63,64), and a non-invasive procedure with isolation of fetal DNA from maternal blood analogous to fetal D genotyping (65) is under study.

The diagnosis is straightforward when a maternal antibody with a corresponding parental antigen incompatibility are present. If the father is heterozygous for the considered antigen or if the paternity is uncertain, the infant's platelet typing should be performed to confirm the diagnosis.

Difficulties in making the diagnosis may be caused by:

- absence of maternal antibody (43)
- presence of maternal autoantibodies (44)
- antibody detectable only by a specific technique, antigenic epitope lost during platelet storage (24,66), or antibody identification depending on a specific monoclonal antibody being used in the capture-antigen assay (42).
- rare, private, or new antigen implicated (16)

Such difficulties should not delay therapy especially when there is a risk of life-threatening hemorrhage and there are sufficient grounds for a provisional diagnosis.

In any ambiguous case and if the diagnosis of FMAIT is highly suspected, the testing should be pursued; repeat samples should be obtained from the family after a reasonable delay (usually between 1 and 3 months after birth). It is known that the kinetics of the maternal alloantibody disappearance after delivery is highly variable. We have observed that the antibody could persist for months or years, which led to the diagnosis of epilepsy linked with FMAIT in a 9-year-old girl when neonatal ICH was found retrospectively (personal observation). On the other hand, the antibody could disappear in a few weeks. It is helpful to combine a number of different sensitive techniques to detect or characterize a weak antibody and at least include DNA sequencing in case a role for private antigens may be suspected. It is important that the diagnosis should be confirmed or refuted before the next pregnancy to enable the best management to be planned. If no conclusion can be reached, it is important to retest early in the next pregnancy. During a subsequent pregnancy, when there is platelet antigen incompatibility and the initial detection of maternal antibody is negative, we suggest retesting for maternal antibody once a trimester.

In summary, establishing the diagnosis of suspected fetal thrombocytopenia or neonatal thrombocytopenia is important for the management of the index case and of a subsequent pregnancy to avoid the deleterious consequence of severe thrombocytopenia.

NEONATAL THERAPY

Most of the cases of FMAIT are unexpected and therefore diagnosed after birth. Therapy depends on the presence of bleeding and the severity of thrombocytopenia at birth. If treatment is required, it must not be delayed because of difficulties in ascertaining the diagnosis, as the infant is at risk of hemorrhage throughout the severe thrombocytopenic period.

For the Infant with Bleeding or Severe Thrombocytopenia (Platelet Counts Below 30.10^9/L) During the First 24 Hours of Life

The optimal therapy is the transfusion of platelets that will not be destroyed by the maternal alloantibody present in the infant circulation. The best donor is the mother. However, logistic problems can arise depending on physical maternal conditions, results of pre-donation testing, the mother's location and the availability of apheresis facilities (67). Moreover, the platelets must be washed to remove the maternal alloantibody, and irradiated to prevent graft versus host disease. At least matched platelets for rare or private antigens can be obtained from family members.

Lack of facilities to prepare maternal platelets has led to alternatives, like development of a registry of suitable donors HPA-1b/1b and HPA-5a/5a (National Blood Service in England) (68); most FMAIT encountered in Caucasian population is linked with anti HPA-1a or 5b immunization. However, establishing a panel of accredited donors is a huge task. After screening 60,000 blood donations, 45 HPA-1a negative donors were found who were CMV negative and without immunization against HPA, HLA, granulocytes antigens. Donation is done upon request (69), and depending on blood donation pre-testing certification, there may be a delay before the platelet concentrates are available for treating the neonate. Another approach has been developed in France with provision of compatible frozen-thawed platelet concentrates. The concentrates may be stored up to three year and after thawing and washing may be delivered within a reasonable time period (70).

In an urgent situation when compatible platelets are not immediately available, it has been suggested that a random-donor platelet concentrate should be given. However, the results are controversial with some good responses being reported (71), but low increases in the median platelet counts have also been observed in a literature review (52).

In our practice in an emergency when there is no other alternative, we recommend transfusion of random platelets combined with perfusion of polyclonal immunoglobulins (IvIgG)(0.8 to 1 g/kg/d for 2 days).

It must be underlined that IvIgG must not be considered as an alternative to platelet transfusion because of the delayed response 12 to 18 hr after injection (72), as the infant is at risk of significant bleeding.

Exchange transfusion which partly removes the circulating antibody and can be followed by matched platelets transfusion is no longer in use.

For Infants Without Bleeding and Platelet Counts Above 30.10^9/L

In this setting, close monitoring is necessary. Usually the platelet counts will increase rapidly as the maternal alloantibody is removed from the infant's circulation and no therapy is required. If there is a drop in platelet count, IvIgG (0.8–1 g/kg/day for 2 days) may be considered to raise the platelet count.

Outcome

Recovery (platelet count $>150\times10^9$/L) is seen within 8 days of birth in the majority of cases, depending on the rate of removal of maternal alloantibody from the neonatal circulation. The outcome depends on antenatal or intranatal occurrence of ICH, the severity of thrombocytopenia at birth, and prompt diagnosis and therapy. The mortality rate was estimated to be 10% of cases and neurological sequelae up to 20% of cases in retrospective studies of anti HPA-1a NAIT (20,73). In a large literature review (52), the mortality rate for an affected untreated case was reported to be 16.3% and 67.4% of cases not receiving treatment were neurologically normal. Close monitoring of affected children is required with a platelet count performed daily until a safe level of 50×10^9/L has been reached. Ultrasound examination or magnetic resonance imaging is recommended to detect clinically silent ICH and appropriate clinical follow-up of the children is mandatory.

The effect of breastfeeding on the outcome has not been fully addressed although one report suggests the absence of any deleterious effect (74).

ANTENATAL MANAGEMENT OF HIGH-RISK PREGNANCIES

Management of Subsequent Pregnancies

Owing to the rate of recurrence and the risk of equally if not more severe clinical manifestations, especially ICH (75), the management of subsequent pregnancies with an incompatible fetus is therefore exacting and must be done in a referral center. The optimal management strategy to reduce mortality and morbidity is controversial and a recent international forum has shown the absence of standardization (76). In any case, the pregnant women should be provided with information concerning the different options for antenatal therapy, their risks and benefits, and be advised to avoid vigorous exercise and drug ingestion interfering with the platelet functions (e.g. aspirin, antibiotics).

With regard to subsequent pregnancies, up to now it has not been possible to predict the onset or severity of thrombocytopenia from clinical or laboratory parameters and there are no reliable methods for assessment of the fetal status without invasive methods, such as FBS.

FBS has been justified both to determine the fetal status and to monitor the therapy. However, due to the risks of this procedure itself [1.4–2.1% of fetal loss (77,78)], establishing that the fetus is at risk is of critical importance. Therefore, if the father is heterozygous for the implicated antigen or if the paternity is uncertain, fetal genotyping should be performed as described above. Once the fetus at risk is identified, we have to deal with the following questions: which fetuses will be affected, which ones will be severely affected, what therapeutic option may be proposed, and which fetuses will respond?

Which Fetuses Will be Affected?

Controversy exists concerning the prediction of fetal thrombocytopenia by monitoring the maternal antiplatelet alloantibodies.

In our experience, no correlation was found between the antibody level and the severity of the fetal thrombocytopenia. Moreover, 15–20% of women with affected infants had no detectable anti-HPA-1a antibodies (46). This condition was also found in a prospective study in 9/237 infants born to HPA-1b mothers without alloantibodies and no other risk factors (43). Another previous study has not found any correlation between titer or IgG subclass and the level of neonatal thrombocytopenia (79). Most pregnant women with an anti-HPA-5b antibody do not deliver a thrombocytopenic child (80).

Alternatively, other data are in favor of considering the maternal alloantibody titer as a predictive factor for fetal thrombocytopenia: a significant association between the existence of a severe neonatal thrombocytopenia and high levels of maternal alloantibodies ($> 1/32$) during the third trimester of pregnancy was found (43). An obvious relation between the antibody level at the time of delivery and the severity of the neonatal thrombocytopenia due to anti-HPA-1a maternal immunization has also been observed (81).

In conclusion, the published data have not shown maternal alloantibodies to correlate consistently with the existence or the degree of fetal or neonatal thrombocytopenia. It will be most valuable to have larger prospective studies relating these two parameters in order to reach a definite conclusion.

Which Fetuses Will be Severely Affected?

The severity of thrombocytopenia may depend on the ability of the fetus to compensate for platelet destruction and on the inhibition of megakaryocytopoietic progenitors by the maternal alloantibodies. Data suggest that the response to platelet destruction could be lower in the fetus and neonate than in adults as reduced megakaryocytic differentiation has been observed in cord blood when compared to bone marrow progenitors from healthy volunteers (82). The level of thrombopoietin (TPO) which is the main hematopoietic growth factor for the megakaryocytic lineage has been evaluated in fetuses with FMAIT. In two studies, the median TPO concentration was significantly elevated in severe thrombocytopenia (83,84), but no significant correlation was found between TPO concentration and platelet counts. In another study (85), no difference was found between thrombocytopenic and non-thrombocytopenic fetuses or healthy neonates. Further information concerning the TPO levels in fetuses during pregnancy is needed before a definite conclusion can be reached, as it has also been observed that anti-HPA-1a alloantibodies caused inhibition of HPA-1a fetal and neonatal colony-forming unit megakaryocytes (86). A recent publication concerning the suppression of in vitro megakaryocyte production by antiplatelet autoantibodies observed with plasma from patients with chronic autoimmune thrombocytopenic purpura, suggesting that a similar effect could occur in vivo, may also be taken into account to support the view that antiplatelet antibodies do not only induce platelet destruction but may also affect platelet production (87).

The recurrence rate of ICH in the subsequent offspring of women with a history of FMAIT with ICH is high ($\sim$79%) and the risk of ICH in a subsequent pregnancy without past history of ICH has been estimated to be 7% (75).

In the European collaborative study, it has been shown that fetuses with severely affected siblings had significantly lower pretreatment platelet counts than others; 92% of fetuses with a sibling history of ICH had a platelet count $<20\times10^9$/L at a median gestation term of 24 weeks (88). No relationship between sibling history and the platelet count at initial FBS was found in another study, but the data are not strictly comparable (89).

What Are the Therapeutic Options?

Available options include maternal therapy with IvIgG alone or in combination with corticosteroids, or fetal therapy with repeated in utero platelet transfusions.

Repeated in utero platelet transfusion, although effective in preventing ICH in severely affected cases (90), appears to be an invasive option with serious complications. Due to the short half-life of the platelets, approximately 1 week, this treatment would have to be performed weekly. The cumulative risk of 8.3% per pregnancy of the procedure (91) is associated with the risk of in utero transfusion: fetal anemia has been recorded with prophylactic platelet transfusion apparently due to ABO incompatibility from transfused platelets (92). Theoretically, repeated FBS would also increase maternal immunization. In utero transfusion may affect fetal immunity, but this has not been studied in platelet transfusion (93).

Maternal treatment with IvIgG with or without corticosteroids is a less invasive therapy and is the most widely proposed antenatal therapy, but the costs of such therapy must not be underestimated. The mechanism of action of IvIgG is uncertain. In vitro experiments with an isolated perfused lobule of human placenta showed that IvIgG inhibited the transfer of maternal alloantibody to the fetal circulation (94). IvIgG might increase the antibody catabolism (95), and modify the fetal and maternal immune response. Corticosteroids may play a role in immunomodulation of the maternal response.

The effects of maternal therapy on fetal platelet counts is usually monitored with FBS. Evaluation of the results is complex and has utilized different criteria such as improvement or minimal decline in the platelet counts and/or the absence of ICH. There are no randomized controlled trials due to ethical issues. Until recently it was reported that better results have been obtained in North America compared with Europe. However, if the platelet count $>50\times10^9$/L is used to define a response to therapy, then three studies gave comparative results (88,96,97): response to therapy occurred in $\sim$70% of pregnancies.

Low-dose corticosteroids as sole therapy have been given to a limited number of mothers with FMAIT and response to therapy was highly variable.

Which Fetuses Will Respond?

There is no parameter predictive of the fetal response to therapy. The efficacy of therapy could only be evaluated by FBS, but exsanguinations have been reported as a result of FBS (98); therefore, transfusion of compatible platelets was proposed at each FBS by some teams and not by others due to such adverse effects as prolonged bradycardia.

An initial FBS had been considered as a prognostic value for the response to IvIgG in a series of 74 cases. If the platelet count was $>20\times10^9$/L, the response rate was 89% improvement or minimal decline, versus 51% when the platelet count was $<20\times10^9$/L (89). In a previous study, we observed that therapeutic failure occurred more frequently in families with a severely affected sibling (97).

Ongoing Protocols

Most of the recent published studies are in favor of maternal treatment as first line therapy and stratification on the basis of the sibling history. The recent international forum has shown that FBS for the initial assessment of the fetal status and for monitoring the effect of therapy is still a matter of debate; FBS was either performed routinely or because of additional factors such as a previously affected child or a sibling with ICH (76).

Maternal therapy may be considered before or from 16 weeks of gestation [earliest report of ICH (99)] for cases with severely affected siblings and later on (~20 weeks of gestation) in the absence of ICH history, with initial FBS carried out either before therapy in the low risk cases, or 6–8 weeks after initiation of therapy in other cases.

Usually IvIgG is administered at 1 g/kg/wk; nonetheless 2 g/kg/wk have been proposed in very severe cases. Further management depends on the fetal platelet count. In case of therapeutic failure, salvage therapy consists in adding corticosteroids to IvIgG (prednisone 0.5 mg/kg/day), or increasing the dose of IvIgG to 2 g/kg/wk. In case of very severe cases without response to any therapeutic regimen, weekly in utero transfusion has been proposed.

The negative side effects of FBS (1.1% fetal loss and 3.2 to 5.3% emergency C-section (100,101)) warrant consideration of a less invasive strategy for FMAIT without high risk siblings, and propose maternal therapy with IvIgG administered blindly and/or FBS prior to delivery followed by in utero transfusion in case of severe thrombocytopenia (100). This strategy has been applied without an increased incidence of ICH. However, the absence of knowledge of the fetal status is the main disadvantage of the blind therapy.

A pre-delivery FBS is considered by some teams. This allows a fetal transfusion in cases of severe thrombocytopenia which offers better protection against ICH even after an elective C-section (102,103). Vaginal delivery, depending of the obstetrical conditions, is offered if the fetal platelet count is above 50×10^9/L. In the absence of a late FBS, most centers propose C-section and a cord blood platelet count performed at birth and even a post-natal transfusion.

ROUTINE ANTENATAL SCREENING

FMAIT is usually diagnosed after birth, when bleeding has occurred. This raises the question of the role of routine screening.

Prospective studies for anti-HPA-1a FMAIT have been undertaken with different strategies: screening pregnant women or screening newborns (30,43). It has been shown that screening neonates is more cost-effective than screening primiparous women. However, neonatal screening is too late for antenatal management to prevent fetal death or disability during the course of the index pregnancy. It may, however, detect platelet disorders and asymptomatic thrombocytopenic newborns who would otherwise be missed. The major limitation of screening pregnant women is the absence of predictive parameters concerning the fetal status. Further research is required to identify severely affected cases without a previous history of FMAIT and so focus antenatal management on those fetuses at risk. Until these "at risk" cases are identified, maternal screening has low sensitivity. Furthermore, implementation of routine screening for a general population is hampered by the controversies concerning the optimal antenatal management.

However, it is important to identify high-risk women among sisters of a woman who has given birth to a thrombocytopenic child and the family should be counseled. In our experience, when a sister is found to be at risk, we propose testing for alloantibodies once every two to three months, and if alloantibodies are present, we propose antenatal management as described in the above section "Ongoing Protocols."

CONCLUSIONS

FMAIT is a frequently serious fetal and neonatal affection. Significant progress has been made in the understanding of FMAIT, in particular the diagnosis and management of affected infants. However, questions remain unanswered concerning the mechanisms leading to maternal immunization and cellular interactions leading to the fetal platelet destruction. The main issues to be investigated are the definition of high-risk patients and standardization for antenatal management with the less invasive methods. It is probably only after additional progress is made concerning antenatal management that routine antenatal screening could be considered a viable public health issue.

ACKNOWLEDGMENTS

I would like to thank Pr. Alan Waters for reviewing the manuscript.

REFERENCES

1. Harrington WJ, Sprague CC, Minnich V, et al. Immunologic mechanisms in neonatal and thrombocytopenic purpura. Ann Intern Med 1953; 38:433–469.

2. Moulinier J. Alloimmunisation maternelle antiplaquettaire "Duzo". Proc 6th Congr Soc Haematol 1953;817–820.
3. Shulman NR, Marder VJ, Hiller MC, Collier EM. Platelet and leukocyte isoantigens and their antibodies. Serologic, physiologic and clinical studies. In: Moore CV, Brown EB, eds. Progress in Hematology. New-York: Grune and Stratton, 1964:222–304.
4. Davoren A, McParland P, Barnes CA, Murphy WG. Neonatal alloimmune thrombocytopenia in the Irish population: a discrepancy between observed and expected cases. J Clin Pathol 2002; 55:289–292.
5. Sharon R, Amar A. Maternal anti-HLA antibodies and neonatal thrombocytopenia. Lancet 1981; 1:1313.
6. Skacel PO, Contreras M. Neonatal alloimmune thrombocytopenia. Blood Rev 1989; 3:174–179.
7. Taaning E. HLA antibodies and fetomaternal alloimmune thrombocytopenia: myth or meaningful? Transfu Med Rev 2000; 14:275–280.
8. Koyama N, Ohama Y, Kaneko K, Itakura Y, Nakamura T. Association of neonatal thrombocytopenia and maternal anti-HLA antibodies. Acta Paediatr Jpn 1991; 33:71–76.
9. Tanaka T, Umesaki N, Nishio J, et al. Neonatal thrombocytopenia induced by maternal anti-HLA antibodies: a potential side effect of allogenic leukocyte immunization for unexplained recurrent aborters. J Reprod Immunol 2000; 46:51–57.
10. Waters AH, Murphy M, Hambley H, Nicolaides K. Management of alloimmune thrombocytopenia in the fetus and neonate. In: Nance S, ed. Clinical and Basic Science Aspects of Immunohematology. Arlington,VA: American Association of Blood Banks, 1991:155–177.
11. Curtis BR, Edwards JT, Hessner MJ, Klein JP, Aster RH. Blood group A and B antigens are strongly expressed on platelets of some individuals. Blood 2000; 96:1574–1581.
12. van Loghem JJ, Dorfmeijer H, van der Hart M, Schreuder F. Serological and genetical studies on a platelet antigen (Zw). Vox Sang 1959; 4:161–169.
13. von dem Borne AEGKr, Decary F. Nomenclature of platelet specific antigens. Br J Haematol 1990; 74:239–240.
14. Newman PJ. Nomenclature of human platelet alloantigens: a problem with the HPA system? Blood 1994; 83:1447–1451.
15. von dem Borne AEGKr, Kaplan C, Minchinton R. Nomenclature of human platelet alloantigens. Blood 1995; 85:1409–1410.
16. Metcalfe P, Watkins NA, Ouwehand WH, et al. Nomenclature of human platelet antigens. Vox Sang 2003; 85:240–245.
17. Simsek S, Faber NM, Bleeker PM, et al. Determination of human platelet antigen frequencies in the Dutch population by immunophenotyping and DNA (allele-specific restriction enzyme) analysis. Blood 1993; 81:835–840.
18. Liu TC, Shih MC, Lin CL, Lin SF, Chen CM, Chang JG. Gene frequencies of the HPA-1 to HPA-8w platelet antigen alleles in Taiwanese, Indonesian, and Thai. Ann Hematol 2002; 81:244–248.
19. Halle L, Bach KH, Martageix C, et al. Eleven human platelet systems studied in the Vietnamese and Ma'ohis Polynesian populations. Tissue Antigens 2004; 63:34–40.

20. Mueller-Eckhardt C, Kiefel V, Grubert A, et al. 348 cases of suspected neonatal alloimmune thrombocytopenia. Lancet 1989; 1:363–366.
21. Kaplan C, Morel-Kopp MC, Kroll H, et al. HPA-5b (Br[a]) neonatal alloimmune thrombocytopenia: Clinical and immunological analysis of 39 cases. Br J Haematol 1991; 78:425–429.
22. Glade-Bender J, McFarland JG, Kaplan C, Porcelijn L, Bussel JB. Anti-HPA-3a induces severe neonatal alloimmune thrombocytopenia. J Pediatr 2001; 138:862–867.
23. Kroll H, Kiefel V, Santoso S. Clinical aspects and typing of platelet alloantigens. Vox Sang 1998; 74(S2):345–354.
24. Berry JE, Murphy CM, Smith GA, et al. Detection of Gov system antibodies by MAIPA reveals an immunogenicity similar to the HPA-5 alloantigens. Br J Haematol 2000; 110:735–742.
25. Jallu V, Meunier M, Brement M, Kaplan C. A new platelet polymorphism Duv($^{a+}$), localized within the RGD binding domain of glycoprotein IIIa, is associated with neonatal thrombocytopenia. Blood 2002; 99:4449–4456.
26. Santoso S, Kiefel V, Richter IG, et al. A functional platelet fibrinogen receptor with a deletion in the cysteine-rich repeat region of the beta(3) integrin: the Oe(a) alloantigen in neonatal alloimmune thrombocytopenia. Blood 2002; 99:1205–1214.
27. Hann IM. Development of blood in the fetus. In: Hann IM, Gibson BES, Letsky E, eds. Fetal and Neonatal Haematology. London: Bailliere Tindall, 1991:1–28.
28. Pahal GS, Jauniaux E, Kinnon C, Thrasher AJ, Rodeck CH. Normal development of human fetal hematopoiesis between eight and seventeen weeks'gestation. Am J Obstet Gynecol 2000; 183:1029–1034.
29. Forestier F, Daffos F, Galacteros F, Bardakjian J, Rainaut M, Beuzard Y. Hematological values of 163 normal fetuses between 18 and 30 weeks of gestation. Pediatr Res 1986; 20:342–346.
30. Durand-Zaleski I, Schlegel N, Blum-Boisgard C, et al. Screening primiparous women and newborns for fetal/neonatal alloimmune thrombocytopenia: a prospective comparison of effectiveness and costs. Am J Perinatol 1996; 13:423–431.
31. Valentin N, Vergracht A, Bignon JD, et al. HLA-DRw52a is involved in alloimmunization against PL-A1 antigen. Hum Immunol 1990; 27:73–79.
32. Decary F, L'Abbe D, Tremblay L, Chartrand P. The immune response to the HPA-1a antigen: association with HLA-DRw52a. Transfus Med 1991; 1:55–62.
33. L'Abbe D, Tremblay L, Filion M, et al. Alloimmunization to platelet antigen HPA-1a (Pl^{A1}) is strongly associated with both HLA-DR3*0101 and HLA-DQB1*0201. Hum Immunol 1992; 34:107–114.
34. Kuijpers RWAM, von dem Borne AEGKr, Kiefel V, et al. Leucine33-proline33 substitution in human platelet glycoprotein IIIa determines HLA-DRw52a (Dw24) association of the immune response against HPA-1a (Zwa/PlA1) and HPA-1b (Zwb/PlA2). Hum Immunol 1992; 34:253–356.
35. Maslanka K, Yassai M, Gorski J. Molecular identification of T cells that respond in a primary bulk culture to a peptide derived from a platelet glycoprotein implicated in neonatal alloimmune thrombocytopenia. J Clin Invest 1996; 98:1802–1808.

36. Wu S, Maslanka K, Gorski J. An integrin polymorphism that defines reactivity with alloantibodies generates an anchor for MHC class II peptide binding: a model for unidirectional alloimmune responses. J Immunol 1997; 158:3221–3226.
37. Semana G, Zazoun T, Alizadeh M, Morel-Kopp MC, Genetet B, Kaplan C. Genetic susceptibility and anti-human platelet antigen 5b alloimmunization. Role of HLA class II and TAP genes. Hum Immunol 1996; 46:114–119.
38. Westman P, Hashemi-Tavoularis S, Blanchette V, et al. Maternal DRB1*1501, DQA1*0102, DQB1*0602 haplotype in fetomaternal alloimmunization against human platelet alloantigen HPA-6b (GP IIIa-Gln489). Tissue Antigens 1997; 50:113–118.
39. Valentin N, Visentin GP, Newman PJ. Involvement of the cystein-rich domain of glycoprotein IIIa in the expression of the human platelet alloantigen, PlA1: evidence for heterogeneity in the humoral response. Blood 1995; 85:3028–3033.
40. Barron-Casella EA, Nebbia G, Rogers OC, King KE, Kickler TS, Casella JF. Construction of a human platelet alloantigen-1a epitope(s) within murine glycoprotein IIIa: identification of residues critical to the conformation of the antibody binding site(s). Blood 1999; 93:2959–2967.
41. Watkins NA, Schaffner-Reckinger E, Allen DL, et al. HPA-1a phenotype-genotype discrepancy reveals a naturally occrring Arg93Gln substitution in the platelet b3 integrin that disrupts the HPA-1a epitope. Blood 2002; 99:1833–1839.
42. Morel-Kopp MC, Daviet L, McGregor J, Kaplan C. Drawbacks of the MAIPA technique in characterising human antiplatelet antibodies. Blood Coagul Fibrinolysis 1996; 7:144–146.
43. Williamson LM, Hackett G, Rennie J, et al. The natural history of fetomaternal alloimmunization to the platelet-specific antigen HPA-1a (PLA1, Zwa) as determined by antenatal screening. Blood 1998; 92:2280–2287.
44. Dreyfus M, Kaplan C, Verdy E, et al. Frequency of immune thrombocytopenia in newborns: a prospective study. Blood 1997; 89:4402–4406.
45. Hohlfeld P, Forestier F, Kaplan C, Tissot JD, Daffos F. Fetal thrombocytopenia: a retrospective survey of 5194 fetal blood samplings. Blood 1994; 84:1851–1856.
46. Kaplan C, Daffos F, Forestier F, et al. Management of alloimmune thrombocytopenia: antenatal diagnosis and in utero transfusion of maternal platelets. Blood 1988; 72:340–343.
47. Govaert P, Bridger J, Wigglesworth J. Nature of the brain lesion in fetal alloimmune thrombocytopenia. Dev Med Child Neurol 1995; 37:485–495.
48. Sharif U, Kuban K. Prenatal intracranial hemorrhage and neurologic complications in alloimmune thrombocytopenia. J Child Neurology 2001; 16:838–842.
49. Dale ST, Coleman LT. Neonatal alloimmune thrombocytopenia: antenatal and postnatal imaging findings in the pediatric brain. Am J Neuroradiol 2002; 23:1457–1465.
50. de Vries LS, Connell J, Bydder GM, et al. Recurrent intracranial haemorrhages in utero in an infant with alloimmune thrombocytopenia. Case report. Br J Obstet Gynaecol 1988; 95:299–302.
51. Giovangrandi Y, Daffos F, Kaplan C, Forestier F, Mac Alleese J, Moirot M. Very early intracranial haemorrhage in alloimmune fetal thrombocytopenia. Lancet 1990; 336:310.

52. Spencer JA, Burrows RF. Feto-maternal alloimmune thrombocytopenia: a literature review and statistical analysis. Aust N Z J Obstet Gynaecol 2001; 41:45–55.
53. Friedman JM, Aster RH. Neonatal alloimmune thrombocytopenic purpura and congenital porencephaly in two siblings associated with a "new" maternal antiplatelet antibody. Blood 1985; 65:1412–1415.
54. Sherer DM, Anyaegbunam A, Onyeije C. Antepartum fetal intracranial hemorrhage, predisposing factors and prenatal sonography: a review. Am J Perinatol 1998; 15:431–441.
55. Murphy MF, Hambley H, Nicolaides K, Waters AH. Severe fetomaternal alloimmune thrombocytopenia presenting with fetal hydrocephalus. Prenat Diagn 1996; 16:1152–1155.
56. Stanworth SJ, Hackett GA, Williamson LM. Fetomaternal alloimmune thrombocytopenia presenting antenatally as hydrops fetalis. Prenat Diagn 2001; 21:423–424.
57. Kaplan C, Dreyfus M, Proulle V, Tchernia G. Thrombocytopenia in childhood. In: Gresele P, Page CP, Vermylen J, Fuster V, eds. Platelets in thrombotic and non-thrombotic disorders: pathophysiology, pharmacology and therapeutics. Cambridge: Cambridge University Press, 2002:556–568.
58. Beadling WV, Herman JH, Stuart MJ, Keashen-Schnell M, Miller JL. Fetal bleeding in neonatal alloimmune thrombocytopenia mediated by anti-PlA1 is not associated with inhibition of fibrinogen binding to platelet GPIIb-IIIa. Am J Clin Pathol 1995; 103:636–641.
59. Kiefel V, Santoso S, Weisheit M, Mueller-Eckhardt C. Monoclonal antibody-specific immobilization of platelet antigens (MAIPA): a new tool for the identification of platelet-reactive antibodies. Blood 1987; 70:1722–1726.
60. Kaplan C. Evaluation of serological platelet antibody assays. Vox Sang 1998; 74(S2):355–358.
61. Goldman M, Trudel E, Richard L. Report on the Eleventh International Society of Blood Transfusion Platelet Genotyping and Serology Workshop. Vox Sang 2003; 85:149–155.
62. Jones DC, Bunce M, Fuggle SV, Young NT, Marshall SE. Human platelet alloantigens (HPAs): PCR-SSP genotyping of a UK population for 15 HPA alleles. Eur J Immunogenet 2003; 30:415–419.
63. Bugert P, Lese A, Meckies J, Zieger W, Eichler H, Klüter H. Optimized sensitivity of allele-specific PCR for prenatal typing of human platelet alloantigen single nucleotide polymorphisms. Biotechniques 2003; 35:170–174.
64. Hurd C, Lucas G. Human platelet antigen genotyping by PCR-SSP in neonatal/fetal alloimmune thrombocytopenia. In: Goulden NJ, Steward CG, eds. Pediatric Hematology: Methods and Protocols. Totowa, NJ: Humana Press Inc, 2004:71–78.
65. Finning KM, Martin PG, Soothil PW, Avent ND. Prediction of fetal D status from maternal plasma: introduction of a new noninvasive fetal RHD genotyping service. Transfusion 2002; 42:1079–1085.
66. Harrison CR, Curtis BR, McFarland JG, Huff RW, Aster RH. Severe neonatal alloimmune thrombocytopenia caused by antibodies to human platelet antigen 3a (Baka) detectable only in whole platelet assays. Transfusion 2003; 43:1398–1402.
67. Murphy MF, Verjee S, Greaves M. Inadequacies in the postnatal management of fetomaternal alloimmune thrombocytopenia (FMAIT). Br J Haematol 1999; 105:123–126.

68. Win N, Ouwehand WH, Hurd C. Provision of platelets for severe neonatal alloimmune thrombocytopenia. Br J Haematol 1997; 97:930–932.
69. Ranasinghe E, Walton JD, Hurd CM, et al. Provision of platelet support for fetuses and neonates affected by severe fetomaternal alloimmune thrombocytopenia. Br J Haematol 2001; 113:40–42.
70. Lee K, Beaujean F, Bierling P. Treatment of severe fetomaternal alloimmune thrombocytopenia with compatible frozen-thawed platelet concentrates. Br J Haematol 2002; 117:480–483.
71. Win N. Provision of random-donor platelets (HPA-1a Positive) in neonatal alloimmune thrombocytopenia due to anti HPA-1a alloantibodies. Vox Sang 1996; 71:130–131.
72. Massey GV, McWilliams NB, Mueller DG, Napolitano A, Maurer HM. Intravenous immunoglobulin in treatment of neonatal isoimmune thrombocytopenia. J Pediatr 1987; 111:133–135.
73. Kaplan C, Daffos F, Forestier F, Morel MC, Chesnel N, Tchernia G. Current trends in neonatal alloimmune thrombocytopenia: diagnosis and therapy. In: Kaplan-Gouet C, Schlegel N, Salmon Ch, Mac Gregor J, eds. Platelet Immunology: Fundamental and Clinical Aspects. Paris: John Libbey-Eurotex/ed.INSERM, 1991:267–278.
74. Reese J, Raghuveer TS, Dennington PM, Barfield CP. Breast feeding in neonatal alloimmune thrombocytopenia. J Paediatr Child Health 1994; 30:447–449.
75. Radder CM, Brand A, Kanhai HH. Will it ever be possible to balance the risk of intracranial haemorrhage in fetal or neonatal alloimmune thrombocytopenia against the risk of treatment strategies to prevent it? Vox Sang 2003; 84:318–325.
76. Engelfriet CP, Reesink HW, Kroll H, et al. International forum: prenatal management of alloimmune thrombocytopenia of the fetus. Vox Sang 2003; 84:142–149.
77. Ghidini A, Sepulveda W, Lockwood CJ, Romero R. Complications of fetal blood sampling. Am J Obstet Gynecol 1993; 168:1339–1344.
78. Hickok DE, Mills M, the western collaborative perinatal group. Percutaneous umbilical blood sampling: results from a multicenter collaborative registry. Am J Obstet Gynecol 1992; 166:1614–1618.
79. Proulx C, Filion M, Goldman M, et al. Analysis of immunoglobulin class, IgG subclass and titre of HPA-1a antibodies in alloimmunized mothers giving birth to babies with or without neonatal alloimmune thrombocytopenia. Br J Haematol 1994; 87:813–817.
80. Panzer S, Auerbach L, Cechova E, et al. Maternal alloimmunization against fetal platelet antigens: a prospective study. Br J Haematol 1995; 90:655–660.
81. Jaegtvik S, Husebekk A, Aune B, Oian P, Dahl LB, Skogen B. Neonatal alloimmune thrombocytopenia due to anti HPA-1a antibodies:the level of maternal antibodies predicts the severity of thrombocytopenia in the newborn. BJOG 2000; 107:691–694.
82. Miyazaki R, Ogata H, Iguchi T, et al. Comparative analyses of megakaryocytes derived from cord blood and bone marrow. Br J Haematol 2000; 108:602–609.
83. Sainio S, Javela K, Kekomäki R, Teramo K. Thrombopoietin levels in cord blood plasma and amniotic fluid in fetuses with alloimmune thrombocytopenia and healthy controls. Br J Haematol 2000; 109:330–335.
84. Cremer M, Dame C, Schaeffer HJ, Giers G, Bartmann P, Bald R. Longitudinal thrombopoietin plasma concentrations in fetuses with alloimmune thrombocytopenia treated with intrauterine PLT transfusions. Transfusion 2003; 43:1216–1222.

85. Porcelijn L, Folman CC, de Haas M, et al. Fetal and neonatal thrombopoietin levels in alloimmune thrombocytopenia. Pediatr Res 2002; 52:105–108.
86. Warwick RM, Vaughan J, Murray N, Lubenko A, Roberts I. In vitro culture of colony forming unit-megakaryocyte (CFU-MK) in fetal alloimmune thrombocytopenia. Br J Haematol 1994; 88:874–877.
87. McMillan R, Wang L, Tomer A, Nichol J, Pistillo J. Suppression of in vitro megakaryocyte production by antiplatelet autoantibodies from adult patients with chronic ITP. Blood 2004; 103:1364–1369.
88. Birchall JE, Murphy MF, Kaplan C, Kroll H, on behalf of the European Fetomaternal Alloimmune Thrombocytopenia Study Group. European collaborative study of the antenatal management of feto-maternal alloimmune thrombocytopenia. Br J Haematol 2003; 122:275–288.
89. Gaddipati S, Berkowitz RL, Lembet AA, Lapinski R, McFarland JG, Bussel JB. Initial fetal platelet counts predict the response to intravenous gammaglobulin therapy in fetuses that are affected by PLA1 incompatibility. Am J Obstet Gynecol 2001; 185:976–980.
90. Murphy MF, Pullon HW, Metcalfe P, et al. Management of fetal alloimmune thrombocytopenia by weekly in utero platelet transfusions. Vox Sang 1990; 58:45–49.
91. Overton TG, Duncan KR, Jolly M, Letsky E, Fisk NM. Serial aggressive platelet transfusion for fetal alloimmune thrombocytopenia: platelet dynamics and perinatal outcome. Am J Obstet Gynecol 2002; 186:826–831.
92. Yeast JD, Plapp F. Fetal anemia as a response to prophylactic platelet transfusions in the management of alloimmune thrombocytopenia. Am J Obstet Gynecol 2003; 189:874–876.
93. Viëtor HE, Hawes GE, van den Oever C, et al. Intrauterine transfusions affect fetal T-cell immunity. Blood 1997; 90:2492–2501.
94. Morgan CL, Cannell GR, Addison RS, Minchinton RM. The effect of intravenous immunoglobulin on placental transfer of a platelet-specific antibody: anti-Pl^{A1}. Transfus Med 1991; 1:209–216.
95. Yu Z, Lennon VA. Mechanism of intravenous immune globulin therapy in antibody-mediated autoimmune diseases. N Engl J Med 1999; 340:227–228.
96. Bussel JB, Berkowitz RL, Lynch L, et al. Antenatal management of alloimmune thrombocytopenia with intravenous gamma-globulin: a randomized trial of the addition of low-dose steroid to intravenous gamma-globulin. Am J Obstet Gynecol 1996; 174:1414–1423.
97. Kaplan C, Murphy MF, Kroll H, Waters AH. Feto-maternal alloimmune thrombocytopenia: antenatal therapy with IvIgG and steroids-more questions than answers. Br J Haematol 1998; 100:62–65.
98. Paidas MJ, Berkowitz RL, Lynch L, et al. Alloimmune thrombocytopenia: fetal and neonatal losses related to cordocentesis. Am J Obstet Gynecol 1995; 172:475–479.
99. Murphy MF, Waters AH, Doughty HA, et al. Antenatal management of fetomaternal alloimmune thrombocytopenia—report of 15 affected pregnancies. Transfus Med 1994; 4:281–292.
100. Radder CM, Brand A, Kanhai HH. A less invasive treatment strategy to prevent intracranial hemorrhage in fetal and neonatal alloimmune thrombocytopenia. Am J Obstet Gynecol 2001; 185:683–688.

101. Silver RM, Porter TF, Branch DW, Esplin MS, Scott JR. Neonatal alloimmune thrombocytopenia: antenatal management. Am J Obstet Gynecol 2000; 182:1233–1238.
102. Daffos F, Forestier F, Kaplan C, Cox W. Prenatal diagnosis and management of bleeding disorders with fetal blood sampling. Am J Obstet Gynecol 1988; 158:939–946.
103. Moïse KJ, Jr. Intrauterine transfusion with red cells and platelets. West J Med 1993; 159:318–324.
104. Shulman NR, Aster RH, Leithner A, Hiller MC. Immunoreactions involving platelets. V. Post-transfusion purpura due to a complement-fixing antibody against a genetically controlled platelet antigen. A proposed mechanism for thrombocytopenia and its relevance in "autoimmunity". J Clin Invest 1961; 40:1597–1620.
105. Saji H, Maruya E, Fujii H, et al. New platelet antigens, Sib[a], involved in platelet transfusion refractoriness in a Japanese man. Vox Sang 1989; 56:283–287.
106. Ishida F, Saji H, Maruya E, Furihata K. Human platelet-specific antigen, Siba, is associated with the molecular weight polymorphism of glycoprotein Ib-alpha. Blood 1991; 78:1722–1729.
107. von dem Borne AE, von Riesz E, Verheugt FW, et al. Baka, a new platelet specific antigen involved in neonatal alloimmune thrombocytopenia. Vox Sang 1980; 39:113–120.
108. Lyman S, Aster RH, Visentin GP, Newman PJ. Polymorphism of human platelet membrane glycoprotein IIb associated with the Baka/Bakb alloantigen system. Blood 1990; 75:2343–2348.
109. Djaffar I, Vilette D, Pidard D, Wautier JL, Rosa JP. Human platelet antigen 3 (HPA-3): localization of the determinant of the alloantibody Lek[a] (HPA-3a) to the C-terminus of platelet glycoprotein IIb heavy chain and contribution of O-linked carbohydrates. Thromb Haemost 1993; 69:485–489.
110. Wang R, Newman PJ. Adhesive and signaling properties of a naturally occuring allele of glycoprotein IIIa with an amino acid substitution within the ligand binding domain—The Pen[a]/Pen[b] platelet alloantigenic epitopes. Blood 1998; 92:3260–3267.
111. Furihata K, Nugent DJ, Bissonette A, Aster RH, Kunicki TJ. On the association of the platelet-specific alloantigen. Pen[a], with glycoprotein IIIa. Evidence for heterogeneity of glycoprotein IIIa. J Clin Invest 1987; 80:1624–1630.
112. Kiefel V, Santoso S, Katzmann B, Mueller-Eckhardt C. The Bra/Brb alloantigen system on human platelets. Blood 1989; 73:2219–2223.
113. Santoso S, Kiefel V, Mueller-Eckhardt C. Immunochemical characterization of the new platelet alloantigen system Bra/brB. Br J Haematol 1989; 72:191–198.
114. McFarland JG, Blanchette V, Collins J, Newman PJ, Wang R, Aster RH. Neonatal alloimmune thrombocytopenia due to a new platelet-specific alloantibody. Blood 1993; 81:3318–3323.
115. Kekomäki R, Jouhikainen T, Ollikainen J, Westman P, Laes M. A new platelet alloantigen. Tu[a], on glycoprotein IIIa associated with neonatal alloimmune thrombocytopenia in two families. Br J Haematol 1993; 83:306–310.
116. Wang R, McFarland JG, Kekomäki R, Newman PJ. Amino acid 489 is encoded by a mutational "hot spot" on the beta-3 integrin chain: the CA/TU human platelet alloantigen system. Blood 1993; 82:3386–3391.

117. Kuijpers RW, Simsek S, Faber NM, Goldschmeding R, van Wermerkerken RK, von dem Borne AE. Single point mutation in human glycoprotein IIIa is associated with a new platelet-specific alloantigen (Mo) involved in neonatal alloimmune thrombocytopenia. Blood 1993; 81:70–76.
118. Kroll H, Kiefel V, Santoso S, Mueller-Eckhardt C. Sra, a private platelet antigen on glycoprotein IIIa associated with neonatal alloimmune thrombocytopenia. Blood 1990; 76:2296–2302.
119. Santoso S, Kalb R, Kroll H, et al. A point mutation leads to an unpaired cysteine residue and a molecular weight polymorphism of a functional platelet beta 3 integrin subunit. The Sra alloantigen system of GPIIIa. J Biol Chem 1994; 269:8439–8444.
120. Noris P, Simsek S, de Bruijne-Admiraal LG, et al. Max^{a}, a new low-frequency platelet-specific antigen localized on glycoprotein IIb, is associated with neonatal alloimmune thrombocytopenia. Blood 1995; 86:1019–1026.
121. Reviron D, Mercier P, Dabanian C, Kekomäki R, Morel-Kopp MC, Kaplan C. La^{a}: a new platelet-specific alloantigen on glycoprotein IIIa, involved in neonatal alloimmune thrombocytopenia. Platelets 1994; 5:289.
122. Peyruchaud O, Bourre F, Morel-Kopp MC, et al. HPA-10w^{b} (La^{a}): genetic determination of a new platelet-specific alloantigen on glycoprotein IIIa and its expression in cos-7 cells. Blood 1997; 89:2422–2428.
123. Simsek S, Vlekke AB, Kuijpers RW, Goldschmeding R, von dem Borne AE. A new private platelet antigen, Gro^{a}, localized on glycoprotein IIIa, involved in neonatal alloimmune thrombocytopenia. Vox Sang 1994; 67:302–306.
124. Simsek S, Folman C, van der Schoot CE, von dem Borne AE. The Arg633His substitution responsible for the private platelet antigen Gro^{a} unravelled by SSCP analysis and direct sequencing. Br J Haematol 1997; 97:330–335.
125. Kiefel V, Vicariot M, Giovangrandi Y, et al. Alloimmunization against Iy a low-frequency antigen on platelet glycoprotein Ib/IX as a cause of severe neonatal alloimmune thrombocytopenic purpura. Vox Sang 1995; 69:250–254.
126. Sachs UJ, Kiefel V, Bohringer M, Afshar-Kharghan V, Kroll H, Santoso S. Single amino acid substitution in human platelet glycoprotein Ibbeta is responsible for the formation of the platelet-specific alloantigen Iy(a). Blood 2000; 95:1849–1855.
127. Santoso S, Amrhein J, Hofmann HA, et al. A point mutation Thr(799)Met on the alpha(2) integrin leads to the formation of new human platelet alloantigen Sit(a) and affects collagen-induced aggregation. Blood 1999; 94:4103–4111.
128. Smith JW, Hayward CPM, Horsewood P, Warkentin TE, Denomme GA, Kelton JG. Characterization and localization of the Gov$^{a/b}$ alloantigens to the glycosylphosphatidylinositol-anchored protein CDw109 on human platelets. Blood 1995; 86:2807–2814.
129. Schuh AC, Watkins NA, Nguyen Q, et al. A tyrosine703serine polymorphism of CD109 defines the Gov platelet alloantigens. Blood 2002; 99:1692–1698.
130. Roberts I, Murray NA. Neonatal thrombocytopenia: causes and management. Arch Dis Child Fetal Neonatal Ed 2003; 88:F359–F364.

10

Thrombotic Microangiopathies: Thrombotic Thrombocytopenic Purpura and the Hemolytic Uremic Syndrome

Keith R. McCrae

Division of Hematology-Oncology, Department of Medicine, Case Western Reserve University School of Medicine/University Hospitals of Cleveland, Cleveland, Ohio, U.S.A.

Douglas B. Cines

Department of Pathology and Laboratory Medicine, University of Pennsylvania School of Medicine, Philadelphia, Pennsylvania, U.S.A.

J. Evan Sadler

Department of Medicine and Department of Biochemistry and Molecular Biophysics, Washington University School of Medicine, and Howard Hughes Medical Institute, St. Louis, Missouri, U.S.A.

INTRODUCTION

In 1925, Moschowitz described a young woman who succumbed to an illness with features of microangiopathic hemolytic anemia (MAHA), petechiae, hemiparesis, and fever (1). In 1955, Gasser described a similar disorder characterized by Coombs negative hemolytic anemia, thrombocytopenia, and renal failure (2). Today, these disorders, which share the common features of MAHA, thrombocytopenia, and microvascular thrombi are termed thrombotic thrombocytopenic purpura (TTP) and the hemolytic uremic syndrome (HUS), respectively, and are included in the family of thrombotic microangiopathies (3,4).

The clinical and pathologic features of TTP and HUS sometimes overlap so extensively that they may be difficult to distinguish, leading some to suggest that they be considered collectively as TTP–HUS (3). However, TTP and HUS may

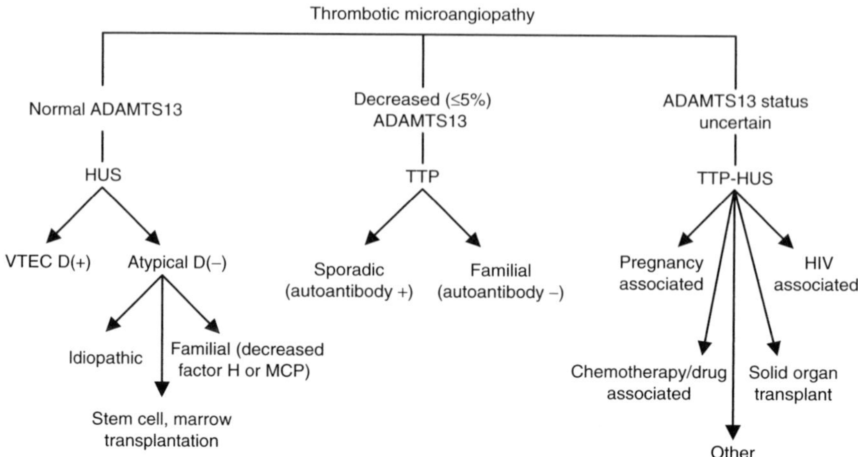

Figure 1 Proposed scheme for integrating clinical and pathophysiological aspects of thrombotic microangiopathies. A scheme such as this has distinct limitations. Moreover, we do not advocate that ADAMTS13 levels be used for diagnostic purposes at this point in time, as not all patients with clinically diagnosed TTP have very low or absent ADAMTS13 levels. Similarly, not all patients with VTEC-related thrombotic microangiopathy have preceding diarrhea, i.e., some cases are VTEC(+) D(−). *Source*: Adapted from Ref. 11.

also have distinct clinical presentations and pathophysiologies, as suggested by the high incidence of severe deficiency of ADAMTS13, the von Willebrand factor (VWF) cleaving protease, in TTP but not HUS (5–7), and a deficiency of complement regulatory proteins in familial HUS (8,9). Moreover, the frequency with which TTP and HUS affect specific organ systems differs, and while plasma exchange is effective therapy for TTP (10–12), it is usually less so for HUS (13). A classification scheme for thrombotic microangiopathies is depicted in Figure 1.

THROMBOTIC THROMBOCYTOPENIC PURPURA (TTP)

Clinical Manifestations

TTP occurs with an annual incidence of 3.7 cases per million with a peak incidence in the fourth decade, and is more common in females (female/male ratio 3:2) (14,15). Other risk factors include African ancestry and obesity (16,17).

The classic pentad of symptoms in TTP includes MAHA, thrombocytopenia, neurologic symptoms, fever, and renal dysfunction (15). However, only approximately 40% of patients display all of these, while 75% present with MAHA, neurologic symptoms, and thrombocytopenia (15,18). If present at diagnosis, renal dysfunction is generally mild, usually limited to hematuria, proteinuria, and granular or red cell casts in the urine (19). A minority of patients experience prodromal symptoms of an upper respiratory tract infection.

Neurological symptoms range from headache and confusion to seizures, aphasia, or coma (15,18–20). Thrombocytopenia may be severe, with platelet counts below 20,000/μl, and may be accompanied by mucocutaneous bleeding (15,18,20). The prothrombin time, partial thromboplastin time, and fibrinogen levels are usually normal, though mild elevations in fibrin(ogen) degradation products occur in one half of patients, and more sensitive assays may demonstrate activation of coagulation and fibrinolytic pathways. MAHA, as demonstrated by the presence of fragmented red cells on the peripheral blood film (Fig. 2), occurs in the microvasculature, and is the cardinal characteristic of TTP; nucleated red blood cells accompany reticulocytosis in most patients. Elevated levels of plasma lactate dehydrogenase (LDH) occur in all patients, reflecting hemolysis and tissue ischemia (21).

Two primary forms of TTP have been recognized, an inherited and an acquired form. Schulman (22) and Upshaw (23) first identified an autosomal recessive, inherited form of TTP in neonates. Patients with this disorder may develop recurrent episodes of thrombotic microangiopathy during early childhood (24,25), sometimes in association with infection, surgery, or vaccinations. Perhaps one half of patients, however, remain asymptomatic until early adulthood, and occasionally into their fourth or fifth decade. The acquired variant of TTP is associated in most cases with low levels of ADAMTS13 due to inhibitory antibodies and is described below.

Pathogenesis

Moake (26) first demonstrated the presence of "unusually large" VWF multimers (ULVWF) in the plasma of patients with the Upshaw–Schulman syndrome.

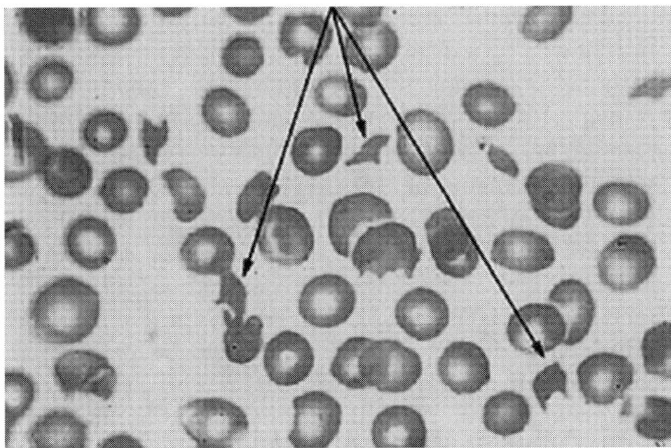

Figure 2 A peripheral blood film from a patient with thrombotic thrombocytopenic purpura demonstrating abundant schistocytes (*arrows*). *Source*: Copyright 2001 by the American Scoeity of Hematology, courtesy of ASH Image Bank.

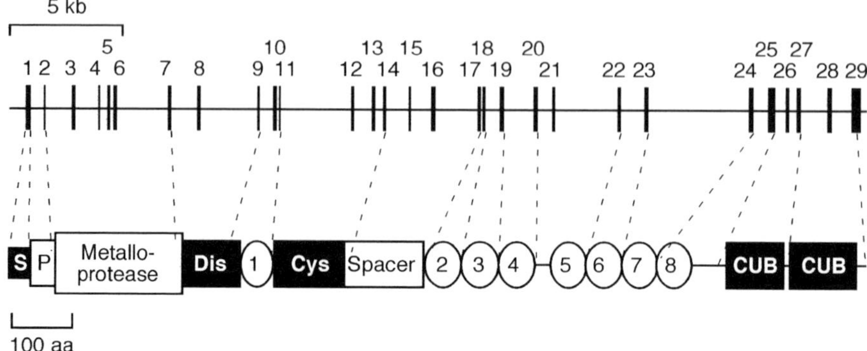

Figure 3 Structure of ADAMTS13. The *ADAMTS13* gene spans 37 kb on chromosome 9q34, and spans 29 exons. Dashed lines show the relationship between the gene structure and domains of the ADAMTS13 protein. The 1427 amino acid ADAMTS13 precursor contains a signal peptide (S), propeptide (P), metalloprotease, disintegrin domain (Dis), thrombospondin type 1 repeats (numbered 1–8), cysteine-rich domain (Cys), spacer domain, and CUB domains. *Source*: Adapted from Ref. 112.

He proposed that these patients lacked a plasma protease or reductase that cleaves these multimers and that intact ULVWF caused intravascular platelet aggregation. A plasma metalloprotease was subsequently discovered that degrades VWF multimers by cleaving the Tyr^{1605}–Met^{1606} bond (27,28), and patients with the Upshaw–Schulman Syndrome were found to lack this protease (29), denoted ADAMTS13. ADAMTS13 is a member of the ADAMTS family, where "ADAMTS" stands for "a disintegrin-like and metalloprotease with thrombospondin type 1 motif" (Fig. 3). The primary translation product consists of 1427 amino acids, and is synthesized in the liver. ADAMTS13 has a metalloprotease domain followed by a disintegrin domain, a thrombospondin-1 repeat, and a cysteine-rich and spacer domain followed by 7 thrombospondin-1 repeats and two CUB domains. Upshaw–Schulman Syndrome has been shown to be caused by mutations in the *ADAMTS13* gene on chromosome 9q34 (30), and occur in almost all structural domains of ADAMTS13. Characterization of ADAMTS13 has allowed development of a model to explain the role of this protease in regulation of VWF-mediated platelet adhesion under normal and pathologic conditions (31).

Following the association of ADAMTS13 deficiency with familial TTP, patients with nonfamilial, acquired TTP were also found to be deficient in ADAMTS13, most often due to IgG inhibitors (6,32). The presence of ADAMTS13 inhibitors in patients with TTP has been confirmed by numerous groups, though the exact prevalence of ADAMTS13 deficiency in these patients remains controversial (16,33), perhaps due to different patient selection criteria and/or intralaboratory variability in ADAMTS13 measurements. While an ADAMTS13 level of $<5\%$ is believed to be specific for TTP (7,34), mild to moderately decreased levels of ADAMTS13 occur in several settings (35), such as liver disease and pregnancy. Hence the sensitivity of ADAMTS13 assays for diagnosis of TTP is uncertain, though a low ADAMTS13 level has been shown to predict a good response to plasma exchange (36).

Inhibitory antibodies against ADAMTS13 have been reported in 59% to 100% of patients with TTP and acquired severe ADAMTS13 deficiency (6,16,32,33), reflecting the variable sensitivity of inhibitor assays, and the fact that some non-inhibitory antibodies induce ADAMTS13 deficiency by promoting its clearance, and are not detected in functional assays. In a recent study, 55% of patients with severe deficiencies of ADAMTS13 were found to have plasmatic inhibitors. Inhibitors were found more commonly in patients with manifestations of an underlying immune disorder such as polyarthritis, skin rashes, and discoid lupus, and were often accompanied by other positive immune serologies including antinuclear, anti-double-stranded DNA, and anticardiolipin antibodies (37). Inhibitors in all patients reported to date recognize the ADAMTS13 spacer domain or a region containing the cysteine-rich and spacer domains. Some patients also have antibodies against other domains including CUB domains, TSP repeats 2–8, or the propeptide (38,39). These results are consistent with other biochemical data that indicate that the spacer region is required for efficient cleavage of VWF by ADAMTS13 (40).

Both congenital and acquired ADAMTS13 deficiency are characterized by unpredictable periods of stability between relapses, which probably reflects a role of stress in exacerbating the disease by activating or damaging endothelium, increasing the release of ULVWF, and triggering microvascular platelet thrombosis. Several other mechanisms may be involved in the pathogenesis of TTP, as well as HUS. These include alterations in pro- and anti-fibrinolytic factors, the effects of vasoregulatory substances such as endothelin and prostacyclin, excessive procoagulant activity induced by circulating endothelial microparticles, or mutations or deficiencies of naturally occurring anticoagulant mechanisms.

Therapy

The mortality rate of TTP exceeds 90% without therapy, but with plasma exchange, long term survival exceeds 80% (3,12,41).

The results of a prospective trial reported in 1991 demonstrated that plasma exhange is superior to plasma infusion in the treatment of patients with TTP; six months after initiation of therapy, complete remissions were seen in 78% of patients treated with exchange versus 31% treated with plasma infusion (42). Thus, unless a genetic deficiency of ADAMTS13 has been documented, plasma infusion should be used only in situations in which exchange is not immediately available.

Plasma exchange is initiated with the goal of exchanging 1–1.5 plasma volumes daily (12). Cryosupernatant, which lacks VWF, offers a theoretical benefit over plasma, although its clinical superiority is controversial.

Neurological improvement usually occurs most rapidly, sometimes within hours (19). Serum LDH level typically falls by 50% within three days, and the platelet count begins to rise in approximately five days, though normalization may take weeks. Renal function is usually last to improve. Daily plasma exchange should be continued until neurological symptoms have resolved and a normal serum LDH and platelet count have been maintained for at least 2–3 days (3,12); the benefits of tapering plasma exchange versus abrupt termination are uncertain. At least 30% of patients experience exacerbations, defined as recurrent symptoms within 30 days of discontinuing plasma exchange (3), or relapses. Plasma exchange is associated with complications in up to 30% of patients, though most of these relate to central venous catheter insertion (43).

Corticosteroids are often used as an adjunct to plasma exchange or in patients who fail to respond adequately (3); though there is no convincing evidence that corticosteroids improve the response to plasma exchange, their immunosuppressive activity provides a rationale for their use in patients with ADAMTS13 inhibitors (12). Splenectomy is generally reserved for refractory patients, with variable response rates reported (44), and may reduce the incidence of relapses (45). Antiplatelet agents have little efficacy as single agents (41) and do not increase the response to plasma exchange (3,42). The efficacy of intravenous immunoglobulin, vincristine, and other immunosuppressive therapies such as azathioprine, cyclophosphamide, cyclosporine, and staphyloccal protein A immunoadsorption has been suggested, but not convincingly confirmed. Accumulating evidence suggests a potentially valuable role for Rituximab in the therapy of TTP, particularly in patients with documented ADAMTS13 inhibitors. To date, there are at least 14 reports of patients with TTP treated with Rituximab, with generally good responses. Approximately 33 patients with active disease have been treated, with 29 complete responses, one delayed relapse, one partial response, and two non-responses (46–59). In addition, six patients in clinical remission, but with persistence of ADAMTS13 inhibitors have received Rituximab therapy, with disappearance or a substantial decrease in the inhibitor level in each (58,59). The frequency of subsequent relapses appears to have been diminished in these patients, at least when compared to their previous clinical course prior to receiving Rituximab.

Commencement of low-dose aspirin (81 mg daily) upon platelet recovery (platelet count $>50{,}000/\mu L$) has been recommended, particularly in patients who experience a rapid rise in the platelet count (12). Folate supplementation and administration of hepatitis B vaccine should be considered routine supportive care (12). Platelet transfusion is relatively contraindicated, and has been associated with dramatic worsening of the disease course in some patients.

HEMOLYTIC UREMIC SYNDROME

Classification of HUS may be confusing, as there are several variants. HUS occurs most commonly in an epidemic form in children due to infection with verotoxin producing *E. coli*. This disorder usually presents with a prodrome of bloody diarrhea, and therefore is often referred to as D(+), typical or childhood HUS (60). A second variant, sporadic HUS, is also characterized by MAHA, thrombocytopenia, and renal failure, but develops in the absence of obvious precipitating factors. This variant is most common in adults, is usually not associated with bloody diarrhea or a specific precipating factor, and is referred to as D(−) or adult HUS (though it may account for up to 10% of HUS cases in children). Thrombotic microangiopathies that complicate bone marrow transplantation, immunosuppressive medication, pregnancy, and chemotherapy generally resemble D(−) HUS most closely (60). Finally, inherited HUS may result from genetic deficiencies of complement regulatory proteins, and present as a familial disorder (61).

Familial HUS

Familial HUS may exhibit autosomal dominant or recessive inheritance (60). Some patients with this disorder display low levels of complement due to a homozygous or heterozygous deficiency of complement factor H (62). Factor H regulates complement activation in plasma and on cell surfaces, including the endothelium. HUS in these patients runs a chronic, relapsing course complicated by hypertension and renal insufficiency (62). Siblings with homozygous factor H deficiency may develop HUS at different times, or sometimes not at all (63).

Plasma exchange (64) or infusions (65) may sometimes slow the progression of renal failure in these patients, but does not induce remissions. HUS due to factor H deficiency often recurs in a transplanted kidney. One patient appears to have been cured by combined kidney and liver transplantation (66).

Deficiency or dysfunction of factor H may also account for 20% of sporadic HUS cases (67), though it accounts for only 10–20% of familial HUS. These findings indicate that other predisposing gene defects have yet to be identified in patients with familial HUS.

Sporadic HUS

Sporadic HUS may be preceded by non-specific prodromal symptoms suggestive of an upper respiratory tract infection, as well as fatigue and malaise. Neurological manifestations are usually less frequent and severe than in TTP. All patients have MAHA, accompanied by an elevated LDH, though thrombocytopenia is usually less severe than in TTP. Renal involvement often dominates the clinical course, and as many as 60% of patients may require dialysis. Due to its rarity, overlap in symptomatology with some cases of TTP, and the inclusion of patients with sporadic HUS in series comprised mostly of patients with idiopathic TTP, or pregnancy, cancer, or chemotherapy-associated microangiopathic hemolytic disorders, the optimal management of patients with sporadic HUS is not well defined. Specifically, the frequency of response to plasma exchange and other management approaches that are used in TTP is difficult to assess, though a trial of plasma exchange is reasonable in patients able to tolerate the procedure (3,12). Sporadic HUS is associated with a poor prognosis, with a mortality rate of 25%, and chronic renal failure occurring in 50% of survivors (68).

Verotoxin-Associated Thrombotic Microangiopathy [D(+)HUS]

Although the incidence of D(+) HUS is greatest in children under 5 years, the disorder can develop at any age (4,69). In a recent study, the median age of patients with D(+) HUS was 4 years, with 88% of patients age 17 or younger and only 6% above age 45 (70). The association of D(+) HUS with verotoxin-producing *E. coli* has been established. The major reservoir of verotoxin-producing *E. coli* is domestic cattle, and outbreaks of VTEC-associated HUS occur most commonly after ingestion of inadequately cooked ground beef (70,71). Person-to-person transmission may contribute to outbreaks of epidemic HUS in day care centers and nursing homes. The disease occurs more frequently during summer months in temperate climates.

VTEC were first implicated in the development of HUS after their detection in stools of 11 of 15 Canadian children with HUS (72). Additional studies demonstrated an association of HUS with other verotoxin-producing strains of *E. coli* (70,73). The disease begins with the sudden onset of abdominal pain and watery diarrhea 1 to 9 days after toxin exposure. Bloody diarrhea generally follows on the second day, sometimes accompanied by nausea and vomiting (70). Fever is generally absent or mild. Colonoscopy shows an edematous colonic mucosa, with occasional ulceration and pseudomembrane formation. Thumbprinting in the distal ascending and proximal transverse colon, reflecting ischemic colitis caused by endotoxin-induced thrombi in the bowel wall microvasculature, may be evident on barium enema (4). This syndrome of *E. coli*-associated hemorrhagic gastroenteritis is followed by HUS in 8–20% of cases, though in approximately 25% a preceding history of hemorrhagic gastroenteritis is not obtained (4). Patients present a median of 5–6 days after the onset of bloody diarrhea with oliguria or other manifestations of renal insufficiency (4,70); 50% of patients require dialysis. The extent of MAHA varies, though most patients require transfusion. Thrombocytopenia is common, with a median platelet count of 30,000/μl in one study, but may be mild or absent in up to 30% of patients. Neurological manifestations such as irritability, somnolence, confusion, paresis, and seizures occur in 25% (70).

Demonstration of a fourfold or greater rise in antibody titer to either Shiga-like toxins or 0157 lipopolysaccharide confirms a diagnosis of VTEC-associated HUS. Positive stool cultures are obtained in only half of those in whom the diagnosis is confirmed serologically, and must be obtained within 7 days of the onset of diarrhea (70). *E. coli* 0157:H7 ferment sorbitol slowly, and appear as colorless colonies on sorbitol-MacConkey agar. Methods to detect Shiga-like toxins or their genes improve diagnostic sensitivity (73).

The capacity of enteropathic E. coli to cause HUS is due to their expression of either of two 70-kD bacterial exotoxins, named verotoxins. Verotoxin-1 is homologous to Shigella toxin and is sometimes referred to as Shiga-like toxin 1 (SLT-1). Many strains of pathogenic *E. coli* produce a second toxin, SLT-2. The toxins bind to Gala1-4Galb (galabiose) residues primarily on globosyltriaosylceramide (Gb_3; also known as CD77 and the human blood group P^k antigen) (74). Receptor-bound toxin is internalized, and the cleaved A subunit binds the 60s ribosomal subunit and cleaves adenosine from ribosomal RNA (75), thereby preventing elongation factor 1-dependent binding of aminoacyl tRNA (76) and inhibiting protein synthesis. The predilection of children exposed to verotoxin to develop renal disease may involve higher levels of Gb_3 expression by glomerular capillary endothelium in children compared to adults (77), as well as the greater expression of Gb_3 by glomerular microvascular endothelium compared with other vascular beds.

Though verotoxin-associated HUS is the most common cause of acute renal failure in children (78), it is usually self-limited with a mortality rate of less than 5%. However, up to 60% of children may require dialysis (70). Renal insufficiency usually resolves within 2–3 weeks, though some patients have prolonged anuria. Many children with VTEC-associated HUS develop chronic renal insufficiency over ensuing decades (79), and complete recovery and long-term preservation of renal function occurs in only 50–60% (80). In randomized trials, neither plasma infusion nor exchange has shown benefit in children with VTEC-associated HUS, though in a single study of older children, all patients requiring long-term dialysis were in the nontreatment group (81). There is also no conclusive evidence that plasma exchange improves outcomes in adults (12), though an empiric trial should be considered given the difficulty in distinguishing some cases of TTP from HUS. Antimotility agents delay clearance of *E. coli* from the gastrointestinal tract, and may increase the risk of developing HUS (82). Likewise, treatment of bloody diarrhea with antibiotics may increase the risk of progression to HUS due to the propensity of subinhibitory concentrations of certain antibiotics to induce toxin production (83).

MISCELLANEOUS CAUSES OF THROMBOTIC MICROANGIOPATHY

Transplantation

Thrombotic microangiopathies occur commonly in the post-transplant setting. The most frequent scenarios involve the development of a disorder most closely resembling sporadic HUS: (1) in association with the use of cyclosporine A (CyA), (2) as recurring disease after renal transplantation for HUS-associated renal failure, or (3) in the setting of marrow transplantation.

Cyclosporine A is the most common cause of drug-induced thrombotic microangiopathy. Thrombotic microangiopathy occurs in 1–5% of CyA-treated renal transplant recipients (84), as well as in occasional patients who have undergone cardiac (85) or liver (86) transplantation. CyA-induced thrombotic microangiopathy generally presents with unexplained renal insufficiency (87). MAHA and thrombocytopenia are generally mild and occur in only half of the patients with this disorder. Renal biopsy may be required to distinguish CyA-induced thrombotic microangiopathy from acute tubular necrosis or rejection (88). The pathogenesis of this disorder appears to involve direct toxic effects of CyA on endothelial cells (89), particularly in association with the effects of pro-inflammatory cytokines.

CyA-induced thrombotic microangiopathy usually responds to a reduction of the dose or discontinuation of CyA, and treatment involves discontinuation of the drug. The role of plasma exchange is uncertain. Though some patients may develop permanent renal failure, the prognosis is generally good. In some patients, other immunosuppresives such as tacrolimus have been substituted successfully, though this agent has also precipitated thrombotic microangiopathy.

In some patients with end stage renal failure due to HUS, thrombotic microangiopathy can recur in a transplanted kidney, even in the absence of CyA. This is least common in children with renal failure due to VTEC-associated HUS (90), and most common in patients with familial HUS, in whom it may occur in 50% of cases (91). Hence, a very careful and detailed multigenerational history must be taken to exclude the possibility of familial thrombotic microangiopathy when a living related donation is considered.

Thrombotic microangiopathy also develops in approximately 6% of patients who undergo allogeneic, and 1% of patients who undergo autologous marrow or stem cell transplantation (92–94). Achieving a diagnosis in this setting may be difficult, as schistocytes and thrombocytopenia occur commonly after hematopoietic cell transplantation (95). The pathogenesis of this disorder presumably involves endothelial cell injury due to a variety of factors including the preconditioning regimen; most reports suggest that a severe deficiency of ADAMTS13 is uncommon (36). Risk factors include use of an unrelated or mismatched donor (94), total body irradiation, CyA post-transplant, and graft-versus-host disease, among others. Treatment involves withdrawal of cyclosporine A; plasma exchange may be considered but is generally not effective (96). Mortality rates may exceed 50% (94). Defibrotide has been used successfully in a few cases.

Cancer and Chemotherapy

Thrombotic microangiopathies may be a terminal event in some patients with advanced malignancies, particularly those of gastrointestinal tract origin (20,97). Patients generally present with moderate to severe MAHA and thrombocytopenia, though renal insufficiency and neurologic manifestations occur less commonly than in idiopathic thrombotic microangiopathies (98). Elevated levels of fibrin(ogen) degradation products occur in 25–80% of patients; however, DIC as the sole cause of this syndrome is unlikely, and additional factors involving abnormalities of the tumor microvasculature may contribute. The role of ADAMTS13 deficiency remains uncertain (99,100), and a role for plasma exchange has not been determined. The only effective therapy is reduction of the tumor burden.

In addition to cancer per se, certain cancer chemotherapeutic agents have been implicated in the development of thrombotic microangiopathy (98). Most patients who develop this disorder have received therapy for an underlying adenocarcinoma within the preceding 4 months, making the risk attributable to the neoplasm versus the treatment difficult to discern (97,101). Patients who develop chemotherapy-associated thrombotic microangiopathy generally do not carry a large tumor burden, and some are in remission (20). Mitomycin-C is the agent most strongly associated with this disorder, but other drugs including cis-platininum, bleomycin, gemcitabine, docetaxel and carboplatin have been implicated (20).

Patients with chemotherapy-associated thrombotic microangiopathy present with moderate to severe MAHA and thrombocytopenia and significant renal dysfunction (97), and a minority develop neurologic manifestations. An event unique to this disease is the development of noncardiogenic pulmonary edema in over 50% of patients in some series. Chemotherapy-associated thrombotic microangiopathies are presumed to result directly from toxicity of these agents toward the endothelium. Less than 20% of patients respond to plasma exchange and corticosteroids, and more than one half die within 2 months (97,102). Anecdotal responses to immunopheresis with staphylococcal protein A columns (ProSorba) have been reported (103).

Miscellaneous Drugs Associated with Thrombotic Microangiopathies

More than 50 drugs, including penicillins, ciprofloxacin, clarithromycin, H_2 receptor antagonists, and the Norplant® contraceptive, have been implicated in the development of thrombotic microangiopathies, but for only a few of these does sufficient information exist to strongly support an association. Cyclosporine A and mitomycin C (see above) have been most strongly implicated; while thrombotic microangiopathy appears to develop after cumulative exposures to these agents, it may develop as an idiosyncratic response to drugs such as ticlopidine, clopidogrel, and ciprofloxacin.

Several reports suggest an association of quinine with a thrombotic microangiopathic syndrome resembling HUS (104); this disorder may develop after ingestion of quinine tablets, or less commonly after exposure to quinine in beverages such as tonic water. The pathogenesis of quinine-associated thrombotic microangiopathy may involve quinine-dependent antibodies reactive with platelet glycoproteins IIb/IIIa and Ib/IX, and related antigens on endothelial cells and neutrophils (104). Patients present with severe MAHA and thrombocytopenia, and renal insufficiency that often requires dialysis (105). Unique to this syndrome is the development of granulocytopenia and lymphopenia in some patients. Though in early reports the prognosis of this disorder was considered favorable after discontinuation of the drug, a recent study reported that more than 50% of affected patients died or were left with chronic renal failure (106).

The incidence of TTP associated with ticlopidine has ranged from 1:600 to 1:4000 patient exposures (84); some cases were associated with concurrent antibodies against ADAMTS13 (107). Due to the frequency of drug-associated TTP, ticlopidine has largely been replaced by clopidogrel. Although TTP was subsequently described in patients treated with clopidogrel, its incidence appears to be substantially lower, ranging from 4 per 1,000,000 to 1 per 8500 to 26,000 (84).

HIV-Associated Thrombotic Microangiopathy

An association between HIV infection and thrombotic microangiopathy has been recognized for many years, and in reports from areas where HIV infection is prevalent, 15–50% of patients with thrombotic microangiopathies have been infected (108,109). The diagnosis of thrombotic microangiopathy in HIV-infected patients may be difficult due to the common occurrence of anemia, fever, thrombocytopenia, nephropathy, neurologic disease, and elevated LDH levels related to other manifestations of HIV infection (110). Thrombotic microangiopathy may occur at any time during the course of infection, but is uncommon in patients with hemophilia. The pathogenesis of HIV-associated thrombotic microangiopathy may involve damage to the microvascular endothelium by infection with opportunistic organisms or HIV, drugs such as fluconazole or valacyclovir, and alterations in plasma cytokine levels. Inhibitory anti-ADAMTS13 antibodies have been reported (111). HIV-associated thrombotic microangiopathy responds to plasma exchange, as well as anti-retroviral therapy in some cases (109). The prognosis is dependent on the severity of the underlying syndrome, and survival exceeding several years has been reported in patients treated aggressively with plasma exchange and anti-retrovirals.

REFERENCES

1. Moschcowitz E. An acute febrile pleiochromic anemia with hyaline thrombosis of the terminal arterioles and capillaries. Arch Intern Med 1925; 36:89–98.
2. Gasser C, Gautier C, Steck A, Seibenmann RE, Deschlin R. Haemolytic-uramische syndromes bilaterale Nierenrindennekrosen bei akuten erworbenchen hamolytischen Anamien. Schwiez Med Wochenschchr 1955; 85:905–909.
3. George JN. How I treat patients with thrombotic thrombocytopenic purpura-hemolytic uremic syndrome. Blood 2000; 96:1223–1229.

4. Ruggenenti P, Noris M, Remuzzi G. Thrombotic microangiopathy, hemolytic uremic syndrome and thrombotic thrombocytopenic purpura. Kidney Int 2001; 60:831–846.
5. Furlan M, Robles R, Galbusera M, et al. von Willebrand factor-cleaving protease in thrombotic thrombocytopenic purpura and the hemolytic-uremic syndrome. N Engl J Med 1998; 339:1578–1584.
6. Tsai H-M, Lian ECY. Antibodies to von Willebrand factor-cleaving protease in acute thrombotic thrombocytopenic purpura. N Engl J Med 1998; 339:1585–1594.
7. Bianchi V, Robles R, Alberio L, Furlan M, Lämmle B. von Willebrand factor-cleaving protease (ADAMTS13) in thrombocytopenic disorders: a severely deficient activity is specific for thrombotic thrombocytopenic purpura. Blood 2002; 100:710–713.
8. Richards A, Kemp EJ, Liszewski MK, et al. Mutations in human complement regulator, membrane cofactor protein (CD46), predispose to development of familial hemolytic uremic syndrome. Proc Natl Acad Sci USA 2003; 100:12966–12971.
9. Noris M, Brioschi S, Caprioli J, et al. Familial haemolytic uremic syndrome and an MCP mutation. Lancet 2003; 362:1542–1547.
10. Moake JL. Thrombotic microangiopathies. N Engl J Med 2002; 347:589–600.
11. Liu J, Hutzler M, Li C, Pechet L. Thrombotic thrombocytopenic purpura (TTP) and the hemolytic uremic syndrome (HUS): the new thinking. J Thromb Thrombolysis 2001; 11:261–272.
12. Allford SL, Hunt BJ, Rose P, Machin SJ. Haemostasis and Thrombosis Task Force of the British Committee for Standards in Haematology: guidelines on the diagnosis and management of the thrombotic microangiopathic haemolytic anaemias. Br J Haematol 2003; 120:556–573.
13. Dundas S, Murphy J, Soutar RL, Jones GA, Hutchinson SJ, Todd WTA. Effectiveness of therapeutic plasma exchange in the Lanarkshire Escherichia coli 0157: H7 outbreak. Lancet 1999; 354:1327–1330.
14. Torok TJ, Holman RC, Chorba TL. Increasing mortality from thrombotic thrombocytopenic purpura in the united states—analysis of national mortality data, 1968–1961. Am J Hematol 1995; 5084:90.
15. Ridolfi RL, Bell WR. Thrombotic thrombocytopenia purpura: report of 25 cases and a review of the literature. Medicine 1981; 60:413–428.
16. Vesely SK, George JN, Lämmle B, et al. ADAMTS13 activity in thrombotic thrombocytopenic purpura-hemolytic uremic syndrome: relation to presenting features and clinical outcomes in a prospective cohort of 142 patients. Blood 2003; 102:60–68.
17. Nicol KK, Shelton BJ, Knovich MS, Owen J. Overweight individuals are at increased risk for thrombotic thrombocytopenic purpura. Am J Hematol 2003; 74:170–174.
18. Amarosi EL, Ultmann JE. Thrombotic thrombocytopenic purpura. Report of 16 cases and review of the literature. Medicine 1966; 45:139–159.
19. Thompson CE, Damon LE, Ries CA, Linker CA. Thrombotic microangiopathies in the 1980s: clinical features, response to treatment, and the impact of the human immunodeficiency virus epidemic. Blood 1992; 80:1890–1895.
20. Nabhan C, Kwaan HC. Current concepts in the diagnosis and management of thrombotic thrombocytopenic purpura. Hematol/Oncol Clin N Am 2003; 17:177–199.

21. Cohen JD, Brechter ME, Bandarenko N. Cellular source of serum lactate dehydrogenase elevation in patients with thrombotic thrombocytopenic purpura. J Clin Apheresis 1998; 13:16–19.
22. Schulman I, Pierce M, Lukens A, Currimbhoy Z. Studies on thrombopoiesis. I. A factor in normal human plasma required for platelet production; chronic thrombocytopenia due to its deficiency. Blood 1960; 16:943–947.
23. Upshaw JD, Jr. Congenital deficiency of a factor in normal plasma that reverses microangiopathic hemolysis and thrombocytopenia. N Engl J Med 1978; 298:1350–1352.
24. Furlan M, Lämmle B. Aetiology and pathogenesis of thrombotic thrombocytopenic purpura and haemolytic uremic syndrome: the role of von Willebrand factor cleaving protease. Best Pract Res Clin Haematol 2001; 14:437–454.
25. Veyradier A, Obert B, Haddad E, et al. Severe deficiency of the specific von Willebrand factor-cleaving protease (ADAMTS 13) activity in a subgroup of children with atypical hemolytic uremic syndrome. J Pediatr 2003; 142: 310–317.
26. Moake JL, Rudy CK, Troll JH, et al. Unusually large plasma factor VIII: von Willebrand factor multimers in chronic relapsing thrombotic thrombocytopenic purpura. N Engl J Med 1982; 307:1432–1435.
27. Tsai H-M. Physiologic cleavage of von Willebrand factor by a plasma protease is dependent on its conformation and requires calcium ion. Blood 1996; 87:4235–4244.
28. Furlan M, Robles R, Lammle B. Partial purification and characterization of a protease from human plasma cleaving von Willebrand factor to fragments produced by in vivo proteolysis. Blood 1996; 87:4223–4229.
29. Furlan M, Robles R, Solenthaler M, Wassmer M, Sandoz P, Lammle B. Deficient activity of von Willebrand factor-cleaving protease in chronic relapsing thrombotic thrombocytopenic purpura. Blood 1997; 89:3097–3103.
30. Levy GG, Nichols WC, Lian EC, et al. Mutations in a member of the ADAMTS gene family cause thrombotic thrombocytopenic purpura. Nature 2001; 413:488–494.
31. Sadler JE. A new name in thrombosis, ADAMTS13. Proc Natl Acad Sci USA 2002; 99:11552–11554.
32. Furlan M, Robles R, Solenthaler M, Lämmle B. Acquired deficiency of von Willebrand factor-cleaving protease in a patient with thrombotic thrombocytopenic purpura. Blood 1998; 91:2839–2846.
33. Veyradier A, Obert B, Houllier A, Meyer D, Girma J-P. Specific von Willebrand factor-cleaving protease in thrombotic microangiopathies: a study of 111 cases. Blood 2001; 98:1765–1772.
34. Tsai H-M. Is severe deficiency of von Willebrand factor cleaving protease (ADAMTS-13) specific for thrombotic thrombocytopenic purpura? Yes J Thromb Haemost 2003; 1:625–631.
35. Mannucci PM, Vanoli M, Forza I, Canciani MT, Scorza R. Von Willebrand factor cleaving protease (ADAMTS-13) in 123 patients with connective tissue diseases (systemic lupus erythematosus and systemic sclerosis). Haematologica 2003; 88:914–918.

36. Zheng XL, Kaufman RM, Goodnough LT, Sadler JE. Effect of plasma exchange on plasma ADAMTS13 metalloprotease activity, inhibitor level, and clinical outcome in patients with idiopathic and nonidiopathic thrombocytopenic purpura. Blood 2004; 103:4043–4049.
37. Coppo P, Bengoufa D, Veyradier A, et al. Reseau d'Etude des Microangiopathies Thrombotique de l'Adulte: Severe ADAMTS13 deficiency in adult idiopathic thrombotic microangiopathies defines a subset of patients characterized by various autoimmune manifestations, lower platelet count, and mild renal involvement. Medicine (Baltimore) 2004; 83:233–244.
38. Klaus C, Plaimauer B, Studt JD, et al. Epitope mapping of acquired ADAMTS13 autoantibodies in acquired thrombotic thrombocytopenic purpura. Blood 2004; 103:4514–4519.
39. Luker BM, Turenhout EAM, Hulstein JJJ. The spacer domain of ADAMTS13 contains a major binding site for antibodies in patients with thrombotic thrombocytopenic purpura. Thromb Haemost 2005; 93:267–274.
40. Soejima K, Matsumoto M, Kokame K, et al. ADAMTS-13 cysteine-rich/spacer domains are functionally essential for von Willebrand factor cleavage. Blood 2003; 102:3232–3237.
41. Kwaan HC, Soff GA. Management of thrombotic thrombocytopenic purpura and hemolytic uremic syndrome. Semin Hematol 1997; 34:159–166.
42. Rock GA, Shumak KH, Buskard NA, et al. Comparison of plasma exchange with plasma infusion in the treatment of thrombotic thrombocytopenic purpura. N Engl J Med 1991; 325:393–397.
43. McMinn JR, Thomas IA, Terrell DR, Duvall D, Vesely SK, George JN. Complications of plasma exchange in thrombotic thrombocytopenic purpura-hemolytic uremic syndrome: a study of 78 additional patients. Transfusion 2003; 43:415–416.
44. Essein FA, Ojeda HF, Salameh JR, Baker KR, Rice L, Sweeney JF. Laparoscopic splenectomy for chronic recurrent thrombotic thrombocytopenic purpura. Surg Laparoscopic Endosc Percutaneous Tech 2003; 13:218–221.
45. Crowther MA, Heddle N, Hayward CPM, Warkentin T, Kelton JG. Splenectomy done during hematologic remission to prevent relapse in patients with thrombotic thrombocytopenic purpura. Ann Intern Med 1996; 125:294–296.
46. Zheng X, Pallera AM, Goodnough LT, Sadler JE, Blinder MA. Remission of chronic thrombotic thrombocytopenic purpura after treatment with cyclophosphamide and rituximab. Ann Intern Med 2003; 138:105–108.
47. Tsai H-M, Shulman K. Rituximab induces remission of cerebral ischemia caused by thrombotic thrombocytopenic purpura. Eur J Haematol 2003; 70:183–185.
48. Yomtovian R, Niklinski W, Silver B, Sarode R, Tsai HM. Rituximab for chronic recurring thrombotic thrombocytopenic purpura: a case report and review of the literature. Br J Haematol 2004; 787:795.
49. Gutterman LA, Kloster B, Tsai HM. Rituximab therapy for refractory thrombotic thrombocytopenic purpura. Blood Cells Mol Dis 2002; 28:385–391.
50. Chemnitz J, Draube A, Scheid C, et al. Successful treatment of severe thrombotic thrombocytopenic purpura with the monoclonal antibody rituximab. Am J Hematol 2002; 71:105–108.
51. Sallah S, Husain A, Wan JY, Nguyen NP. Rituximab in patients with refractory thrombotic thrombocytopenic purpura. J Thromb Haemost 2004; 2:834–836.

52. Fakhouri F, Teixeira L, Delarue R, Grunfeld JP, Veyradier JP. Responsiveness of thrombotic thrombocytopenic purpura to rituximab and cyclophosphamide. Ann Intern Med 2004; 140:314–315.
53. Stein GY, Zeidman A, Fradin Z, Varon M, Cohen A, Mittelman M. Treatment of resistant thrombotic thrombocytopenic purpura with rituximab and cyclophosphamide. Int J Haematol 2004; 80:94–96.
54. Ahmad A, Aggarwal A, Sharma D, et al. Rituximab for treatment of refractory/relapsing thrombotic thrombocytopenic purpura (TTP). Am J Hematol 2004; 77:171–176.
55. Koulova L, Alexandrescu D, Dutcher JP, O'Boyle KP, Eapen S, Weirnik PH. Rituximab for the treatment of refractory idiopathic thrombocytopenic purpura (ITP) and thrombotic thrombocytopenic purpura (TTP): report of three cases. Am J Hematol 2005; 78:49–64.
56. Reddy PS, Deauna-Limayo D, Cook JD, et al. Rituximab in the treatment of relapsed thrombotic thrombocytopenic purpura. Ann Hematol 2005; 84:232–235.
57. Ruiz J, Koduri PR, Valdivieso M, Shah PC. Refractory post-pancreatitis thrombotic thrombocytopenic purpura: response to rituximab. Ann Haematol 2005; 84:267–268.
58. Fakhouri F, Vernant JP, Veyradier JP, et-al. Efficiency of curative and prophylactic treatment with rituximab in ADAMTS13 deficient-thrombotic thrombocytopenic purpura: a study of 11 cases. Blood 2005; 106:1932–1937.
59. Galbusera M, Bresin E, Noris M, et-al. Rituximab prevents recurrence of thrombotic thrombocytopenic purpura: a case report. Blood (epub April 2005).
60. Berns JS, Kaplan BS, Mackow RC, Hefter LG. Inherited hemolytic uremic syndrome in adults. Am J Kidney Dis 1992; XIX:331–334.
61. Neild G. The haemolytic uraemic syndrome: a review. Q J Med 1987; 241:367–376.
62. Taylor CM. Hemolytic uremic syndrome and complement factor H deficiency: clinical aspects. Semin Thromb Haemost 2001; 27:185–190.
63. Pichette V, Querin S, Schurch W, Brun G, Lehner-Netsch G, Delage JM. Familial hemolytic uremic syndrome and homozygous factor H deficiency. Am J Kidney Dis 1994; 24:936–941.
64. Warwicker P, Donne RL, Goodship JA, et al. Familial relapsing haemolytic uraemic syndrome and complement factor H deficiency. Nephrol Dial Transplant 1999; 14:1229–1233.
65. Gerber A, Kirchoff-Moradpour AH, Obieglo S, et al. Successful (?) therapy of hemolytic-uremic syndrome with factor H abnormality Pediatr Nephrol 2003; 18:952–955.
66. Remuzzi G, Ruggenenti P, Codazzi D, et al. Combined kidney and liver transplantation for familial haemolytic uraemic syndrome. Lancet 2002; 359:1671–1672.
67. Donne RL, Abbs I, Barany P, et al. Recurrence of hemolytic uremic syndrome after live related renal transplantation associated with subsequent de novo disease in the donor. Am J Kidney Dis 2002; 40:E22.
68. Remuzzi G. The hemolytic uremic syndrome. Kidney Int 1995; 47:2–19.
69. Griffin PM, Tauxe RV. The epidemiology of infections caused by *E. Coli* 0157:H7, other enterohemorrhagic *E Coli*, and the associated hemolytic uremic syndrome. Epidemiol Rev 1991; 13:60–98.

70. Banatvala N, Griffin PM, Greene KD, et al. Hemolytic Uremic Syndrome Study Investigators: The United States national prospective hemolytic uremic syndrome study: microbiologic, serologic, clinical and epidemiologic findings. J Inf Dis 2001; 183:1063–1070.
71. Acheson DWK, Wolf LE, Park CH. *Escherichia coli* and the hemolytic uremic syndrome. N Engl J Med 1997; 336:515.
72. Karmali MA, Steele BT, Petrie M, Lim C. Sporadic cases of haemolytic uraemic syndrome associated with faecal cytotoxin and cytotoxin producing Escherichia coli in stools. Lancet 1983;619–620.
73. Gianvita A, Tozzi AE, De Petris L, et al. Risk factors for poor renal prognosis in children with hemolytic uremic syndrome. Pediatr Nephrol 2003; 18:1229–1235.
74. Lindberg AA, Brown E, Stromberg N, Westling-Ryd M, Schultz JE, Karlsson KA. Identification of the carbohydrate receptor for shiga toxin produced by *Shigella dysenteriae* type 1. J Biol Chem 1987; 262:1779–1785.
75. Brigotti M, Alfieri R, Sestili P, et al. Damage to nuclear DNA induced by Shiga toxin 1 and ricin in human endothelial cells. FASEB J 2002; 16:365–372.
76. Obrig TG, Moran TP, Brown JE. The mode of action of Shiga toxin on peptide elongation of eukaryotic protein synthesis. Biochem J 1987; 244:287–294.
77. Obrig TG, Louise CB, Lingwood CA, Boyd B, Barley-Maloney L, Daniel TO. Endothelial heterogeneity in Shiga toxin receptors and responses. J Biol Chem 1993; 268:15484–15488.
78. Repetto HA. Epidemic hemolytic-uremic syndrome in children. Kidney Int 1997; 52:1708–1719.
79. Gagnadoux MF, Habib R, Gubler MC, Bacri JL, Broyer M. Long-term (15–25 years) outcome of childhood hemolytic–uremic syndrome. Clin Nephrol 1996; 46:39–41.
80. Gordjani N, Sutor AH, Zimmerhackl LB, Brandis M. Hemolytic uremic syndrome in childhood. Semin Thromb Hemost 1997; 23:281–293.
81. Gianvita A, Perna A, Caringella A, et al. Plasma exchange in children with hemolytic–uremic syndrome at risk of poor outcome. Am J Kidney Dis 1993; 22:264–266.
82. Safdar N, Said A, Gangnon E, Maki DG. Risk of hemolytic uremic syndrome after antibiotic treatment of *Escherichia coli* 0157:H7 enteritis: a meta analysis. J Am Med Assoc 2002; 288:966–1001.
83. Mølbak K, Mead PS, Griffin PM. Antimicrobial therapy in patients with *Escherichia coli* 0157:H7 infection. J Am Med Assoc 2003; 288:1014–1016.
84. McCrae KR, Sadler JE, Cines DB. Thrombotic thrombocytopenic purpura and the hemolytic uremic syndrome. In: Hoffman R, Benz EJ, Jr., Shattil SJ, et al., eds. Hematology: Basic Principles and Practice, 2005:2287–2304.
85. Galli FC, Damon LE, Tomlanovich SJ, Keith F, Chatterjee K, Demarco T. Cyclosporine-induced hemolytic uremic syndrome in a heart transplant recipient. J Heart Lung Transplant 1993; 12:440–444.
86. Dzik WH, Georgi BA, Khettry U, Jenkins RL. Cyclosporine-associated thrombotic thrombocytopenic purpura following liver transplantation—successful treatment with plasma exchange. Transplant 1987; 44:570–572.
87. Zent R, Katz A, Quaggin S, et al. Thrombotic microangiopathy in renal transplant recipients treated with cyclosporin A. Clin Nephrol 1997; 47:181–186.

88. Wolfe JA, McCann RL, Sanfilippo F. Cyclosporine-associated microangiopathy in renal transplantation: A severe but potentially reversible from of early graft injury. Transplant 1986; 41:541–543.
89. Zoja C, Furci L, Ghilardi F, Zilio P, Benigni A, Remuzzi G. Cyclosporin-induced endothelial cell injury. Lab Investig 1986; 55:455–462.
90. Quan A, Sullivan EK, Alexander SR. Recurrence of hemolytic uremic syndrome after renal transplantation in children: a report of the North American Pediatric Renal Transplant Cooperative Study. Transplant 2001; 72:742–745.
91. Lahlou A, Lang P, Charpentier B, et al. Hemolytic uremic syndrome. Recurrence after renal transplantation. Groupe Cooperatif de l'Ile-de-France (GCIF). Medicine 2000; 79:90–102.
92. Elliott MA, Nichols WL, Plumhoff EA, et al. Posttransplantation thrombotic thrombocytopenic purpura: a single-center experience and a contemporary review. Mayo Clin Proc 2003; 78:421–430.
93. Fuge R, Bird JM, Fraser A, et al. The clinical features, risk factors and outcome of thrombotic thrombocytopenic purpura occurring after bone marrow transplantation. Br J Haematol 2001; 113:58–64.
94. Roy V, Rizvi MA, Vesely SK, George JN. Thrombotic thrombocytopenic purpura-like syndromes following bone marrow transplantation: an analysis of associated conditions and clinical outcomes. Bone Marrow Transplant 2001; 27:641–646.
95. Moake JL, Byrnes JJ. Thrombotic microangiopathies associated with drugs and bone marrow transplantation. Hematol/Oncol Clin N Am 1996; 10:485–487.
96. Ruutu T, Hermans J, Niederwiser D, et al. EBMT Chronic Leukemia Working Party: thrombotic thrombocytopenic purpura after allogeneic stem cell transplantation: a survey of the European Group for Blood and Marrow Transplantation (EBMT). Br J Haematol 2002; 118:1112–1119.
97. Kwaan HC, Gordon LI. Thrombotic microangiopathy in the cancer patient. Acta Haematol 2001; 106:52–56.
98. Gordon LI, Kwaan HC. Cancer- and drug-associated thrombotic thrombocytopenic purpura and hemolytic uremic syndrome. Semin Hematol 1997; 34:140–147.
99. Amiral J. Antigens involved in heparin-induced thrombocytopenia. Semin Hematol 1999; 36:7–11.
100. Forman RB, Benkel SA, Novik Y, Tsai HM. Presence of ADAMTS13 activity in a patient with metastatic cancer and thrombotic microangiopathy. Acta Haematol 2003; 109:150–152.
101. Fuchs S, Clark JW, Ryan DP, et al. A phase II trial of gemcitabine in patients with advanced hepatocellular carcinoma. Cancer 2002; 94:3186–3191.
102. von Baeyer H. Plasmapheresis in thrombotic microangiopathy-associated syndromes: review of outcome data derived from clinical trials and open studies. Ther Apheresis 2002; 6:320–328.
103. Snyder HW, Jr., Mittelman A, Oral A, et al. Treatment of cancer chemotherapy-associated thrombotic thrombocytopenic purpura/hemolytic uremic syndrome by protein A immunoadsorption of plasma. Cancer 1993; 71:1882–1892.
104. Gottschall JL, Elliott W, Lianos E, McFarland JG, Wolfmeyer K, Aster RH. Quinine-induced immune thrombocytopenia associated with hemolytic uremic syndrome: a new clinical entity. Blood 1991; 77:306–310.

105. Gottschall JL, Neahring B, McFarland JG, Wu GG, Weitekamp LA, Aster RA. Quinine-induced immune thrombocytopenia with hemolytic uremic syndrome: clinical and serological findings in nine patients and review of literature. Am J Hematol 1994; 47:283–289.
106. Kojouri K, Vesely SK, George JN. Quinine-associated thrombotic thrombocytopenic purpura-hemolytic uremic syndrome: frequency, clinical features, and long term outcomes. Ann Intern Med 2001; 135:1047–1051.
107. Tsai H-M, Rice L, Sarode R, Chow TW, Moake JL. Antibody inhibitors to von Willebrand factor metalloproteinase and increased binding of von Willebrand factor to platelets in ticlopidine-associated thrombotic thrombocytopenic purpura. Ann Intern Med 2000; 132:794–799.
108. Ucar A, Fernandez HF, Byrnes JJ, Lian ECY, Harrington WJ. Thrombotic microangiopathy and retroviral infections: a 13 year experience. Am J Hematol 1994; 45:304–309.
109. Hymes KB, Karpatkin S. Human immunodeficiency virus infection and thrombotic microangiopathy. Semin Hematol 1997; 34:117–125.
110. Perkocha LA, Rodgers GM. Hematologic aspects of human immunodeficiency virus infection: laboratory and clinical considerations. Am J Hematol 1988; 29:94–105.
111. Gruszecki AC, Wehrli G, Ragland BD, et al. Management of a patient with HIV infection-induced anemia and thrombocytopenia who presented with thrombotic thrombocytopenic purpura. Am J Hematol 2002; 69:228–231.
112. Zheng X, Chung D, Takayama TK, et al. Structure of von Willebrand factor-cleaving protease (ADAMTS13), a metalloprotease involved in thrombotic thrombocytopenic purpura. J Biol Chem 2001; 276:41059.

11

Thrombocytopenia in Pregnancy

Keith R. McCrae

Division of Hematology-Oncology, Department of Medicine, Case Western Reserve University School of Medicine/University Hospitals of Cleveland, Cleveland, Ohio, U.S.A.

INTRODUCTION

In uncomplicated pregnancies, the platelet count decreases by an average of 10% by term, though most pregnant patients do not become thrombocytopenic (defined as a platelet count below 150,000/μl) (1). However, in approximately 7% of pregnant individuals, the platelet count falls below this threshold, making thrombocytopenia the second most common hematologic complication of pregnancy, following anemia (2). A wide array of disorders, listed in Table 1, may cause thrombocytopenia in pregnant patients, and the clinical manifestations of some of these overlap so extensively that it may be difficult, if not impossible, to distinguish them. Nevertheless, since the management of pregnancy-associated thrombocytopenia is dependent upon defining its cause as accurately as possible, familiarity with the more common causes of thrombocytopenia in this population is essential for physicians who care for pregnant patients. In this review, we provide an overview of these disorders. For additional discussion of pregnancy-associated thrombocytopenia, the reader is referred to recent reviews (3–8).

CAUSES OF THROMBOCYTOPENIA IN PREGNANCY

Gestational Thrombocytopenia

Gestational or "incidental" thrombocytopenia is the most common cause of thrombocytopenia in pregnancy, affecting almost 6% of pregnant women and

Table 1 Causes of Thrombocytopenia in Pregnancy

Pregnancy-specific	Not pregnancy-specific
Gestational (incidental) thrombocytopenia	Immune thrombocytopenic purpura
Preeclampsia	Thrombotic microangiopathies
HELLP syndrome	Thrombotic thrombocytopenic purpura
Acute fatty liver of pregnancy	Hemolytic uremic syndrome
	Systemic lupus erythematosus
	Viral infection (HIV, CMV, EBV)
	Antiphospholipid antibodies
	Disseminated intravascular coagulation
	Bone marrow dysfunction
	Nutritional deficiencies
	Drug-induced thrombocytopenia
	Type IIb von Willebrand disease
	Congenital
	Hypersplenism

accounting for at least 75% of cases of pregnancy-associated thrombocytopenia (2,6,9–11). Women with this disorder usually develop mild thrombocytopenia in the late second or third trimester, with platelet counts remaining above ~110,000/μl, and by definition above ~70,000/μl. Patients with gestational thrombocytopenia are otherwise healthy, with no history of immune thrombocytopenic purpura (ITP) or other autoimmune disorders. The pathogenesis of gestational thrombocytopenia may involve hemodilution and/or accelerated platelet clearance in the placental circulation (9,11). Patients with gestational thrombocytopenia are not at increased risk for poor pregnancy outcomes or delivery of thrombocytopenic offspring (2,6,9–12), and for this reason, evaluation of an otherwise healthy pregnant woman with mild thrombocytopenia occurring beyond the mid second trimester may be limited to careful assessment for the presence of hypertension and/or proteinuria (13). A cardinal feature of gestational thrombocytopenia is that unlike many cases of ITP, it remits spontaneously following delivery.

Immune Thrombocytopenia Purpura

ITP is characterized by the presence of circulating antiplatelet antibodies that cause accelerated clearance of platelets by the reticuloendothelial system, primarily the spleen (14), though diminished platelet production may also contribute in some patients (15,16). ITP affects approximately one of every 1000 pregnancies, accounts for 5% of cases of pregnancy-associated thrombocytopenia, and is the most common cause of isolated thrombocytopenia in the first trimester (3,6,11,15). A history of prior thrombocytopenia, autoimmune disease or severe thrombocytopenia (platelet count <50,000/μl) makes the diagnosis of ITP more likely (18). Contemporary antiplatelet glycoprotein antibody assays, though not commonly employed and relatively insensitive, may be diagnostically useful if positive (14).

Cases of ITP associated with mild thrombocytopenia may be indistinguishable from gestational thrombocytopenia. Routine laboratory testing is not helpful in discerning these disorders. Though ITP may occur at any time during pregnancy, from a practical perspective a platelet count below 100,000/μl in the first trimester, with continued decline as pregnancy progresses, is most consistent with this disorder (19), while mild thrombocytopenia developing in the second or third trimester that is not associated with hypertension or proteinuria usually results from gestational thrombocytopenia.

Therapy for pregnant patients with ITP should be dictated based on the maternal platelet count. Through the first and second trimesters, patients with a platelet count above 20,000–30,000/μl, who are not bleeding, do not require treatment (13,20). As term approaches, more aggressive therapy may be indicated to raise the platelet count to a level that allows safe administration of epidural anesthesia and minimizes the risk of hemorrhage during delivery. Many experts consider a platelet count of >50,000/μl adequate for vaginal delivery, and some believe this sufficient for caesarean section as well. However, others recommend a higher platelet count (>80,000/μl), particularly if epidural anesthesia is employed (8,13).

Though most physicians employ corticosteroids as first line therapy for ITP in pregnancy, these agents are associated with unique pregnancy-associated toxicities such as gestational diabetes, pregnancy-induced hypertension, and perhaps premature rupture of the fetal membranes (19). These considerations have led some to advocate the use of high dose (2 gm/kg) intravenous immunoglobulin as initial therapy for ITP pregnant women (17). However, though 70–80% of both pregnant and non-pregnant patients with ITP respond to IVIg, these responses are often transient, and multiple courses of therapy may be required to maintain an adequate platelet count. Thus, though the optimal first line therapy for ITP in pregnancy remains controversial, it is agreed that corticosteroids should be used judiciously, and IVIg considered if patients require prolonged therapy with an unacceptably high maintenance dose of corticosteroid (>7.5 mg/day of prednisone) (8). Intravenous anti-D has been used successfully and safely in a small number of Rh(D)-positive pregnant patients who have not been splenectomized (21). Presumably, complete adsorption of anti-D to circulating maternal red cells minimizes its transplacental passage, and thus its potential to cause immune hemolytic anemia in the fetus. However, a larger experience is required to unequivocally establish the safety of this agent in pregnancy (3).

Patients who fail to respond adequately to corticosteroids and/or IVIg are usually referred for splenectomy, which is associated with an initial response rate of 75–85% in pregnant and non-pregnant patients. The second trimester has been considered as the optimal time for splenectomy, as procedures earlier in pregnancy may be associated with a high incidence of premature labor, and at later points the surgical field may be obscured by the gravid uterus (8). However, it has recently been argued that the gestational age at which splenectomy is performed may not be as important as once believed (22), and hence the issue remains unsettled. Laparoscopic splenectomy may be performed safely during pregnancy.

In occasional patients, ITP proves refractory to corticosteroids, IVIg, and splenectomy. Some of these individuals may respond to high dose corticosteroids (methylprednisolone, 1 gm IV) and IVIg (2 gm/kg) in combination. For those with severe thrombocytopenia who do not respond to this approach, additional immunosuppressive and cytotoxic agents may be considered (8). Rituximab has been shown to induce complete or partial remissions in 50% of non-pregnant patients with ITP (23), but there is little experience with its use in pregnancy.

Due to the transplacental passage of antiplatelet antibodies, maternal ITP may cause fetal and neonatal thrombocytopenia. Approximately 10–20% of the offspring of mothers with ITP will be born with a platelet count <50,000/μl, and 5% will be severely thrombocytopenia with platelet counts <20,000/μl (24). However, in contrast to neonatal alloimmune thrombocytopenia, platelet counts rarely fall below 10,000/μl, and although 25–50% of severely thrombocytopenic neonates experience bleeding during delivery, intracranial hemorrhage is rare (<0.5%) (12). Unfortunately, there exists no non-invasive means to determine which neonates will be born thrombocytopenic, since neither the maternal platelet count nor the level of platelet-associated IgG predicts neonatal thrombocytopenia. The best predictor may be a history of neonatal thrombocytopenia in a sibling (19,25).

The inability to determine the fetal platelet count non-invasively has led to debate concerning the use of percutaneous umbilical cord blood sampling (PUBS) to determine the fetal platelet count, with the aim of delivering neonates with platelet counts <50,000/μl by caesarian section. PUBS is associated with a neonatal morbidity (bleeding and/or fetal bradycardia requiring emergent caesarean section) of 0–1%, which is equal to or greater than that of fetal intracranial hemorrhage during vaginal delivery (24). Moreover, though an irremediable low risk of fetal intracranial hemorrhage exists with any delivery method, there is no evidence that this risk is reduced by caesarean section (26). Based on this consideration, most perinatologists in the United States advocate the use of cesarean section for maternal indications only (27).

The actual risk of neonatal intracranial hemorrhage in the offspring of patients with ITP may be greatest in the first few days after delivery, as platelet counts may fall further during this period. Thus, close monitoring of the platelet count and treatment of worsening thrombocytopenia may be indicated in these children, and some authorities recommend routine cranial ultrasounds for severely thrombocytopenic infants (8).

Preeclampsia and the HELLP Syndrome

Preeclampsia affects 6–10% of all first pregnancies and remains a major cause of maternal morbidity and mortality (28,29). This disorder primarily affects nulliparas of less than 20 or greater than 30 years of age. The diagnostic criteria for preeclampsia include hypertension (blood pressure of $\geq$140/90 mmHg) and proteinuria ($\geq$300 mg/24 hr) developing after 20 weeks of gestation. Patients with severe preeclampsia have a higher blood pressure ($\geq$160/110 mmHg), more proteinuria ($\geq$5 g/24 hr), and/or a number of other manifestations (30). Eclampsia is defined by the occurrence of grand mal seizures in patients with preeclampsia. Both paternal and maternal genetic factors contribute to the development of preeclampsia (31). Recent reports also suggest an association of preeclampsia with genetic or acquired abnormalities that predispose to thrombosis, though this remains controversial.

Though the clinical manifestations of preeclampsia usually do not appear until the third trimester, the pathophysiology of this disorder involves deficient remodeling of the maternal uterine vasculature early in pregnancy (32). Resulting fetoplacental hypoxia presumably leads to the imbalanced production of vasoactive substances and enhanced lipid peroxidation that contribute to the endothelial dysfunction and platelet activation characteristic of preeclampsia.

Approximately 20–50% of patients with preeclampsia develop thrombocytopenia, the degree of which is usually proportional to the severity of disease (1). In some cases, thrombocytopenia may precede other manifestations of preeclampsia, and incipient preeclampsia must be considered in the differential diagnosis of isolated third trimester thrombocytopenia.

The HELLP (Hemolysis, Elevated Liver function tests, Low Platelets) syndrome is considered by some as a variant of preeclampsia, since it may develop in 20% of patients with severe preeclampsia (33). HELLP is defined by: (1) microangiopathic hemolytic anemia (MAHA), (2) SGOT >70 U/L, and (3) thrombocytopenia, with a platelet count below 100,000/µl (34). HELLP occurs most commonly in multiparous Caucasians greater than 25 years of age. Patients with HELLP characteristically present with right upper quadrant and epigastric pain, and may be mistakenly diagnosed with a primary gastrointestinal disorder, particularly since HELLP need not be accompanied by hypertension and/or proteinuria. Like preeclampsia, HELLP is associated with significant maternal and neonatal morbidity (35).

The offspring of patients with preeclampsia or HELLP may also have mild thrombocytopenia, though this may not develop until after delivery. The pathogenesis of neonatal thrombocytopenia in these individuals, though often attributable to routine causes such as sepsis, may involve impaired platelet production (1).

Management of preeclampsia or HELLP is usually supportive and focused on stabilizing the patient for definitive treatment—delivery of the fetus. Though some have argued for conservative management of mildly affected patients or patients of less than approximately 34 weeks gestation, the only reason to delay delivery in patients with severe preeclampsia or HELLP is to allow time for fetal lung maturation to occur after administration of betamethasone (28). Though platelet survival is reduced in these disorders, platelet transfusion may be used to temporarily raise the platelet count in order to allow epidural anesthesia and/or cesarean section, and antepartum corticosteroids may raise the platelet count in some individuals and enhance their candidacy for regional anesthesia (36). Disseminated intravascular coagulation (DIC) should be suspected in patients with bleeding from multiple sites, a prolonged prothrombin time, and elevated levels of fibrin(ogen) degradation products and/or decreased fibrinogen, and may be managed through judicious use of fresh frozen plasma. Significant hypofibrinogenemia is uncommon, but if present may be treated using cryoprecipitate. Though, by definition, preeclampsia or HELLP, and the associated thrombocytopenia remit within several days after delivery, occasional patients may experience worsening disease or develop these disorders post-partum. In such individuals who develop significant organ dysfunction and deteriorating clinical status, or in whom less severe illness continues to progress beyond the period of expected resolution, plasma exchange and/or corticosteroids may hasten improvement (37,38).

Thrombotic Thrombocytopenic Purpura (TTP) and the Hemolytic Uremic Syndrome (HUS)

The thrombotic microangiopathies TTP and HUS are characterized by MAHA and thrombocytopenia. These disorders are not specific to pregnancy, though their incidence appears to be increased in pregnant patients (4,39).

The classic pentad of symptoms associated with these syndromes includes MAHA, thrombocytopenia, neurologic dysfunction, fever, and renal failure. Classically, neurologic dysfunction is considered to be more common and severe in TTP, while renal failure is more prominent in HUS. While one study observed that the peak incidence of TTP occurred in the second trimester, other series have described its frequent development near term (5). HUS occurs primarily in the postpartum period (1). However, in some cases the manifestations of these disorders may overlap so extensively that they may be impossible to distinguish from one another and patients with otherwise unexplained MAHA and thrombocytopenia should be presumptively treated for TTP or HUS. These thrombotic microangiopathies may also be difficult if not impossible to distinguish from preeclampsia or HELLP, though careful consideration of specific clinical manifestations and laboratory results may be helpful (1).

Many cases of TTP are associated with deficiency of a specific protease, ADAMTS13, which cleaves von Willebrand factor (vWF). Patients with congenital TTP have a genetic basis for the deficiency (40), while many of those with acquired TTP may have antibodies against the protease (41,42). In either case, ultra-large vWF multimers with increased avidity for platelets may circulate, causing platelet agglutination in the microvasculature. In contrast to TTP, ADAMTS13 deficiency is uncommon in HUS. Though levels of ADAMTS13 decrease during normal pregnancy (43), whether this contributes to the increased incidence of TTP in pregnancy is uncertain (39).

Unlike preeclampsia and HELLP, delivery of the fetus does not lead to resolution of thrombotic microangiopathies. Approximately 90% of pregnant and non-pregnant patients with TTP respond to plasma exchange without undergoing therapeutic abortion. Plasma exchange is recommended for individuals with HUS as well, particularly in light of the difficulty distinguishing these disorders, though its efficacy in classical HUS appears to be lower than in TTP. Both TTP and HUS are associated with poor fetal outcomes, and even successfully-treated mothers with HUS suffer long term morbidity, including hypertension and renal insufficiency. The incidence with which TTP or HUS recurs in subsequent pregnancies is controversial, with estimates of 18–100% (44).

Other Causes of Pregnancy-Associated Thrombocytopenia

Other causes of pregnancy-associated thrombocytopenia, though uncommon, should be appreciated (1). Acute fatty liver of pregnancy is characterized by cholestatic liver dysfunction, hypoglycemia, diabetes insipidus, and decreased levels of antithrombin and fibrinogen. Thrombocytopenia is generally mild. DIC may cause thrombocytopenia in several pregnancy-related disorders, including retained fetal products, amniotic fluid embolism, and uterine rupture. HIV infection may induce thrombocytopenia through immune and non-immune mechanisms, and should be considered in patients with risk factors. Thrombocytopenia may complicate up to 25% of cases of systemic lupus erythematosus. Approximately 10% of patients with antiphospholipid antibodies develop thrombocytopenia, and some patients with these antibodies develop microangiopathic syndromes resembling TTP, HUS, or HELLP. Drug-induced thrombocytopenia must be considered in any thrombocytopenic patient exposed to a potential offending medication such as quinine, heparin or trimethoprim-sulfamethoxazole, among others. Congenital macrothrombocytopenias, such as the May-Hegglin anomaly, may occasionally escape recognition until adulthood—the presence of large platelets on the peripheral blood film should alert the clinician to the possibility of these disorders (45 46). Patients with type II von Willebrand disease express a mutant vWF molecule that causes agglutination and enhanced clearance of circulating platelets, and the increased levels of this protein that occur in pregnancy may lead to the development or worsening of thrombocytopenia (47). Primary hematologic disorders such as leukemias or myelodysplastic syndromes may occasionally present with isolated thrombocytopenia, and patients with chronic liver disease leading to portal hypertension may sequester platelets in the spleen. Finally, while uncommon in the United States, deficiencies of nutrients such as vitamin B12 and folic acid may lead to pancytopenia in pregnant patients.

REFERENCES

1. McCrae KR. Thrombocytopenia in pregnancy: differential diagnosis, pathogenesis and management. Blood Rev 2003; 17:7–14.
2. Burrows RF, Kelton JG. Thrombocytopenia at delivery: a prospective survey of 6715 deliveries. Am J Obstet Gynecol 1990; 162:731–734.
3. McCrae KR, Bussel JB, Mannucci PM, Remuzzi G, Cines DB. Platelets: an update on diagnosis and management of thrombocytopenic disorders. Hematology (Am Soc Hematol Educ Program) 2001;282–305.
4. McCrae KR, Cines DB. Thrombotic microangiopathy during pregnancy. Sem Hematol 1997; 34:148–158.
5. McMinn JR, George JN. Evaluation of women with clinically suspected thrombotic thrombocytopenic purpura-hemolytic uremic syndrome during pregnancy. J Clin Apheresis 2001; 16:202–209.
6. Crowther MA, Burrows RF, Ginsberg J, Kelton JG. Thrombocytopenia in pregnancy: diagnosis, pathogenesis and managment. Blood Rev 1996; 10:8–18.
7. Kelton JG. Idiopathic thrornbocytopenic purpura complicating pregnancy. Blood Rev 2002; 16:43–46.
8. Provan D, Newland A, Norfolk D, et al. Guidelines for the investigation and managment of idiopathic thrombocytopenic purpura in adults, children and in pregnancy. Br J Haematol 2003; 120:574–596.
9. Shehata N, Burrows RF, Kelton JG. Gestational thrombocytopenia. Clin Obstet Gynecol 1999; 42:327–334.
10. Burrows RF, Kelton JG. Incidentally detected thrombocytopenia in healthy mothers and their infants. N Engl J Med 1988; 319:142–145.
11. McCrae KR, Samuels P, Schreiber AD. Pregnancy-associated thrombocytopenia: pathogenesis and management. Blood 1992; 80:2697–2714.
12. Burrows RF, Kelton JG. Fetal thrombocytopenia and its relation to maternal thrombocytopenia. N Engl J Med 1993; 329:1463–1466.
13. Letsky EA, Greaves M. Guidelines on the investigation and management of thrombocytopenia in pregnancy and neonatal alloimmune thrombocytopenia. Br J Haematol 1996; 95:21–36.
14. Cines DB, Blanchette VS. Immune thrombocytopenic purpura. N Engl J Med 2002; 346:13–995.
15. Chang M, Nakagawa PA, Williams SA, et al. Immune thrombocytopenic purpura (ITP) plasma and purified ITP monoclonal autoantibodies inhibit megakaryocytopoiesis in vitro. Blood 2003; 102:887–895.
16. McMillan R, Wang L, Tomer A, Nichol J, Pistillo J. Suppression of in vitro megakaryocyte production by antiplatelet autoantibodies from adult patients with chronic ITP. Blood 2004; 103:1364–1369.
17. Gill KK, Kelton JG. Management of idiopathic thrombocytopenic purpura in pregnancy. Sem Hematol 2000; 37:275–283.
18. Webert KE, Mittal R, Siguoin C, Heddle NM, Kelton JG. A retrospective 11-year analysis of obstetric patients with idiopathic thromobocytopenic purpura. Blood 2003; 102:4306–4311.
19. Fujimura K, Harada Y, Fujimoto T, et al. Nationwide study of idiopathic thrombocytopenic purpura in pregnant women and the clinical influence on neonates. Int J Haematol 2002; 75:426–433.

20. George JN, Woolf SH, Raskob GE, et al. Idiopathic thrombocytopenic purpura: a practice guideline developed by explicit methods for the American Society of Hematology. Blood 1996; 88:3–40.
21. Michel M, Novoa MV, Bussel JB. Intravenous anti-D as a treatment for immune thrombocytopenic purpura (ITP) during pregnancy. Br J Haematol 2003; 123:142–146.
22. Gottlieb P, Axelsson O, Bakos O, Rastad J. Splenectomy during pregnancy: an option in the treatment of autoimmune thrombocytopenic purpura. Br J Obstet Gynaecol 1999; 106:373–375.
23. Cooper N, Stasi R, Cunningham-Rundles S, et al. The efficacy and safety of B-cell depletion with anti-CD20 monoclonal antibody in adults with chronic immune thrombocytopenic purpura. Br J Haematol 2004; 125:232–239.
24. Burrows RF, Kelton JG. Pregnancy in patients with idiopathic thrombocytopenic purpura: assessing the risks for the infant at delivery. Obst Gynecol Surv 1993; 48:781–788.
25. Godelieve C, Christiaens ML, Nieuwenhuis HK, Bussel JB. Comparison of platelet counts in first and second newborns of mothers with immune thrombocytopenic purpura. Obstet Gynecol 1997; 90:546–552.
26. Payne SD, Resnik R, Moore TR, Hedriana HL, Kelly TF. Maternal characteristics and risk of severe neonatal thrombocytopenia and intracranial hemorrhage in pregnancies complicated by autoimmune thrombocytopenia. Am J Obstet Gynecol 1997; 177:149–155.
27. Peleg D, Hunter SK. Perinatal management of women with immune thrombocytopenic purpura: survey of United States perinatologists. Am J Obstet Gynecol 1999; 180:645–650.
28. Lain KY, Roberts JM. Contemporary concepts of the pathogenesis and management of preeclampsia. J Am Med Assoc 2002; 287:3183–3186.
29. Zhang J, Meikle S, Trumblc A. Severe maternal morbidity associated with hypertensive disorders in pregnancy in the United States. Hypertens Preg 2003; 2003:203–212.
30. American College of Obstetrics and Gynecology. ACOG practice bulletin: diagnosis and management of preeclampsia in pregnancy. Obstet Gynecol 2002; 99:159–167.
31. Esplin MS, Fausett MB, Fraser A, et al. Paternal and materal components of the predisposition to preeclampsia. N Engl J Med 2001; 344:867–872.
32. Goldman-Wohl D, Yagel S. Regulation of trophoblast invasion: from normal implantation to preeclampsia. Mol Cell Endocrinol 2002; 187:233–238.
33. Curtin WM, Weinstein L. A review of the HELLP syndrome. J Perinatol 1999; 19:138–143.
34. Sibai BM. The HELLP syndrome (hemolysis, elevated liver enzymes, and low platelets): Much ado about nothing? Am J Obstet Gynecol 1990; 162:311–316.
35. Sibai BM. Diagnosis, controversies and management of the syndrome of hemolysis, elevated liver enzymes, and low platelet count. Obstet Gynecol 2004; 103:981–991.
36. Rose CH, Thigpen BD, Bofill JA, Cushman J, May WL, Martin JN, Jr. Obstetric implications of antepartum corticosteroid therapy for HELLP syndrome. Obstet Gynecol 2004; 104:1011–1014.

37. Martin JN, Jr., Perry KG, Blake PG, May WA, Moore A, Robinette L. Better maternal outcomes are achieved with dexamethasone therapy for postpartum HELLP (hemolysis, elevated liver enzymes, and thrombocytopenia) syndrome. Am J Obstet Gynecol 1997; 177:1011–1017.
38. Martin JN, Jr., Files JC, Blake PG, Perry KG, Jr., Morrison JC, Norman PH. Postpartum plasma exchange for atypical preeclampsia-eclampsia as HELLP (hemolysis, elevated liver enzymes and low platelets syndrome). Am J Obstet Gynecol 1995; 172:1107–1112.
39. George JN. The association of pregnancy with thrombotic thrombocytopenic purpura-hemolytic uremic syndrome. Curr Opin Hematol 2003; 10:339–344.
40. Levy GG, Nichols WC, Lian EC, et al. Mutations in a member of the ADAMTS gene family cause thrombotic thrombocytopenic purpura. Nature 2001; 413:488–494.
41. Furlan M, Robles R, Galbusera M, et al. von Willebrand factor-cleaving protease in thrombotic thrombocytopenic purpura and the hemolytic-uremic syndrome. N Engl J Med 1998; 339:1578–1584.
42. Tsai H-M, Lian ECY. Antibodies to von Willebrand factor-cleaving protease in acute thrombotic thrombocytopenic purpura. N Engl J Med 1998; 339:1585–1594.
43. Mannucci PM, Canciani T, Forza I, Lussana F, Lattuada A, Rossi E. Changes in health and disease of the metalloprotease that cleaves von Willebrand factor. Blood 2001; 98:2730–2735.
44. Vesely SK, McMinn JR, Terrell DR, George JN. Pregnancy outcomes after recovery from thrombotic thrombocytopenic purpura-hemolytic uremic syndrome. Transfusion 2004; 44:1149–1158.
45. Cines DB, Bussel JB, McMillan RB, Zehnder JL. Congenital and acquired thrombocytopenia. Hematology (Am Soc Hematol Educ Program) 2004;390–406.
46. Ramasamy I. Inherited bleeding disorders: disorders of platelet adhesion and aggregation. Crit Rev Oncol Hematol 2004; 49:1–35.
47. Hepner DL, Tsen LC. Severe thrombocytopenia, type 2B von Willebrand disease and pregnancy. Anesthesiol 2004; 101:1465–1467.

12

Platelet Transfusion: Indications and Adverse Effects

Janice McFarland
Department of Pathology and Medicine, Medical College of Wisconsin, and BloodCenter of Wisconsin, Milwaukee, Wisconsin, U.S.A.

INTRODUCTION

The beneficial effect of platelets in the control and prevention of thrombocytopenic hemorrhage was first noted early in the last century. In 1910, Duke showed that the platelets contained in transfused whole blood decreased the bleeding time and controlled bleeding (1). In 1962 Gaydos et al. first documented the relationship between platelet count and hemorrhage in patients with leukemia (2). Hemorrhage was not observed until the platelet count fell to less than 50,000/ul and at counts under 5000/ul, 90% of patients had some form of bleeding. Slichter later showed that blood loss in stable patients with aplastic anemia accelerated only when the count fell to less than 10,000/ul, and markedly increased at counts under 5000/ul (3).

The demonstration that the platelet count was inversely related to the risk of hemorrhage led to the practice of infusing platelet-rich plasma and later, platelet concentrates (PCs), in order to increase the platelet count in thrombocytopenic patients. A number of observational studies, some utilizing autopsy data from patients who died of acute leukemia, found that morbidity or death due to hemorrhage was significantly more common among patients who did not receive platelet transfusion therapy compared to those who did (4–6).

In the five decades since platelet levels were recognized to be important in preventing hemorrhage, the practice of platelet transfusion has developed into an essential part of treating patients whose diseases or associated treatments cause severe reductions in either the numbers or function of circulating platelets. This chapter will review available platelet products, address the currently accepted indications and contraindications for both therapeutic and prophylactic platelet transfusions, and provide guidance for acceptable platelet transfusion practice. Finally, adverse events associated with platelet transfusions will be discussed.

PLATELET PRODUCTS

Preparations of platelets for transfusions are available either as pools of PCs derived from whole blood donations from several different donors or as platelets collected from single donors using apheresis techniques.

Whole Blood–Derived Platelet Concentrates

In the United States, these platelet products are prepared from whole blood donations using the platelet rich plasma (PRP) method (7). In the PRP method, 450–500 mL of citrate-anticoagulated whole blood is separated into PRP and red cells (containing the buffy coat) using low speed centrifugation. The PRP is further separated into a platelet pellet and platelet poor plasma (PPP) using a high-speed centrifugation step. About 50 mL of the PPP is re-added to the platelet pellet, which is then resuspended after a 1–2 hour rest, and constitutes the PC. The PCs derived from individual units of whole blood are stored at 22°C with constant gentle agitation. A longstanding FDA requirement is that PCs be produced using a method that results in a product having a minimum of 5.5×10^{10} platelets, as established by periodic quality control measurements. As a result of improvements in production techniques and equipment, however, a typical PC manufactured today (2004) contains $8.0–9.0 \times 10^{10}$ platelets (7). The PRP method results in a product with roughly between 1 and 5×10^{8} contaminating white blood cells (WBC) which may cause adverse events in the recipient including non-hemolytic febrile transfusion reactions (NHFTRs), alloimmunization to HLA antigens, or CMV infection (see below). While a single PC may provide a sufficient dose of platelets for an infant or small child, generally several (4–6) PCs must be pooled together to provide an adequate dose for an adult patient.

Advantages of PCs include efficiency of manufacture in that they are in essence a by-product of whole blood collections, and lower cost of production compared to apheresis products. Disadvantages are that they must be pooled in order to provide an adequate dose for most patients, thereby increasing donor exposures and risk of viral transmissions and alloimmunization. Additionally, these products contain large numbers of contaminating WBC that can cause FNHTRs, alloimmunization and CMV infection in susceptible patients. WBC reduction is possible, but is costly when each individual PC is filtered prior to storage and pooling. Alternatively, filtration to remove leucocytes can be performed after pooling of the PCs, but this shortens the shelf life of the component to four hours if done using open system techniques. Moreover, post pooling filtration may result in the loss of about 20% of the platelet content of the product, reducing the number of platelets ultimately available to the patient (8).

Apheresis Platelet Concentrates

Large numbers of platelets can be collected from a single donor using an apheresis device. The FDA requires that an apheresis product contain at least 3.0×10^{11} platelets, a dose equivalent to a pool of four PCs, using recent quality control data from U.S. blood product manufacturers. The apheresis devices available today can collect as many as 12×10^{11} platelets from a single donor, depending on the donor's platelet count and the volume of blood processed in the device. Many blood suppliers "split" such collections into two or three products that can be issued to as many different patients.

Many of the shortcomings of whole blood–derived PCs are overcome with apheresis platelets. The latter offer the advantage of collecting large doses of platelets from single donors, thereby reducing donor exposures to recipients and risks of viral transmission and alloimmunization. Moreover, the technologies used today allow integral WBC reduction steps to be taken such that high yield, leukocyte-reduced products are routinely produced. Disadvantages include the cost of the product (usually at least about 50% greater than equivalent doses of non-leukocyte-reduced PCs), and the need to recruit donors to undergo the 1–2 hour procedure—a greater time commitment than for donating whole blood.

Despite their drawbacks (cost and donor inconvenience), apheresis platelets have become the dominant platelet product produced by blood suppliers in the US, comprising 62% of all platelet transfusions given according to a recent nationwide survey (9).

Platelet Storage

Both PCs and apheresis platelets can be stored for up to five days at room temperature. Although viability of platelets stored for up to seven days in current bag systems has been demonstrated, the risk of bacterial contamination has prevented blood component manufacturers from extending the storage period for either product beyond five days. In the future, monitoring of platelet products for bacterial contamination (see below), methods for viral and bacterial inactivation, and development of plasma-free platelet storage solutions will likely result in the ability to store viable platelet products for much longer periods (10–12).

Modification of Platelet Products

Leukocyte Reduction of Platelet Products

Contaminating leukocytes are responsible for many of the adverse effects associated with platelet transfusion. These complications include FNHTRs, alloimmunization to HLA antigens, and CMV infection. Preceded by European programs of universal leukodepletion of blood products, many U.S. blood providers established programs to achieve similar goals in the late 1990's. In order for products to be labeled leukocyte-reduced, the FDA requires that fewer than 5.0×10^6 contaminating WBC be present. The FDA can license only leukoreduced *apheresis* platelets for shipment across state lines. Currently accepted indications for leukocyte-reduced platelets are: (1) for the prevention of FNHTRs, (2) for the prevention or reduction of alloimmunization (to HLA), and (3) to reduce the risk of CMV transmission in susceptible patients. The latter include low birth weight infants ($<$ 1200 gms), patients with compromised immune systems secondary to either hematopoietic stem cell transplantation (HSCT) or solid organ transplantation, and those with severe congenital immunodeficiency syndromes (e.g., SCID, Wiscott-Aldrich syndrome).

Volume-Reduced Platelet Products

The typical volume of a pool of 4–6 PCs is about 200–300 mL while the volume of a single donor apheresis platelet collection can range from 200–400 mL. An optimal platelet storage environment (in plasma) is dependent on adequate oxygen entering the bag, bicarbonate, and substrate to maintain oxidative metabolism and minimize glycolysis (7,12). Plasma can be removed from the product before issuing for transfusion. This requires centrifugation and resuspension of the platelets. Such volume-reduced products are sometimes required for patients with congestive heart failure, severe renal failure, or in small children.

A special circumstance in which platelet product modification is required is the collection of maternal platelets for transfusion to an infant who has neonatal alloimmune thrombocytopenia (NATP). In this case, plasma is removed from the apheresis platelet product in order to reduce the amount of maternal antiplatelet antibody. A common procedure involves centrifugation of the platelets and expression of the plasma, followed by resuspension of the platelets in normal saline. The procedure is repeated and the platelets issued at a concentration of approximately 10^9/mL, resuspended in saline (13).

Gamma Irradiation

Transfusion-induced graft-vs-host disease (GVHD) is a rare complication of blood component transfusion and can be prevented by treating the component with gamma irradiation in order to inactivate donor T-lymphocytes. The current standard for this treatment is to deliver 25 Gy to the midplane of the component (14). Platelets appear to be radio-tolerant, as in vitro measures of platelet function and in vivo recovery and survival are not significantly affected by 50 Gy of gamma irradiation (15). Patients with severe congenital or acquired immunodeficiency states are at risk of transfusion-induced GVHD. In addition, immunologically normal recipients of blood products from blood relatives or HLA matched donors are also at risk for this complication due to the patient's immune system being unable to recognize closely HLA-matched donor lymphocytes as foreign. Therefore, all blood products that may contain even very low levels of WBC (e.g., leukocyte-reduced blood products) should be irradiated for these patients.

Testing for Bacterial Contamination

A recent addition to the required processing of platelet products is demonstration that they are free of contaminating bacteria after collection. For single donor apheresis platelets, aliquots can be collected in a sterile manner at 24 hours after collection and submitted to automated culture systems, e.g., Bac-T-ALERT (Organon Teknika, Durham, NC). After a further 12-24 hours, products linked to aliquots in which there is no evidence of growth can be released for transfusion. In the first year that this requirement was in effect, the rate of detection of bacteria in apheresis platelet components was one in 1000 to one in 3000 (16). Due to the smaller volume of PCs and the fact that they must be pooled together prior to transfusion to a patient, measures to assure sterility in these products have lagged behind those used for apheresis platelets.

INDICATIONS FOR PLATELET TRANSFUSIONS

Therapeutic Platelet Transfusions

In 1986, an NIH-sponsored consensus development conference determined that at platelet counts of 50,000/ul or greater, bleeding is unlikely to be caused by thrombocytopenia (17), while severe, life-threatening hemorrhage is a risk when the count is under 5000/ul. Between 5000/ul and 10,000/ul, there is an increased risk of spontaneous hemorrhage. Between 10,000/ul and 50,000/ul, there is an increased risk of hemorrhage during hemostatic challenges. Similar conclusions were reached at a conference held in the United Kingdom a decade later (18,19).

Active bleeding occurring in patients with platelet counts lower than 50,000/ul is therefore appropriately addressed with platelet transfusions. In the presence of platelet function defects or serious structural lesions, particularly in the CNS, platelet transfusions may also be appropriate at higher platelet count levels.

Prophylactic Platelet Transfusions

Today, most platelet transfusions are administered not to patients who are actively bleeding, but to those who, by virtue of their low platelet counts, are judged to be *at risk* of bleeding. The majority of prophylactic platelet transfusions are given to patients with hematologic or oncologic disorders whose thrombocytopenia is either disease- and/or treatment-related. Another common feature of patients treated with prophylactic transfusions is that the thrombocytopenia is expected to be temporary, if treatment for the underlying disease is successful.

Common clinical practice is to transfuse platelets when the platelet count is at or below a given threshold, formerly 20,000 platelets/uL and more recently

10,000 platelets/uL, in order to prevent spontaneous hemorrhage. Despite its widespread use, however, the practice of prophylactic platelet transfusion has never been shown in randomized controlled clinical trials to be superior to therapeutic platelet transfusion when significant bleeding, or death due to bleeding, have been the outcomes assessed (20,21).

DISEASES IN WHICH PLATELET TRANSFUSIONS ARE INDICATED

Thrombocytopenia

The normal circulating platelet count in the adult is between 150,000 and 450,000 platelets/uL. When platelet counts fall under 50,000/uL, mild bleeding symptoms and signs are common. These include petechial rashes in dependent areas of the body as well as minor epistaxis and gum bleeding with tooth brushing. Patients may also note increased easy bruising with minor trauma. When the platelet count is less than 10,000/uL and certainly less than 5000/uL, the risk of spontaneous serious hemorrhage is increased (see above). More serious bleeding often manifests as hematuria, gastrointestinal hemorrhage, or CNS hemorrhage.

Hypoproliferative Thrombocytopenia (Disorders of Platelet Production)

Conditions in which the marrow's production of platelets is reduced are listed in Table 1. These can be categorized into three broad groups: congenital/familial thrombocytopenias, acquired (disease-related) thrombocytopenias, and treatment-related thrombocytopenia. In these conditions the thrombocytopenia is due largely to the failure to produce sufficient numbers of platelets to maintain

Table 1 Causes of Hypoproliferative Thrombocytopenia

Congenital/familial thrombocytopenia
Acquired thrombocytopenia
Space occupying lesions of the bone marrow
(1) Primary or secondary leukemias
(2) Myelodysplastic syndromes
(3) Metastatic carcinomas
(4) Infections (e.g., tuberculosis)
Diseases that suppress platelet production
(1) Viral infection (HIV, measles, mumps)
(2) Aplastic anemia
(3) Nutritional deficiencies (e.g., B12, folate)
Treatment-related thrombocytopenia
Chemotherapy for leukemia
Chemo-radio therapy for solid tumors
Conditioning therapy for hematopoietic stem cell transplantation (HSCT)

adequate peripheral blood platelet counts. In many patients more than one mechanism of depressed platelet production may be present. In the absence of alloimmunization to HLA antigens or conditions that cause accelerated clearance of circulating platelets, platelet transfusions in hypoproliferative thrombocytopenia should result in predictable platelet count increments and prevention or treatment of spontaneous hemorrhage.

Among congenital thrombocytopenias, patients with Wiskott-Aldrich syndrome, X-linked thrombocytopenia, May-Hegglin anomaly and other MYH9-related thrombocytopenias, Bernard-Soulier Syndrome (BSS), or thrombocytopenia with absent radii (TAR) syndrome, may require platelet transfusions to treat hemorrhage or to prevent bleeding during operative procedures. In general, such patients with life-long thrombocytopenia are not candidates for vigorous prophylactic platelet transfusions due to the eventual risk of alloimmunization and refractoriness to platelet transfusions.

Platelet transfusion therapy was initially attempted in patients with acute leukemia and aplastic anemia. Early studies demonstrated the benefit of treating active bleeding with platelet transfusions (4,5) and introduction of prophylactic platelet transfusions in such patients led to a marked reduction in major hemorrhage when platelet counts were less than 5000/uL. The clear benefit of prophylactic vs. therapeutic transfusions was less apparent at platelet counts higher than this level (5000–20,000/uL), however (22).

The advent of more potent anti-leukemic drugs, while improving the rates of complete remission in this disease, also meant longer periods of marrow aplasia requiring prolonged platelet transfusion support. In patients undergoing allogeneic HSCT for leukemia, the period of aplasia is typically between two and four weeks (23,24). Some patients with lymphoma or multiple myeloma are candidates for autologous HSCT, a procedure that results in a shorter period of aplasia and fewer platelet transfusions (24).

Disorders of Platelet Consumption

Disorders of platelet consumption result in the accelerated clearance of circulating platelets such that the patient is unable to maintain a normal peripheral blood platelet count level, despite increased production of platelets by the bone marrow (Table 2). These conditions can be divided into two broad categories: immune-mediated and non-immune-mediated. Immune-mediated platelet consumption occurs when an antibody(ies) reactive with autologous platelets is present and binds to the platelets. The antibody-coated platelets are sequestered via receptors in the reticulo-endothelial system (spleen, liver, bone marrow) and are destroyed. Immune-mediated platelet destruction occurs in acute and chronic idiopathic (autoimmune) thrombocytopenia (ITP) and in drug-induced thrombocytopenia due to drug-dependent platelet-reactive antibodies.

Generally, platelet transfusions, especially prophylactic transfusions, are contraindicated in both acute and chronic ITP. An exception is if life-threatening

Table 2 Diseases Causing Increased Platelet Consumption

Immune
Autoimmune thrombocytopenic purpura (ITP)
Post transfusion purpura (PTP)
Drug-induced immune thrombocytopenia
Non-immune
Disseminated intravascular coagulation (DIC)
Thrombotic thrombocytopenic purpura (TTP)
Infection
Hemangioma-thrombocytopenia (Kasabach-Merritt) syndrome
Severe burns
Turbulent circulation (cardiopulmonary bypass, severe aortic stenosis, etc.)

hemorrhage occurs, or in the context of splenectomy, particularly if the platelet transfusions can be withheld until after the splenic vessels are clamped. In cases in which the platelet count is severely depressed and/or bleeding symptoms are present and unresponsive to medical therapy, the provision of platelet transfusions after infusion of high dose intravenous immunoglobulin (IVIG) may allow a transient elevation of the platelet count so as to provide a margin of safety for completion of the operative procedure (25).

A special category of immune-mediated thrombocytopenia is post transfusion purpura (PTP). This syndrome is characterized by severe thrombocytopenia 5 to 10 days following a blood transfusion in a patient who has had a remote exposure to platelet antigens either through pregnancy or transfusion. Coincident with the severe thrombocytopenia (usually less than 10,000/uL) is the development of a potent platelet specific alloantibody, usually anti-HPA-1a (anti - Pl^{A1}). Subsequent platelet-typing of the patient demonstrates invariably that the patient lacks the platelet alloantigen to which the alloantibody is directed. Although PTP was first recognized nearly five decades ago, a consensus has developed only recently regarding the cause of autologous platelet destruction in this disease. Increasing evidence points to the development of a platelet autoantibody along with the alloantibody during the acute phase of the disease (26,27). With appropriate therapy (IVIG or plasma exchange), the patient's autologous platelets recover and only the alloantibody remains detectable. As is the case in ITP, platelet transfusions are generally not indicated, despite the severity of the thrombocytopenia. This recommendation is modified for impending or active serious hemorrhage, however. In this case, there is some evidence that while transfused platelet increments and survivals are severely reduced regardless of the platelet phenotype used, the transfusion of antigen negative platelets (e.g., HPA-1b/b) may afford somewhat better short term hemostasis than antigen positive transfusions (28,29).

Non-immune-mediated platelet consumption complicates many serious medical conditions and can be attributed to a number of etiologies. Disseminated intravascular coagulation (DIC) is a common complication arising in severe infection, trauma, or surgery in which there is abnormal exposure of the coagulation system to tissue factor, precipitating massive thrombin generation. This in turn consumes both clotting factors and platelets leading to a risk of hemorrhage, or alternatively, to thrombosis. In general, the appropriate therapy is to diagnose and treat the underlying disorder that is triggering the DIC. Hemostatic therapy, including platelet transfusion, should only be provided for active hemorrhage or severe threat of serious bleeding.

Thrombotic thrombocytopenia purpura (TTP) is a rare disease characterized by microangiopathic hemolytic anemia and thrombocytopenia. TTP is often, but not invariably, accompanied by fever, neurologic symptoms, or renal dysfunction. The pathogenesis relates to the formation of intravascular platelet thrombi that cause "shredding" of red cells as they pass through the affected small vessels. Prior to effective treatment, TTP was almost universally fatal. However, plasma exchange therapy now results in the majority of patients recovering, albeit with a significant rate of relapse (30). Although platelet count levels can be severely depressed in TTP, hemorrhage is, if anything, less common than one would expect at similar platelet count levels in other diseases. Platelet transfusions are generally not indicated, no matter how severe the thrombocytopenia in TTP since they may actually accelerate the process of intravascular thrombi formation (31,32). However, if severe, life-threatening hemorrhage occurs or threatens, particularly in the CNS, platelet transfusions should not be withheld. In a recent report, two patients with active TTP underwent plasma exchange followed by platelet transfusion prior to laparoscopic surgery, and both sustained a platelet count increment with neither hemorrhagic nor thrombotic complications (33).

A number of other clinical settings may be complicated by thrombocytopenia due to increased destruction of platelets, including pregnancy, preeclampsia, burns, ARDS, sepsis, cardiac valve lesions, intravascular prosthetics, and renal vein thrombosis. If hemorrhage occurs in these conditions, platelet transfusions should be considered, particularly if the platelet count is less than 50,000/ul.

Platelet count increments and the survival of transfused platelets given to treat thrombocytopenia due to consumptive platelet disorders are usually less than would be expected in patients whose thrombocytopenia is due to another mechanism since the same process indiscriminately clears both autologous and transfused platelets. It may be necessary to provide larger doses of platelets than would be given a patient without a consumptive process in order to achieve a hemostatic level.

Platelet Sequestration

A third broad cause of thrombocytopenia results from neither production nor destruction abnormalities, but from abnormal sequestration, usually in an enlarged spleen. In individuals with normal spleens, approximately one-third of circulating platelets are present in the splenic parenchyma at any one time. Normal platelet production compensates for this pool to maintain normal peripheral blood platelet counts between 150,000 and 450,000 platelets/uL.

A number of conditions can cause splenic sequestration to increase such that the normal platelet count range is no longer maintained (Table 3). While isolated hypersplenism rarely reduces platelet counts to a level at which either prophylactic or therapeutic platelet transfusions are required, in the presence of platelet production or destruction abnormalities, hypersplenism amplifies the severity of the thrombocytopenia and can necessitate such transfusions.

Disorders of Platelet Function

Disorders of platelet function can be divided into two groups: congenital and acquired. In these disorders, the platelets are often present at normal or near

Table 3 Causes of Splenomegaly and Hypersplenism

Splenomegaly with appropriate hypersplenism
Hereditary hemolytic anemias
Hereditary spherocytosis
Hereditary elliptocytosis
Thalassemia
Sickle cell anemia (infants)
Autoimmune cytopenia
Idiopathic (autoimmune) thrombocytopenia
Warm autoimmune hemolytic anemia
Infections and inflammation
Epstein-Barr virus (mononucleosis)
Subacute bacterial endocarditis
Miliary tuberculosis
Felty's syndrome
Systemic lupus erythematosus
Sarcoidosis
Malaria
Splenomegaly with inappropriate hypersplenism
Congestion (Banti syndrome)
Cirrhosis of the liver with portal hypertension
Portal vein thrombosis
Splenic vein obstruction
Budd-Chiari syndrome
Congestive heart failure
Infiltrative diseases
Lymphomas
Agnogenic myeloid metaplasia
Leukemias, chronic and acute
Polycythemia Rubra Vera
Gaucher disease
Amyloidosis
Tumors and cysts

normal levels. If hemorrhagic signs and symptoms are present, these manifest as easy bruising, mucocutaneous hemorrhage (e.g., menorrhagia), or mucosal hemorrhage (gingival bleeding, epistaxis). Occasionally, severe disorders of platelet function require therapeutic or prophylactic platelet transfusion.

Congenital Disorders of Platelet Function

These platelet disorders are caused by a defect or deficiency in structures that are required for normal platelet adhesion, aggregation, or procoagulant activity (Table 4). Since these are life-long disorders, platelet transfusions should be reserved for therapeutic indications (i.e., active bleeding) or in some cases, as a preventative measure prior to surgery. The autosomal recessive conditions BSS and Glanzmann's thrombasthenia (GT) can result in severe hemorrhage. BSS is characterized by thrombocytopenia, large platelets and a reduction or absence of the GPIb-IX-V complex, which is the site of platelet interactions with von Willebrand factor (vWF) and is therefore essential for proper platelet adhesion. GT patients lack normal levels of the platelet glycoprotein (GP) IIb/IIIa complex, the receptor necessary for fibrinogen binding and key to platelet aggregation. A third platelet membrane defect, platelet type von Willebrand's Disease (vWD), features abnormal GPIb-vWF interactions such that normal levels of high

Table 4 Disorders of Platelet Function—Inherited and Acquired

Inherited (Congenital) Disorders of Platelet Function
Glycoprotein (GP) abnormalities
GPIIb/IIIa—Glanzmann thrombasthenia
GPIb,IX and V—Bernard-Soulier syndrome
GPIb—Platelet type von Willebrand disease
Granule disorders
Delta storage pool deficiency
Gray platelet syndrome (alpha-granules)
Alpha-delta storage pool deficiency
Abnormalities of platelet procoagulant activity
Abnormalities of signal transduction and secretion
Defects in arachidonic acid metabolism
Defects in thromboxane A2 sensitivity, calcium mobilization and calcium responsiveness
Disorders of Platelet Function—Acquired
Uremia
Cardiopulmonary bypass
Myeloproliferative disorders
Dysproteinemias
Drug-induced
Aspirin
Non-steroidal anti-inflammatory drugs
GPIIb/IIIa antagonists
Antibiotics

molecular weight vWF are depleted by interaction with the patient's circulating platelets. This leads to a mild bleeding disorder with a minimal to moderate reduction in the platelet count. Platelet transfusions are rarely indicated for treatment of bleeding in platelet type vWD.

Congenital platelet function defects in which platelet granules are affected can be separated into three groups, depending on the type of granules affected. Gray platelet syndrome is characterized by a deficiency of alpha granules. These granules are also deficient in Hermansky-Pudlak syndrome. In delta or dense granule deficiency, constituents of the dense granules, including ADP, ATP, serotonin, calcium, and phosphate are lacking. Platelets affected by alpha-delta storage pool deficiency lack constituents of both types of granules. These conditions are diagnosed by platelet aggregation studies and occasionally can be defined by electron microscopy. If severe bleeding symptoms are unresponsive to pharmacologic therapy (e.g., DDAVP®), platelet transfusions are an appropriate alternative therapy for platelet storage pool disorders.

Acquired Disorders of Platelet Function

Conditions in which platelet function is disturbed by disease or treatment are more common indications for platelet transfusion therapy than are congenital defects in platelet function (Table 4). Platelet dysfunction is most commonly due to medication, prostaglandin inhibitors such as aspirin (acetylsalicylic acid) being the most prominent example. Aspirin blocks thromboxane A2 synthesis by irreversibly acetylating cyclooxygenase. The latter is responsible for converting arachidonic acid to prostaglandin endoperoxides G2 and H2 (34). In vitro, platelet aggregation responses to epinephrine, ADP, collagen, and arachidonic acid are all reduced or eliminated when platelets have been exposed to aspirin. In contrast, the platelet function defects caused by other non-steroidal anti-inflammatory drugs (NSAIDs), while still mediated through effects on cyclooxygenase, are much milder and reversible (34).

A new class of drug that inhibit the function of the platelet GPIIb/IIIa complex, are extremely potent, causing effective paralysis of platelets in an irreversible manner. Examples of the latter are ticlopidine, abciximab, tirofiban, and eptifibatide. These drugs are useful as adjuncts to coronary angioplasty procedures and are particularly effective in preventing occlusions in coronary artery stents or in reconstructed vessels (35). A recently recognized adverse affect, however is severe thrombocytopenia due to drug-induced platelet-reactive antibodies that further complicate the bleeding risk caused by the drugs' effect on platelet function (36–38). In the event of bleeding occurring after exposure to a GPIIb/IIIa-inhibiting drug, with or without thrombocytopenia, platelet transfusions are indicated as first line therapy (38).

Uremia is an acquired condition in which platelet function is globally affected, with decreased adhesion, aggregation, and procoagulant activity. The risk of bleeding is further complicated by conditions often present in patients with renal failure, including anemia, thrombocytopenia, and the need for anticoagulation to maintain vascular access. The causes of the bleeding tendency in uremia are complex and not clearly related to the level of either serum creatinine or blood urea nitrogen (BUN). Other substances removed by dialysis such as guanidinosuccinic acid may have a greater impact on platelet dysfunction (39). The impact of anemia on bleeding should not be underestimated in uremia, and it appears that maintaining a hematocrit between 25% and 30% either by transfusion or erythropoietin can reduce bleeding (40). A higher hematocrit may displace platelets from the center of the vessel lumen to the periphery, resulting in increased exposure of platelets to the endothelium. Pharmacologic approaches to uremic bleeding such as DDAVP and conjugated estrogen should not be overlooked.

In contrast to congenital platelet function disorders and many drug-induced defects (e.g., aspirin), the platelet function defect caused by uremia affects both transfused as well as autologous platelets. Therefore, particularly in the absence of thrombocytopenia, platelet transfusions are unlikely to have a major impact on bleeding in uremia. Platelet transfusions should be reserved for bleeding symptoms refractory to pharmacologic approaches.

Cardiopulmonary bypass is a major clinical setting requiring platelet transfusions. The combination of medications (aspirin, GPIIb/IIIa inhibitors, heparin), the stress of the extracorporeal circuit, and induced hypothermia combine to cause both intraoperative and postoperative thrombocytopenia and platelet dysfunction. Excessive blood loss traced to microvascular bleeding not amenable to surgical correction is best addressed with platelet transfusions. Similar defects in platelet numbers and function are seen in neonates receiving extracorporeal membrane oxygenation (ECMO), and platelet transfusions are universally used in this setting as well.

A number of other medical conditions, including myeloproliferative disorders (CML, myelofibrosis, essential thrombocytosis, and polycythemia vera), acute leukemia, and dysproteinemias (e.g., multiple myeloma) are associated with multiple, often poorly characterized platelet function disorders. Because many of these conditions are also complicated by thrombocytopenia, the recognition of a defect in platelet function is often not straightforward. The severity of bleeding signs and symptoms out of proportion to the patient's platelet count (e.g., spontaneous hemorrhage at platelet counts above 20,000/ul) is an indication that a platelet function disorder is present in addition to thrombocytopenia. In this situation, provision of platelet transfusions at trigger levels higher than in patients who have thrombocytopenia without evidence of a platelet function disorder should be considered.

CONTRAINDICATIONS TO PLATELET TRANSFUSIONS

While active bleeding in the presence of thrombocytopenia, regardless of the cause, is usually an appropriate indication for transfusing platelets, in the absence of bleeding, platelet transfusions are contraindicated in a number of clinical settings in which even severe thrombocytopenia may be present. In general, platelet transfusions are not appropriate in cases of severe thrombocytopenia associated with states of accelerated platelet destruction, either immune or non-immune-mediated, when bleeding signs or symptoms are absent. As noted above, platelet transfusions given to patients with TTP or heparin-induced thrombocytopenia (HIT) in whom the major clinical presentation involves thrombosis rather than hemorrhage may aggravate the thrombotic processes (31,32,41). In ITP, since the autoantibody reacts with both autologous and allogeneic (transfused) platelets, the recovery and survival of these platelets is significantly reduced. Again, in the absence of bleeding, platelet transfusions are not helpful.

In patients with either congenital or acquired chronic thrombocytopenia that is not likely to resolve with treatment, and who then are likely to experience severely decreased platelet counts over several years, it is often not possible to support a given platelet count level (e.g., 10,000/uL or higher) over a long period of time due to the risk of eventual alloimmunization and refractoriness. Studies show that in stable patients it is feasible to use lower transfusion triggers and greater inter-transfusion intervals (e.g., once per week) and still avoid severe hemorrhagic complications (42). Provision of pharmacological alternatives to platelet transfusion (e.g., DDAVP, Amicar®) can be considered in these patients as well.

TRANSFUSION PRACTICE

Platelet Dosing

"Standard" platelet doses vary widely. In many European centers, a "standard" platelet dose may consist of a pool of 3 or 4 random donor PCs, whereas in many U.S. centers, a pool of 6 to 8 units is common (43). Authors of a clinical trial comparing three different doses of platelets for prophylactic transfusions in hypoproliferative thrombocytopenia suggested an "optimal" dose of 0.07×10^{11} platelets per kg for stable thrombocytopenic patients and 1.5×10^{11}/kg for patients with clinical factors known to result in platelet consumption (44). This compares with an optimal dose of 6×10^{11}/kg for an average size adult, as suggested by Strauss (45). These doses are in the same range as that proposed in the Platelet Transfusion Therapy Consensus Conference guidelines (1 PC per 10 kg body weight) (17), assuming that an average PC contains 7.5×10^{10} platelets.

Although these dose recommendations may produce optimal increments and inter-transfusion intervals, they have not been shown to be superior to smaller, more frequent doses in preventing bleeding (46,47). A recent randomized controlled trial of standard vs. low dose platelet transfusions in patients undergoing autologous HSCT or acute leukemia induction therapy supported the safety of the lower dose regimen, there being no clinically significant increase in hemorrhage in patients assigned to the low dose arm (46). However, reservations concerning the limited numbers of patients enrolled and the statistical analysis performed suggest that the definitive study re the optimal dosing strategy for platelet transfusions is yet to be undertaken (47). A newly established NIH sponsored Transfusion Medicine-Hemostasis Clinical Trials Network has embarked on a study to examine the appropriate platelet dosing strategy using a RCT with three arms: low (0.5×10^{10}/kg), medium (1×10^{10}/kg), and high (2×10^{10}/kg) (47).

In transfusing platelets to address consumptive thrombocytopenias, the dose may need to be increased to achieve the same platelet count increment that a lower dose would achieve if given to a patient with hypoproliferative thrombocytopenia. For instance, in DIC with marked platelet consumption, if platelet transfusions are given for severe thrombocytopenia with risk of or active bleeding, an appropriate dose may be as much as 1 to 2×10^{11} platelets per 10 kg (7). This higher dose recommendation holds also for other consumptive thrombocytopenias (e.g., ITP, TTP) for which platelet transfusions are rarely indicated.

The Transfusion Trigger

In recent years a number of clinical trials have compared platelet transfusion strategies that utilize different platelet count levels to "trigger" prophylactic transfusion. Notably, in 1991, Gmur et al. published a prospective study of patients with newly diagnosed acute leukemia whose platelet transfusions were managed using a stringent algorithm (48). In order for platelet transfusions to be given, the protocol required platelet counts to be 5000/ul or less in stable patients; between 6 and 10,000/uL in those with fresh minor hemorrhage or fever; between 11 and 20,000/uL in the presence of coagulation disorders or on heparin therapy and before bone marrow biopsy or lumbar puncture; and over 20,000/uL in the presence of major bleeding or before minor surgical procedures. While minor bleeding increased progressively according to decreases in the platelet count under 20,000/uL in this study, major bleeding was present on only about 2% of the days when the platelet counts were less than 10,000/uL and was even more rare (0.07% of days) when the platelet count was between 10 and 20,000/uL. The authors concluded that stable thrombocytopenic patients could be safely managed using a transfusion trigger of 5000 platelets/uL. They suggested that in the presence of minor bleeding and/or fever, the trigger should be raised to 10,000/uL. Higher levels (e.g., 20,000/uL) were recommended if coagulation disorders, heparin, or anatomical lesions were present.

Additional trials reported that lowering the trigger to 5000/uL was safe in a cohort of patients receiving high dose chemotherapy for gynecological tumors (49) and for those with severe, chronic aplastic anemia requiring prolonged platelet transfusion support (42). Additional randomized, controlled trials (50–53) have reported comparisons of prophylactic transfusion practices using 10,000 platelets/uL vs. 20,000 platelets/uL. These trials found no increase in either bleeding risk or red cell transfusion requirements when the lower transfusion trigger was used. However, most reported that significantly more platelets were given when the higher level of platelet count was used.

Platelet Transfusion Guidelines

Organizations responsible for granting accreditation to hospitals in the U.S. require that hospitals monitor blood product transfusions for appropriateness. This requires that transfusion guidelines be adopted and promulgated for each type of blood component. Figure 1 provides a current example of a guideline for platelet transfusions.

ADVERSE EVENTS WITH PLATELET TRANSFUSION

Adverse events associated with platelet transfusions occur either primarily with these components or are complications that may arise after transfusion of other blood products as well.

Adverse Events Specific to Platelet Transfusions

HLA Alloimmunization and Platelet Refractoriness

HLA antibodies are the most important cause of alloimmune platelet transfusion refractoriness. Prior to the widespread use of leukocyte-reduced blood products, up to 70% of multitransfused patients developed HLA antibodies (54). There is consensus that primary alloimmunization to HLA is unlikely to occur before 3–4 weeks after the first transfusion in patients receiving multiple transfusions. HLA antibodies detected sooner than this most likely represent secondary immune responses in patients with remote histories of transfusion or pregnancy.

Contaminating WBC in the transfusion products appear to be most responsible for primary HLA alloimmunization. A number of studies in animals and humans demonstrate that when platelets devoid of WBCs are transfused, primary immunization to HLA is very much delayed or does not occur at all, whereas unmodified PCs are associated with high rates of sensitization (55–57). However, data from in vitro studies using murine platelets and leukocytes reveal that platelets in the absence of WBCs can stimulate, albeit slowly, a primary immune response including transformation of T lymphocytes and subsequent programming of B lymphocytes to produce antibody to the major histocompatibility complex. There may then be two possible pathways for the primary immune response to HLA antigens on platelets to develop: one depending on WBCs and another, less efficient mechanism, independent of leukocytes (58).

Although the risk of HLA alloimmunization may be reduced by removing or inactivating contaminating WBC, it has not been eliminated, particularly in those patients who have been sensitized through pregnancy (59). This appears to be the case in a randomized controlled trial of platelet transfusion products, the aim of which was to reduce alloimmune refractoriness, the TRAP trial. In this study, although previously pregnant patients had a lower rate refractoriness, the TRAP trial. of antibody formation when they received leukocyte-reduced

An example of a guideline for platelet transfusion.

Platelet concentrate infusions can be administered to patients without further justification in the following circumstances:

1. Active bleeding and platelet count less than 50,000/uL or platelet function defect *
2. Non bleeding patients with:

a. Temporary myelosuppression due to chemo-radiotherapy or underlying disease in a stable patient with platelet count less than 10,000/uL. Patients with temporary myelosuppression due to chemotherapy or underlying disease (e.g. leukemia) may require prophylactic transfusions at levels between 10,000/uL and 20,000/uL in the presence of fever or minor hemorrhagic signs.

b. Impending surgery or invasive procedures involving the CNS (including ocular), or other critical areas in which microvascular bleeding is harmful and a platelet count of less than 100,000/uL**.

c. Other surgery or invasive procedures where the operative field can be visualized or external pressure can be utilized to maintain hemostasis and a platelet count of less than 50,000/uL**.

d. Surgery or invasive procedure and documented qualitative platelet function defect*. (DDAVP (0.3ug/kg) should be considered for patients with von Willebrand disease or qualitative platelet function defects (e.g. cirrhosis or uremia).

3. Open heart surgery patients with :

a. Microvascular bleeding and platelet count less than 150,000/uL**

b. Microvascular bleeding and nondiagnostic coagulation panel abnormality (e.g. post-operative chest tube drainage greater than 500 mL within 6 hours)

c. Microvascular bleeding and platelet function defect*

4. Active microvascular bleeding with a platelet count of less than 75,000/uL**.

Contraindications for platelet transfusions

1. Platelet transfusions are generally contraindicated in thrombotic thrombocytopenic purpura (TTP) and immune thrombocytopenias including heparin induced thrombocytopenia (HIT) unless life-threatening hemorrhage exists.
2. Prophylactic platelet transfusions are not generally indicated for patients with chronic aplastic anemia or myelodysplastic diseases. Platelet transfusion for symptomatic thrombocytopenia (minor or moderate bleeding) is a more rational approach in such patients.
3. There is no role for prophylactic platelet transfusion in routine primary open heart surgery

* Platelet function defect should be documented by template bleeding time greater than two times the upper limit of normal or greater than 12 minutes or presumed defect based on medication ingestion, hypothermia, or instrumentation affecting platelet function.

** Platelet counts listed represent maximal levels; procedures have been performed at lower levels without hemorrhage.

Outcome indicators: A platelet count should be obtained within 24 hours of transfusion. If refractoriness to platelet transfusion is suspected, it is recommended that a platelet count be performed within one hour after transfusion. Patients receiving HLA matched or cross match compatible platelets should have platelet counts performed ten minutes to six hours after the transfusion.

A single unit of random platelets (i.e. derived from one unit of whole blood) should increase the platelet count 5,000/uL to 10,000/uL in a 70kg recipient.

Figure 1 An example of a guideline for platelet transfusion.

platelets, they experienced a rate of HLA alloimmunization twice that of women who had never been pregnant (62% vs. 33%).

The underlying disease for which transfusions are required also influences the likelihood of HLA alloimmunization. Patients with aplastic anemia have a significantly higher frequency of HLA sensitization compared with those with hematologic malignancies (60). In a like manner, patients undergoing induction therapy for acute myelogenous leukemia (AML) experience a higher rate of alloimmunization than those with acute lymphoblastic leukemia (ALL) (61). The lower sensitization rate in the ALL patients may be due to a decreased immune responsiveness attributable to the underlying disease, or to the immunosuppressive effects of high-dose corticosteroids given to these patients and not to the AML group. Others note that alloimmunization also appears to occur sooner in AML patients than in ALL patients.

A dose-response relationship between donor exposures in platelet transfusion and the rate of HLA alloimmunization is not always evident. One group failed to detect such a relationship in AML patients receiving induction therapy. However, in this study, almost all of the patients received over 20 donor exposures in the course of their platelet transfusion therapy (62). Evidence from animal studies suggests that there may be a rather steep dose-response curve associating alloimmunization to the numbers of different platelet donors (62,63).

As important as they appear to be in determining responses to platelet transfusions, lymphocytotoxic (LCT) antibodies are often a transient finding, disappearing in more than half the patients who develop them. LCT antibodies can be lost despite a patient's continued exposure to random-donor platelet transfusions (64).

A number of factors have changed in the last decade that may have reduced the risk of alloimmunization in the average patient receiving multiple transfusions. More blood products are being leukocyte-reduced and there is a marked shift to supply transfusions as apheresis platelets rather than as pools of PCs (9,65). In addition, the platelet count level at which prophylactic platelet transfusions are given has been lowered in most institutions. These trends—leukocyte reduction, increase in apheresis platelets, and lowering the platelet transfusion trigger—have resulted in lowering donor exposures involved in supporting patients with multiple platelet transfusions. These changes are likely to translate into reduced or at least delayed alloimmunization, particularly in patients without prior exposure to HLA antigens through pregnancy.

ABH Antigens and Platelet Transfusion

The ABH blood group system is also an important antigen system represented on platelets. The amount of ABH substance on platelets varies not only from person to person but also among platelets in the same person (66). This distribution of ABH could explain why, in some platelet transfusions, there is a rapid destruction of a subset of ABO incompatible cells followed by near normal survival of the remaining cells. Important for the purpose of platelet donor selection for recipients with high anti-A or anti-A,B titers, individuals of the subgroup A_2 have no detectable A antigens on their platelets (67), and A_2 platelets can be substituted successfully for group O.

Recently donors with unusually high A or B antigen expression were observed to account for about 7% of non-group O individuals. The differentiation of high and low expression of A and B substances is independent of secretor phenotype and correlates with high levels of glycosyltransferase measured in donor serum. This inherited pattern of high and low ABH expression may offer an additional explanation for the non-uniform refractory response some patients develop to ABO-incompatible platelet transfusions (68,69).

In the aggregate, patients receiving multiple platelet transfusions have been thought to demonstrate a statistically significant but clinically unimportant decrease in platelet recovery after transfusion of ABO-incompatible platelets (especially group A). In a subset, however, as many as 20% of group O patients could develop severe refractoriness to group A platelets (70). Failure to respond to HLA-matched platelet transfusions in the absence of non-immune clinical factors should prompt an examination of the ABO types of the recipient and of the donors to determine whether ABO incompatibility might be responsible for the unexpected poor responses.

The importance of ABO compatibility in platelet transfusions has been the subject of a number of studies over the past two decades. ABO-identical platelet transfusions result in significantly higher post transfusion recoveries, particularly after several transfusions have been given. Platelets that are ABO compatible, but not identical, however, have a reduced recovery, similar to those that are ABO incompatible with the recipient. There appears to be a detrimental effect of incompatible plasma, containing isoagglutinins that interact with recipient ABH antigens, as well as that of incompatible platelets that express ABH antigens to which the recipient has antibodies. ABO non-identical transfusions also appear to predict subsequent alloimmunization and refractoriness to platelet transfusions (71).

The mechanism for platelet destruction in platelet ABO-incompatible transfusions (the recipient has isoagglutinins against donor ABH) relates to IgM and IgG anti-A or anti-B in the recipient interacting with A and B substances on the transfused platelets, resulting in their destruction.

The suboptimal response of the plasma-incompatible transfusions (the donor has isoagglutinins against recipient ABH) may be related to immune complexes of soluble recipient ABH substance and donor anti-A or -B antibodies. These immune complexes may secondarily interact with the transfused platelets via the FcγRIIα receptor, or the complement receptors cC1q-R and gC1q-R, and mediate their destruction (72).

Platelet-Specific Antigens and Platelet Transfusions

Occasionally patients who become refractory to random platelet transfusions develop antibodies to platelet specific antigens, usually in addition to HLA antibodies. In such patients, the failure of HLA-matched platelets may be observed (73).

Although there are a few well-documented cases of transfusion failures attributable to platelet-specific antibodies (74,75), most "platelet-specific reactivity" detected in the sera of refractory recipients does not seem to influence transfusion responses (76–78). This is perhaps due to the fact that many of the platelet-specific antibodies detected in such patients are directed against platelet antigens present on the platelets of a minority of platelet donors (79,80), and are therefore unlikely to cause refractory responses to a majority of attempted platelet transfusions. In the TRAP study (see above), about 8% of study patients developed platelet-specific antibodies during the trial, regardless of assigned treatment arm, and similar to earlier studies, there did not appear to be any significant contribution of these antibodies to refractory responses (59). Alloimmunization to high-frequency platelet-specific antigens would be expected to present a major challenge in finding compatible platelets to support a patient requiring multiple platelet transfusions. Fortunately, these cases are extremely rare (74,75). An exception to this experience may be isoimmunization to GPIV (CD36), and there are now several reports of platelet transfusion refractoriness caused by such antibodies in patients who are GPIV deficient (81,82). These patients are difficult to support since virtually all platelet products available for transfusion would be incompatible (GPIV positive).

Diagnosis of Alloimmune Refractoriness

Clinical diagnosis of refractoriness: The diagnosis of alloimmune refractoriness rests first on demonstrating that platelet transfusions from randomly selected donors are not successful. In adults of average size, the expected increment in platelet count after a platelet transfusion is roughly 5000–10,000/μL per single concentrate (or per 0.75×10^{11}platelets) transfused. Therefore, after a six-donor pool of PCs is transfused, the expected platelet count increment at 1 hr after transfusion is approximately 30,000–60,000/μL. In patients with leukemia or other hematologic malignancies requiring platelet support, the platelet count increment per unit transfused is often not optimal because of non-immune clinical factors that cause increased platelet destruction (fever, sepsis). However, failure to obtain a 1-hour post-transfusion corrected count increment (CCI) of at least 5000 on consecutive transfusions defines a refractory response (59). The CCI is calculated using the following formula:

$$\text{CCI} = \text{Post} - \text{pretransfusion platelet count}(/\mu\text{L}) \\ \times \\ \frac{\text{body surface area}(\text{M}^2)}{\text{Number of platelets transfused} \times 10^{-11}}$$

Although a 1-hour post-transfusion platelet count is often recommended for determination of the CCI, adequate data support using a post-transfusion count taken as early as 10 min after the transfusion (83). This is important because earlier post-transfusion counts facilitate the evaluation of platelet transfusion responses in the outpatient setting.

Early in the course of alloimmunization, the 24-hour platelet recovery often begins to deteriorate before the 1-hour post-transfusion platelet count is affected. If 24-hour post-transfusion increments are consistently poor in the absence of non-immune clinical factors that might explain shortened platelet survival, the possibility of HLA alloimmunization should be considered.

Diagnosis of HLA alloimmunization: Because many clinical factors can influence platelet transfusion success, a laboratory test to help diagnose alloimmune platelet refractoriness is useful. Many centers use periodic (e.g., weekly) LCT antibody screening to predict when patients might be developing a need for HLA-selected platelet transfusions

The standard assay to evaluate platelet transfusion recipients for alloimmunization is lymphocyte cytotoxicity [antiglobulin-enhanced, complement-dependent cytotoxicity (AHG-CDC)]. A standard lymphocyte panel consists of 30–60 frozen cells. The panel reactive antibody score or PRA is calculated by dividing the number of wells containing significant numbers of killed cells by the total number of wells in the assay × 100. Alloimmunization can be defined as at least one well with > 60% of cells killed or at least 2 wells with > 40% cells killed as defined in the TRAP trial (59).

One alternative to the standard AHG-CDC is Flow PRA in which patient serum is incubated with micro-beads coated with class I and Class II antigens (84) that are then analyzed in the flow cytometer. When more than 5% of class I or class II beads exhibit fluorescence above a negative control, the result is positive. Flow PRA appears to be more sensitive and specific in detecting class I and II antibodies than the AHG-CDC and is now recommended as a screening procedure for prospective recipients of renal allografts in order to identify which patients will require pre-transplant cross-match testing with prospective donor lymphocytes (84). Another option for determining whether patients are HLA alloimmunized is a commercially available kit that uses purified Class I HLA molecules derived from a large number of donors. Pooled, purified Class I HLA serves as the target substance in this rapid enzyme-linked immunosorbent assay (ELISA)-based test that can detect broadly reactive HLA antibodies in about 4 hours (85).

Diagnosis of platelet-specific alloimmunization: When patients fail HLA-matched, ABO-compatible platelet transfusions and clinical factors are insufficient to explain the poor response, a platelet-specific antibody should be suspected. Certain specialty laboratories offer platelet antibody detection and identification services. Alternatively, some hospital laboratories offer screening with a solid-phase red cell adherence method. This intact platelet antibody screen cannot distinguish between HLA- and platelet-specific antibodies when untreated target platelets are used, but prior treatment of target platelets with chloroquine may alter HLA structures sufficiently to allow detection of a platelet-specific reaction (86). Newer, commercially available glycoprotein-based platelet antibody detection kits may soon prove to be superior for detecting platelet-specific antibodies in such patients.

Selecting Platelets in the Management of the Alloimmunized Patient

HLA-selected platelet transfusions: A standard approach to supporting a patient who is refractory to random-donor platelet transfusions is to supply

HLA-matched, single-donor PCs (87). Since the primary cause of immune refractoriness is alloimmunization to Class I HLA antigens, it follows that avoidance of incompatible HLA antigens in platelet products should result in more successful responses. In practice, 65–90% of refractory patients benefit from these products (88,89). Moreover, even though HLA-matched apheresis platelets are generally more expensive to provide than either pools of random-donor PCs or random-donor apheresis platelets, provision of well-matched HLA-selected platelets can be more cost-effective in supporting alloimmunized refractory patients than the use of those alternative products (90). A number of community blood centers maintain files of HLA-typed donors for the provision of HLA-matched platelet support to refractory patients.

Certain "private" HLA antigens can be segregated into so-called cross-reactive groups or GREGS, defined by antisera that react with several different but structurally related Class I specificities. The refractory patient's immune system is relatively unable to recognize donor antigens from the same cross-reactive groups as those of the patient's HLA antigens. Selectively mismatching donors to patients using these GREG associations greatly increases the number of potentially successful platelet donors in a given pool, thus reducing the donor pool size necessary to ensure a reasonable chance of finding matched donors for most patients—from 10,000 random donors for sufficient numbers of rigorously HLA-compatible matches to only 500 donors for HLA-matched and selectively mismatched transfusions (Table 5) (91).

An additional approach to providing HLA-matched platelets for these patients is to identify the specificity of their HLA antibodies, if possible, and avoid these in selecting platelet donors. This antibody specificity profile (ASP) method is utilized when large files of HLA-typed donors are not available and patients are not heavily alloimmunized (92).

Table 5 Classification of Donor/Recipient Pairs on the Basis of HLA Match

A	All 4 antigens in donor identical to those in recipient
BIU	Only 3 antigens detected in donor; all present and identical in recipient
BIX	Three donor antigens identical to recipient; fourth antigen cross-reactive with recipient
B2U	Only 2 antigens detected in donor; both present and identical in recipient
B2UX	Only 3 antigens detected in donor; 2 identical with recipient, third crossreactive
B2X	Two donor antigens identical to recipient; third and fourth antigens crossreactive with recipient
C	One antigen of donor not present in recipient and noncrossreactive with recipient
D	Two antigens of donor not present in recipient and noncrossreactive with recipient

In a recent innovation in the use of HLA-typing to find suitable platelet donors for highly alloimmunized refractory patients, Duquesnoy employs a computerized algorithm—HLA Matchmaker—for evaluation of the molecular similarities and differences between HLA class I epitopes (93). The strategy is based on the concept that immunogenic epitopes are represented by amino acid triplets on exposed parts of protein sequences of the class I alloantigens that are accessible to alloantibodies. Using this scheme, many class I HLA antigens that are classified as mismatches to a patient's HLA type have no incompatible exposed amino acid triplets and therefore would not be expected to elicit an antibody response. The pool of potentially compatible HLA selected donors is thereby greatly expanded.

Platelets matched for platelet-specific antigens: In those rare instances in which a platelet-specific antibody reaction is contributing to poor platelet transfusion responses, it is possible to select platelet donors using platelet antigen typing. Antibodies to platelet-specific antigens, even low-incidence antigens, may be a problem with regard to consistent transfusion support in patients who also have broad specificity HLA alloimmunization (94). In these instances, it may be necessary to screen HLA-matched donors for the platelet antigen in question to be more certain of a successful transfusion response. In a single report, GPIV negative platelets were obtained by large-scale screening of donor populations with a higher frequency of GPIV deficiency (African), and transfusion of those platelets resulted in good platelet increments for the patients (95).

Platelet crossmatching: An alternative to selecting platelets that are HLA-matched or selectively mismatched to the patient is to use a platelet crossmatching strategy. Platelet transfusion failures due to immunization can often be predicted with pretransfusion platelet crossmatching assays that test reactions of patient serum with donor platelets. Although virtually any platelet or lymphocyte antibody detection method can be used as a platelet compatibility test, the method that has gained greatest acceptance for this purpose is the commercially available solid-phase red cell adherence (SPRCA) assay (96). First described by Shibata et al. (97) and later by Rachel et al. (96), the test is rapid and sensitive, particularly for detecting HLA antibodies. Clinical trials comparing the adequacy of platelet support of refractory patients with HLA selected vs. crossmatch selected platelets have shown that particularly for moderately alloimmunized patients (PRA $<60\%$), the methods are equivalent. However, when patients are heavily alloimmunized (PRA $>80\%$), well matched HLA selected products are superior (98).

A common approach to using platelet crossmatching is to obtain a recent sample of serum from the patient and crossmatch available single donor (apheresis) platelet products. Those products with negative or lowest reactivity to patient serum are then selected for transfusion.

Reactions Due to the Accumulation of Cytokines

Febrile, nonhemolytic transfusion reactions are the most frequent adverse reactions to platelets, occurring in between 5 and 30% of transfusions (99). Most of the reactions are mild, manifesting fever and chills during or shortly after the product is infused. Occasionally, the reactions can be accompanied by hypo- or hypertension. Until recently, these were thought to be due to the interaction between anti-leukocyte antibodies in the recipient and contaminating WBC in the platelet component. This view was supported by the reduction in FNHTRs resulting from leukocyte depletion of the platelet products (100,101). However, a number of observations challenged this hypothesis: FNHTRs were more frequent with platelet products than with red cell transfusions, despite there being many more contaminating WBC in the latter than the former; the reactions can occur in untransfused male recipients who have had no opportunity to become sensitized to foreign antigens; the reactions tend to be more frequent when platelet products are stored vs. fresh; and finally, post-storage WBC reduction failed to eliminate all reactions. Following up on these observations, the role of supernatant plasma from platelet products in FNHTRs was examined. Standard PCs were separated into their plasma and cellular components and transfused in random order, with patients serving as their own controls. There were significantly more reactions to the plasma supernatant than to the cells. Measurements of interleukin-1β and IL-6 in the plasma supernatant correlated with the risk of reaction, supporting the hypothesis that bio-reactive substances accumulated in the plasma during platelet storage (102). A subsequent study demonstrated that removal of WBC prior to storage was as effective as removing post storage plasma supernatant in preventing these reactions, supporting the hypothesis that contaminating WBC were the source of the reaction-producing substances (103).

Septic Transfusion Reactions

With the dramatic reduction in risk of viral transmission through blood products brought about by improved methods of donor screening by history and infectious disease testing, the most important remaining risk to blood transfusion was bacterial sepsis associated with platelet products, due mainly to the fact that they are stored at room rather than at refrigerated temperature (104). Rates of bacterial contamination of platelets range from 1:1000 to 1:3000 (105). Bacteria and/or their endotoxins are infused in sufficient amounts to cause sepsis or shock. Precise incidence data on clinically apparent sepsis reactions to platelets are lacking. The BaCon Study, in which passively reported reactions to participating transfusion services were investigated, reported clinically significant septic reactions in 1 in 100,000 platelet products transfused, and deaths in 1 in 500,000. Due to this study's strict inclusion criteria and the passive reporting, the true incidence of severe septic reactions is probably underestimated.

The sources of contamination in platelet products are either silent donor bacteremias, in which case gram negative organisms are usually cultured, or inadequate sterile preparation of the skin at the venipuncture site, in which case skin flora (gram positive) are usually isolated. The latter are the most common finding. The risk of septic transfusion reactions to platelets can be reduced by: (1) assuring adequate skin preparation, (2) diversion of an initial aliquot of donor blood from the product such that bacteria associated with any skin plugs do not end up in the product, and (3) monitoring platelet products for bacterial contamination.

The major blood banking organizations in the U.S. have recently added a requirement that blood collecting agencies perform bacterial detection procedures on platelet products prior to issuing for transfusion. Available methods for this include the detection of bacterial growth by automated CO2 detection (Bac-t Alert) or by O2 consumption (106). Currently, it is recommended that apheresis platelets be collected, rest 24 hours, then undergo sampling for bacterial testing. The products can then be either released or held for a further period and released when the cultures remain negative. Bacterial detection of PCs is problematic. Because multiple PC units make up one dose of platelets, sampling requirements and cost remain significant barriers to effectively screening these products for bacterial contamination. The currently available strategies of staining (gram or Wright), or of testing for glucose or pH with urine dipsticks are far less sensitive than the automated culture systems used for apheresis platelets.

Adverse Events Shared with Other Blood Products

In addition to the adverse events that are uniquely associated with platelets, other adverse events associated with other blood products may also occur with platelet transfusions. As noted above, FNHTRs, which can be related to bioreactive substances in platelet supernatants, are also caused by recipient antibody interacting with contaminating WBC in the platelet product. Such reactions can be effectively eliminated by both pre and post storage WBC reduction. Since the former also addresses cytokine related reactions, this is the preferred strategy for removing leukocytes from platelet products

Although platelet products contain very few contaminating RBC, nevertheless, there are sufficient numbers of red cells to pose a risk of sensitization to red cell antigens in some patients. In particular, Rh-negative patients can become sensitized, particularly if they are not immunosuppressed. It is therefore recommended that for Rh(D)-negative girls or young women, Rh(D)-positive platelet products be avoided (107,108).

As with other plasma containing blood products, platelets can elicit allergic or anaphylactic reactions. Recently, transfusion induced lung injury (TRALI) has assumed more importance as second only to bacterial sepsis in transfusion-related deaths. Again, the plasma in platelet products is implicated in these reactions either because it contains WBC reactive antibodies (anti-class I or II

HLA or anti-neutrophil) formed by the donor, or because it contains bioreactive substances, that when transfused, lead to lung injury in susceptible patients (109).

Immunosuppressed patients are at risk of developing graft-versus-host disease (GVHD) caused by T lymphocytes present in platelet transfusions. It is now recommended that all cellular blood products provided to such patients be gamma irradiated to inhibit proliferation of contaminating T lymphocytes (see above). WBC-reduction strategies are considered inadequate for prevention of GVHD.

A rare complication of blood transfusion is PTP in which acute, severe thrombocytopenia develops in a patient 7 to 10 days after a transfusion of a blood product containing platelet antigens. The thrombocytopenia is accompanied by the development of a potent platelet-specific alloantibody in the patient's serum (usually anti-HPA-1a, Pl^{A1}). An underlying autoantibody is thought to mediate the autologous platelet destruction (110). In thrombocytopenic patients who require platelet transfusions, PTP is difficult to differentiate from more straightforward alloimmunization to a platelet antigen that the patient lacks. The response to antigen-negative platelets may help to clarify this situation. In PTP, the response to an antigen-negative transfusion would not be expected to be superior to that to an antigen-positive transfusion, while in alloimmunization, a platelet transfusion compatible with the recipient's antibody should be successful.

As with other blood products, platelet transfusions may also be complicated by viral transmission or fluid overload.

REFERENCES

1. Duke WW. The relation of blood platelets to hemorrhagic disease. Description of a method for determining the bleeding time and the coagulation time. JAMA 1910; 55:1185–1192.
2. Gaydos LA, Freireich EJ, Mantel N. The quantitative relation between platelet count and hemorrhage in patients with acute leukemia. NEJM 1962; 266:905–909.
3. Slichter SJ, Harker LA. Thrombocytopenia: mechanism and management of defects in platelet production. Clin Hematol 1978; 7:523–539.
4. Han T, Stutzman L, Cohen E, Kim U. Effect of platelet transfusion on hemorrhage in patients with acute leukemia. An autopsy study. Cancer 1966; 19:1937–1942.
5. Roy AJ, Jaffe N, Djerassi I. Prophylactic platelet transfusions in children with acute leukemia: a dose response study. Transfusion 1973; 13:283–290.
6. Higby DJ, Cohen E, Holland JF, Sinks L. The prophylactic treatment of thrombocytopenic leukemia patients with platelets: a double blind study. Transfusion 1974; 14:440–446.
7. Murphy S. In: Loscalzq J, Schafer AI, eds. Platelet Transfusion Therapy in Thrombosis and Hemorrhage. 2nd ed. Baltimore: Williams and Wilkins, 1998:1119–1134.

8. Kao KJ, Mickel M, Braine HG, et al. White cell reduction in platelet concentrates and packed red cells by filtration: a multicenter clinical trial. The trap study group. Transfusion 1995; 35:13–19.
9. Sullivan MT, McCullough J, Schreiber GB, Wallace EL. Blood collection and transfusion in the United States in 1997. Transfusion 2002; 42:1253–1260.
10. McCullough J, Vesole DH, Benjamin RJ, et al. Therapeutic efficacy and safety of platelets treated with a photochemical process for pathogen inactivation: the SPRINT trial (MS#2003-12-4443). Blood 2003; 12:4443.
11. Gulliksson H. Platelet storage media. Transfus Apheresis Sci 2001; 24:241–244.
12. Dumont LJ, Vanden Broeke T. Seven-day storage of apheresis platelets: report of an in vitro study. Transfusion 2003; 43:143–150.
13. Blanchette VS, Kuhne T, Hume H, Hellmann J. Platelet transfusion therapy in newborn infants. Transfus Med Rev 1995; 9:215–230.
14. Standards for Blood Banks and Transfusion Services, 23rd ed. Bethesda, MD: American Association of Blood Banks, 2005.
15. Read EJ, Kodis C, Carter CS, Leitman SF. Viability of platelets following storage in the irradiated state. A pair—controlled study. Transfusion 1988; 28:446–450.
16. Centers for Disease Control and Prevention (CDC). Fatal bacterial infections associated with platelet transfusions—United States, 2004. MMWR Morbidity & Mortality Weekly Report, 2005; 54:168–170.
17. NIH Consensus Conference, Platelet Transfusion Therapy. JAMA 1987; 257:1777–1780.
18. Norfolk DR, et al. Consensus conference on platelet transfusion. Royal College of Physicians of Edinburgh, 27-28 November 1997. Br J Haematol 1998; 101:609–617.
19. Contreras M. The appropriate use of platelets: an update for the Edinburgh consensus conference. Br J Haematol 1998; 101:10–12.
20. Murphy S, Litwin S, Herring LM, et al. Indications for platelet transfusion in children with acute leukemia. m J Hematol 1982; 12:347–356.
21. Solomon J, Bofenkamp T, Fahey JL, Chillar RK, Beutler E. Platelet prophylaxis in acute non-lymphoblasticleukemia. Lancet 1978; 1:267.
22. Hirsch EO, Gardner FH. The transfusion of human blood platelets with a note on the transfusion of granulocytes. J Lab Clin Med 1952; 39–56:556–569.
23. Bensinger WI, Martin PJ, Storer B, et al. Transplantation of bone marrow as compared with peripheral-blood cells from HLA-identical relatives in patients with hematologic cancers. N Engl J Med 2001; 344:175–181.
24. Bernstein SH, Nademanee AP, Vose JM, et al. A Multicenter study of platelet recovery and utilization in patients after myeloablative therapy and hematopoietic stem cell transplantation. Blood 1998; 91:3509–3517.
25. Bauman MA, Menitove JE, Aster RH, Anderson T. Urgent treatment of idiopathic thrombocytpenic purpura with single dose gamma-globulin infusion followed by platelet transfusion. Ann Int Med 1986; 104:808–817.
26. Stricker RB, Lewis BH, Corash L, Shuman MA. Posttransfusion purpura associated with an autoantibody directed against a previously undefined platelet antigen. Blood 1987; 69:1458–1463.
27. Minchinton RM, Cunningham I, Cole-Sinclair M, Van der Weyden M, Vaughan S, McGrath KM. Autoreactive platelet antibody in post transfusion purpura. Aust NZ J Med 1990; 20:111–115.

28. Brecher ME, Moore SB, Letendre L. Posttransfusion purpura: the therapeutic value of PlA1-negative platelets. Transfusion 1990; 30:433–435.
29. Loren AW, Abrams CS. Efficacy of HPA-1a (PlA1)-negative platelets in a patient with post-transfusion purpura. Am J Hematol 2004; 76:258–262.
30. Rock GA, Shumak KH, Buskard NA, et al. Comparison of plasma exchange with plasma infusion in the treatment of thrombotic thrombocytopenic purpura. Canadian Apheresis Study Group. N Engl J Med 1991; 325:393–397.
31. Harkness DR, Byrnes JJ, Lian EC, Williams WD, Hensley GT. Hazard of platelet transfusion in thrombotic thrombocytopenic purpura. JAMA 1981; 246:1931–1933.
32. Gordon LI, Kwaan HC, Rossi EC. Deleterious effects of platelet transfusion and recovery in patients with thrombotic microangiopathy. Semin Hematol 1987; 17:1037.
33. Coppo P, Lassoued K, Mariette X, et al. Effectiveness of platelet transfusions after plasma exchange in adult thrombotic thrombocytopenic Purpura: a report of two cases. Am J Hemat 2001; 68:198–201.
34. Catella-Lawson F, Reilly MP, Kapoor SC, et al. Cylooxygenase inhibitors and the antiplatelet effects of aspirin. NEJM 2001; 345:1809–1817.
35. Merritt JC, Bhatt DL. The efficacy and safety of perioperative antiplatelet therapy. J Thromb Thrombolysis 2004; 17:21–27.
36. Bougie DW, Wilker PR, Wuitschick ED, et al. Acute thrombocytopenia after treatment with tirofiban or dptifibatide is associated with antibodies specific for ligand occupied GPIIb/IIIa. Blood 2002; 100:2071–2076.
37. Kereiakes DJ, Essell JH, Abbottsmith CW, Broderick TM, Runyon JP. Abciximab-associated profound thrombocytopenia: therapy with immunoglobulin and platelet transfusion. Am J Cardiol 1996; 78:1161–1163.
38. Curtis BR, Swyers J, Divgi A, McFarland JG, Aster RH. Thrombocytopenia after second exposure to abciximab is caused by antibodies that recognize abciximab-coated platelets. Blood 2002; 99:2054–2059.
39. Noris M, Remuzzi G. Uremic bleeding: closing the circle after 30 years of controversires? Blood 1999; 94:2569–2574.
40. Castillo R, Lozano T, Escolar G, et al. Defective platelet adhesion on vessel subendothelium in uremic patients. Blood 1986; 68:337.
41. Babcock RB, Dumper CW, Scharfman WB. Heparin induced immune thrombocytopenia. NEJM 1976; 295:237–241.
42. Sagmeister M, Oec L, Gmur J. A restrictive platelet transfusion policy allowing long-term support of outpatients with severe aplastic anemia. Blood 1999; 93:3124–3126.
43. Pisciotto PT, et al. Prophylactic vs therapeutic platelet transfusion practices in hematology and/or oncology patients. Transfusion 1995; 35:498–502.
44. Norol R, et al. Platelet transfusion: a dose-response study. Blood 1998; 92:1448–1453.
45. Strauss RG. Clinical perspectives of platelet transfusions: defining the optimal dose. J Clin Apher 1995; 10:124–127.
46. Tinmouth A, Tannock IF, Crump M, et al. Low dose prophylactic platelet transfusions in recipients of an autologous peripheral blood progenitor cell transplant and patients with acute leukemia: a RCT with a sequential Bayesian design. Transfusion 2004; 44:1711–1719.

47. Strauss R. Low-dose prophylactic platelet transfusions: time for further study, but too early for routine clinical practice. Transfusion 2004; 44:1680–1682.
48. Gmur J, Burger J, Schanz U, Fehr J, Schaffner A. Safety of stringent prophylactic platelet transfusion policy for patients with acute leukemia. Lancet 1991; 338:1223–1226.
49. Fanning J, Hilgers RD, Murray KP, Bolt K, Aughenbaugh DM. Conservative management of chemotherapeutic-induced thrombocytopenia in women with gynecologic cancers. Gynecol Oncol 1995; 59:191–193.
50. Zumberg MS, del Rosario ML, Nejame CF, et al. A prospective randomized trial of prophylactic platelet transfusion and bleeding incidence in hematopoietic stem cell transplant recipients: 10,000/ul vs 20,000/ul trigger. Biol Blood Marrow Transplant 2002; 8:569–576.
51. Rebulla P, Finazzi G, Marangoni F, et al. The threshold for prophylactic platelet transfusions in adults with acute myeloid leukemia. NEJM 1997; 337:1870–1875.
52. Wandt H, Frank M, Ehninger G, et al. Safety and cost effectiveness of a 10×10*9/l trigger for prophylactic platelet transfusions compared to the traditional 20×10*9/l: a prospective comparative trial in 105 patients with acute myeloid leukemia. Blood 1998; 91:3601–3606.
53. Heckman KD, Weiner GJ, Davis CS, Strauss RG, Jones MP, Burns CP. Randomized study of prophylactic platelet transfusion threshold during induction therapy for adult acute leukemia: 10,000/ul vs 20,000/ul. JCO 1997; 15:1143–1149.
54. Dzik WH. Leukoreduced blood components: laboratory and clinical aspects. In: Simon TL, Dzik WH, Snyder EL, eds. Rossi's Principles of Transfusion Medicine. 3rd ed. Baltimore: Lippincott, Williams and Wilkins, 2002:270.
55. Claas FH, Smeenk RJ, Schmidt R, et al. Alloimmunization against the MHC antigens after platelet transfusions is due to contaminating leukocytes in the platelet suspension. Exp Hematol 1981; 9:84–89.
56. Brand A, Claas FH, Voogt PJ, et al. Alloimmunization after leukocyte-depleted multiple random-donor platelet transfusions. Vox Sang 1988; 54:160–166.
57. Blajchman M, Bardossy L, Carmen R, et al. An animal model of allogeneic donor platelet refractoriness: the effect of the time of leukodepletion. Blood 1992; 79:1371–1375.
58. Semple JW, Speck ER, Milev YP. Indirect allorecognition of platelets by T helper cells during platelet transfusions correlates with anti-major histocompatibility complex antibody and cytotoxic T lymphocyte formation. Blood 1995; 86:805–812.
59. The Trial to Reduce Alloimmunization to Platelets Study Group. Leukocyte reduction and ultraviolet B irradiation of platelets to prevent alloimmunization and refractoriness to platelet transfusions. N Engl J Med 1997; 337:1861–1869.
60. Holohan TV, Terasaki PI, Deisseroth AB. Suppression of transfusion-related alloimmunization in intensively treated cancer patients. Blood 1981; 58:122–128.
61. Lee EJ, Schiffer CA. Serial measurement of lymphocytotoxic antibody and response to nonmatched platelet transfusions in alloimmunized patients. Blood 1987; 70:1727–1729.
62. Dutcher JP, Schiffer CA, Aisner J, Wiernik PH. Alloimmunization following platelet transfusion: The absence of a dose-response relationship. Blood 1981; 57:395–398.

63. Slichter S, O'Donnell M, Weiden P, et al. Canine platelet alloimmunization: The role of donor selection. Br J Haematol 1986; 63:713–727.
64. McGrath K, Wolf M, Bishop J, et al. Transient platelet and HLA antibody formation in multitransfused patients with malignancy. Br J Haematol 1988; 68:345–350.
65. Blackall DP. The canadian universal leukoreduction program. Current Hematology Reports, 2003; 2:493–494.
66. Dunstan RA, Simpson MB. Heterogenous distribution of antigens on human platelets demonstrated by fluorescence flow cytometry. Br J Haematol 1985; 61:603–609.
67. Skogen B, Rossebo Hansen B, Husebekk A, Havnes T, Hannestad K. Minimal expression of blood group. A antigen on thrombocytes from A_2 individuals. Transfusion 1988; 28:456–459.
68. Ogasawara K, Ueki J, Takenaka M, Furihata K. Study on the expression of ABH antigens on platelets. Blood 1993; 82:993–999.
69. Curtis BR, Edwards JT, Hessner MJ, Klein JP, Aster RH. Blood group A and B antigens are strongly expressed on platelets of some individuals. Blood 2000; 96:1574–1581.
70. Brand A, Sintnicolaas K, Claas FHJ, Eernisse JG. ABH antibodies causing platelet transfusion refractoriness. Transfusion 1986; 26:463–466.
71. Heal JM, Rowe JM, Blumberg N. ABO and platelet transfusion revisited. Ann Hematol 1993; 66:309–314.
72. Heal J, Masel D, Rowe J, Blumberg N. Circulating immune complexes involving the ABO system after platelet transfusion. Br J Haematol 1993; 85:566–572.
73. Novotny VMJ, van Doorn R, Witvliet MD, et al. Occurrence of allogeneic HLA and non-HLA antibodies after transfusion of prestorage filtered platelets and red blood cells: a prospective study. Blood 1995; 85:1736–1741.
74. Taaning E, Jacobsen N, Morling N. Graft derived anti-HPA2b production after allogeneic bone-marrow transplantation. Br J Haematol 1994; 86:651–653.
75. Murata M, Furihata K, Ishida F, et al. Genetic and structural characterization of an amino acid dimorphism in glycoprotein Ib alpha involved in platelet transfusion refractoriness. Blood 1992; 79:3086–3090.
76. Bishop J, McGrath K, Wolf M, et al. Clinical factors influencing the efficacy of pooled platelet transfusions. Blood 1988; 71:383–387.
77. Godeau B, Fromont P, Seror T, et al. Platelet alloimmunization after multiple transfusions: A prospective study of 50 patients. Br J Haematol 1992; 81:395–400.
78. Meenaghan M, Judson P, Yousaf K, et al. Antibodies to platelet glycoprotein V in polytransfused patients with haematological disease. Vox Sang 1993; 64:167–170.
79. Schnaidt M, Northoff H, Wernet D. Frequency and specificity of platelet-specific alloantibodies in HLA immunized haematologic oncologic patients. Transfus Med 1996; 6:111–114.
80. Wernet D, Schnaidt M, Mayer G, Northoff H. Serological screening, using three different test systems of platelet transfused patients with hematologic oncologic disorders. Vox Sang 1993; 65:108–113.
81. Ikeda H, Mitani T, Ohnuma M, et al. A new platelet-specific antigen, Naka, involved in the refractoriness of HLA-matched platelet transfusion. Vox Sanguinis 1989; 57:213–217.

82. Fujino H, Ohta K, Taniue J, et al. Primary refractoriness to platelet transfusion caused by Nak(a) antibody alone. [Erratum appears in Vox Sang 2002 Jan;82(1):53 Note: Taniue A.]. Vox Sang 2001; 81:42–44.
83. O'Connell B, Lee EJ, Schiffer CA. The value of 10-minute posttransfusion platelet counts. Transfusion 1988; 28:66–67.
84. Gebel HM, Bray RA. Sensitization an sensitivity: defining the unsensitized patient. Transplantation 2000; 69:1370–1374.
85. Lucas DP, Paparounis ML, Myers L, Hart JM, Zachary AA. Detection of HLA class I-specific antibodies by the quikscreen enzyme-linked immunosorbent assay. Clin Diagn Lab Immunol 1997; 4:252–257.
86. Freedman J, Hornstein A. Simple method for differentiating between HLA and platelet-specific antibodies by flow cytometry. Am J Hematol 1991; 38:314–320.
87. Yankee RA, Grumet FC, Rogentine GN. Platelet transfusion therapy: the selection of compatible platelet donors for refractory patients by lymphocyte HLA typing. N Engl J Med 1969; 281:1208–1212.
88. Duquesnoy RJ. Donor selection in platelet transfusions therapy of alloimmunized thrombocytopenic patients. In: Greenwalt TJ, Jamieson GA, eds. The Blood Platelet in Transfusion Therapy. New York: Alan R. Liss, 1978:229–243.
89. Dahlke MB, Weiss KL. Platelet transfusion from donors mismatched for cross-reactive HLA antigens. Transfusion 1984; 24:299–302.
90. McFarland JG, Larson EB, Hillman RS, Slichter SJ. Cost benefit analysis of a plateletpheresis program. Transfusion 1986; 26:91–97.
91. Duquesnoy RJ, Filip DJ, Rodey GE, Rimm AA, Aster RH. Successful transfusion of platelets "mismatched" for HLA antigens to alloimmunized thrombocytopenic patients. Am J Hematol 1977; 2:219–226.
92. Petz LD, Garratty G, Calhoun L, et al. Selecting donors of platelets for refractory patients on the basis of HLA antibody specificity. Transfusion 2000; 40:1446–1456.
93. Duquesnoy RJ. HLAMatchmaker: a molecularly based algorithm for histocompatibility determination. I. Description of the algorithm. Hum Immunol 2002; 63:339–352.
94. Schnaidt M, Northoff H, Wernet D. Frequency and specificity of platelet-specific alloantibodies in HLA immunized haematologic oncologic patients. Transfus Med 1996; 6:111–114.
95. Lee K, Godeau P, Fromont P. CD36 deficiency is frequent and can cause platelet immunization in Africans. Transfusion 1999; 39:873–879.
96. Rachel JM, Sinor LT, Tawfek OW, et al. A solid phase red cell adherence test for platelet crossmatching. Med Lab Sci 1985; 42:194–195.
97. Shibata Y, Juji T, Nishizawa Y, Sakamoto H, Ozawa N. Detection of platelet antibodies by a newly developed mixed agglutination with platelets. Vox Sang 1981; 41:25–31.
98. Moroff G, Garratty G, Hal JM, et al. Selection of platelets for refractory patients by HLA matching and prospective crossmatching. Transfusion 1992; 32:633–640.
99. Chambers LA, Kruskall MS, Pacini DG, Donovan LM. Febrile reactions after platelet transfusion: the effect of single versus multiple donors. Transfusion 1990; 30:219–221.
100. Kalmin ND, Orrell JE, Villarreal IG. An effective method for the preparation of leukocyte-poor platelets. Transfusion 1987; 27:281–283.

101. Mangano MM, Chambers LA, Kruskall MS. Limited efficacy of leukopoor platelets for prevention of febrile transfusion reactions. Am J Clin Pathol 1991; 95:733–738.
102. Heddle NM, Klama L, Singer J, et al. The role of the plasma from platelet concentrates in transfusion reactions. NEJM 1994; 331:625–628.
103. Heddle NM, Blajchman MA, Meyer RM, et al. A randomized controlled trial comparing the frequency of acute reactions to plasma removed platelets and prestorage WBC reduced platelets. Transfusion 2002; 42:556–566.
104. Detection of Bacterial Contamination of Platelet Components, Blood Bulletin, Vol.6, Washington, DC:Americas Blood Centers, 2003.
105. Hillyer CD, Josephson CD, Blajchman MA, Vostal JG, Epstein JS, Goodman JL. Bacterial contamination of blood components: risks, strategies, and regulation: joint ASH and AABB educational session in transfusion medicine. Hematology (Am Soc Hematol Educ Program) 2003;575–589.
106. Brecher ME, Means N, Jere CS, Heath D, Rothenberg S, Stutzman LC. Evaluation of an automated culture system for detecting bacterial contamination of platelets an analysis with 15 contaminating organisms. Transfusion 2001; 41:477–482.
107. Goldfinger D, McGinniss MH. Rh-incompatible platelet transfusion-risks and consequences of sensitizing immunosuppressed individuals. NEJM 1971; 284:942–944.
108. Haspel RL, Walsh L, Sloan SR. Platelet transfusion in an infant leading to formation of anti-D: implications for immunoprophylaxis. Transfusion 2004; 44:747–749.
109. Kleinman S, Caulfield T, Chan P, et al. Toward an understanding of transfusion-related acute lung injury: statement of a consensus panel. Transfusion 2004; 44:1774–1789.
110. Watkins NA, Smethurst PA, Allen D, Smith GA, Ouwehand WH. Platelet alphaIIbbeta3 recombinant autoantibodies from the B-cell repertoire of a post-transfusion purpura patient. Br J Haematol 2002; 116:677–685.

Index